# Head and Neck Surgery: Advances in Otolaryngology

# Head and Neck Surgery: Advances in Otolaryngology

Editor: Chad Downs

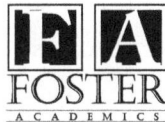

**FA FOSTER**
ACADEMICS

www.fosteracademics.com

www.fosteracademics.com

**FA**
FOSTER
ACADEMICS

Cataloging-in-Publication Data

Head and neck surgery : advances in otolaryngology / edited by Chad Downs.
 p. cm.
Includes bibliographical references and index.
ISBN 978-1-63242-508-9
1. Otolaryngology. 2. Head--Surgery. 3. Neck--Surgery. 4. Head--Diseases. 5. Neck--Diseases.
I. Downs, Chad.
RF46.5 .H43 2017
617.51--dc23

© Foster Academics, 2017

Foster Academics,
118-35 Queens Blvd., Suite 400,
Forest Hills, NY 11375, USA

ISBN 978-1-63242-508-9 (Hardback)

Printed and bound in the United States of America.

# Contents

# Preface

Otolaryngology refers to the surgery of the head and neck region and particularly, the organs of the ear, nose and throat. This book on head and neck surgery elucidates the concepts and innovative models around surgical and restorative procedures that are practiced in this field. It sheds light on the various dimensions of this medical field with special emphasis on its varied techniques of treatment and rehabilitation. For all those who are interested in head and neck surgery, this text can prove to be an essential guide. From theories to research to practical applications, case studies related to all contemporary topics of relevance to this field have been included herein. This book, with its detailed analyses and data, will prove immensely beneficial to professionals and students involved in this area at various levels.

Various studies have approached the subject by analyzing it with a single perspective, but the present book provides diverse methodologies and techniques to address this field. This book contains theories and applications needed for understanding the subject from different perspectives. The aim is to keep the readers informed about the progress in the field; therefore, the contributions were carefully examined to compile novel researches by specialists from across the globe.

Indeed, the job of the editor is the most crucial and challenging in compiling all chapters into a single book. In the end, I would extend my sincere thanks to the chapter authors for their profound work. I am also thankful for the support provided by my family and colleagues during the compilation of this book.

**Editor**

# A different entity: a population based study of characteristics and recurrence patterns in oropharyngeal squamous cell carcinomas

Scott Murray[1*], Michael N. Ha[1], Kara Thompson[2], Robert D. Hart[1,3], Murali Rajaraman[1,4] and Stephanie L. Snow[1,5]

## Abstract

**Background:** Cases of squamous cell carcinoma (SCC) of the oropharynx were compared with other head and neck cancer (HNC) anatomic subsites in patients treated at the provincial referral centre for HNC, the Nova Scotia Cancer Centre (NSCC).

**Methods:** A retrospective chart review was performed on HNC patients assessed at the NSCC between 2010 and 2011. Patient demographics, disease characteristics, treatment details and outcomes, including recurrence rates and survival were collected. Data was collected on new and recurrent cases of HNC. This data was compared between the two types of HNC using chi-square tests for dichotomous categorical variables or Fishers exact test where appropriate. Wald test was used to compare categorical variables with 3 categories. Continuous variables were compared using the non-parametric Wilcoxon test.

**Results:** 318 charts were included in the analysis. 122 (38 %) were oropharyngeal squamous cell carcinomas (OPSCCs). In terms of disease characteristics, OPSCCs were more likely to be poorly differentiated/undifferentiated ($n = 267$, 49(40 %) vs 42(21 %), $p < 0.001$), non-keratinizing ($n = 169$, 25(20 %) vs 17(9 %), $p < 0.001$), greater than 2 cm ($n = 253$, 72(59 %) vs 78(40 %), $p = 0.0061$), stage 4 ($n = 313$, 55(45 %) vs 64(33 %), $p = 0.0315$) and have had locoregional nodal spread ($n = 315$, 103(84 %) vs 55(28 %), $p < 0.001$). In the subset of 57 patients that had p16 testing, OPSCCs were more likely to be p16(+) (37(30 %) vs 1(1 %), $p < .001$). There were no significant differences in terms of Charlson probability of 10 year survival, smoking or alcohol consumption although OPSCC patients were significantly less likely to have COPD as a co-morbidity ($n = 318$, 19(16 %) vs 53(27 %), $p = 0.0175$). Finally, OPSCCs had less chance for relapse than non-OPSCCs in both univariate (2.119 times less, p=0.0034) and multivariate (1.899 times less, p=0.0505) analyses along with a 1.822 times less overall mortality in a multivariae analysis (p=0.0408).

**Conclusions:** This analysis suggests that Nova Scotian OPSCCs should be considered distinct from other HNC lesions, most notably in terms of disease characteristics and prognosis. Specifically, despite a higher association with disease factors traditionally considered to be linked to poor prognosis, outcomes were actually superior in terms of relapse and overall mortality.

**Keywords:** Oropharyngeal squamous cell carcinoma, Human papillomavirus, p16, Head and neck cancer, Staging

* Correspondence: sipmurray@gmail.com
[1]Dalhousie University, Faculty of Medicine, Halifax, Nova Scotia, Canada
Full list of author information is available at the end of the article

## Background

Worldwide there are over 550,000 new cases of head and neck cancer (HNC) reported annually, including an estimated 130,300 oropharyngeal cancers (OPC) [1, 2]. In Canada, the estimated incience of oral and laryngeal cancers alone was 5350 in 2014 [3]. Understanding HNC's characteristics, its causative factors and potential differences among HNC subsites is integral to providing optimal care of HNC patients. Ultimately this would aid in achieving the goals of disease prevention and reduction of associated morbidity and mortality in this population.

It is increasingly apparent that we must consider oropharyngeal squamous cell carcinomas (OPSCCs) separately from other subsites of head and neck squamous cell carcinoma (HNSCC) due to a different biologic and epidemiologic profile. Specifically, the incidence of other subtypes of HNSCC, including the larynx, oral cavity and hypopharynx, is declining whereas the incidence of OPSCCs, particularly in the tonsillar and base of tongue region, have demonstrated a recent increase in incidence in the United States (US), Canada, Australia, Denmark, Japan, Slovakia, the United Kingdom (UK) and Sweden [4–11].

Additionally, the risk factors to develop OPSCC are different from those associated with other HNSCC sites. The principal risk factors for HNC are cigarette smoking and alcohol consumption [12]. In North America there has been a demonstrable decline in both of these cancer-associated activities, most notably in smoking [13, 14]. In Canada, from 1992–2007, these trends have been mirrored by the decline in incidence of oral cavity tumours and other HNSCC tumours including hypopharynx, larynx and nasopharynx tumours [4]. These trends have not been seen in OPSCCs, however, which have shown an increase in incidence in men and women within the same time period [4]. Similar epidemiologic trends have been appreciated in populations around the world [4–11].

Further, the human papilloma virus (HPV) has been recognized as a contributing factor in the development of OPSCCs more frequently than in other HNSCCs, likely accounting for some of the disparity in incidence trends between these two groups [6, 8, 9, 15, 16]. HPV has been established as central to the development of cervical squamous neoplasias, with the virus being detected in as high as 99.7 % of cases [17]. Research has recently shown that in the US, HPV positive (+) tumours have also become the most prominent form of OPSCC, suggesting that HPV exposure has surpassed smoking and alcohol as the most significant risk factor for this subsite [11].

OPSCC is more commonly diagnosed in younger males with a history of high-risk sexual behavior and marijuana use [10, 18]. This stands in contrast to the "classic" HNSCC risk factors of heavy tobacco and alcohol use, along with poor oral hygiene [10, 18]. Further, HPV(+) OPSCC tumours have a different biological disease profile, presenting at earlier T stages with advanced N stages, and pathologically as poorly differentiated, non-keratinizing tumours [19]. Finally, HPV(+) OPSCC tumours have been associated with improved overall survival (OS) as well as disease free survival over other HNSCCs [20–23].

The aim of this population based study was to assess disease patterns and outcomes in OPSCC patients treated at the provincial HNC referral center, the Nova Scotia Cancer Centre (NSCC), between 2010 and 2011 with the intention of comparing provincial trends with those that have been appreciated elsewhere in North America, Europe, Japan and Australia. There have been many studies examining the differences in patient and disease characteristics of HPV(+) versus HPV(-) HNSCCs. Due to the increasing prevalence of HPV(+) SCCs within the oropharynx, our study sought to determine if the Nova Scotian population with HNC demonstrated similar trends as previously studied HPV(+) populations when OPSCCs are grouped together regardless of HPV status and compared to other HNSCCs.

## Methods

Data for this study was collected as part of a Canada-wide study on HNSCCs and HPV incidence currently underway. Capital Health Research Ethics Board approval was attained prior to this study. Following approval, a retrospective chart review was performed for all patients presented at the 2010 and 2011 NSCC's head and neck tumour board rounds. With the NSCC acting as the province-wide HNC referral centre, all Nova Scotia (NS) head and neck oncology cases are discussed within this forum.

Patient inclusion criteria consisted of patients diagnosed between January 2003 and December 2011 within NS with a pathologically confirmed invasive squamous cell carcinoma of the oropharynx, lip/oral cavity, nasopharynx, hypopharynx, larynx, salivary glands, nasal cavity or paranasal sinuses. Patients were excluded if they were diagnosed in another province, presented with a non-SCC HNC, presented with a primary tumour site not specified in the inclusion criteria, or if tissue pathology reports were not included in their charts.

Patient characteristics analyzed included age at diagnosis, sex, ethnicity, birth place, education, occupation, smoking history, alcohol history, illicit drug history, family medical history, height, weight, comorbidities including prior cancer history and ECOG performance status at diagnosis. The prevalidated Charlson Comorbidity Index and Charlson probability of 10 year survival will be used to quantify the comorbidities identified [24]. Disease characteristics included anatomic cancer site, anatomic cancer subsite, stage, grade, histology and p16 staining (the most commonly used surrogate marker for HPV status) [23]. Testing for p16 was performed routinely on primaries of the base of tongue and tonsillar region and at the surgeon/pathologist's discretion otherwise. Primary treatment details (treatment within the first 5 months of therapy initiation) and outcomes, including recurrence rates and survival within the follow- up period were also collected, with follow-up defined as the last clinical encounter prior to September 2013. Patients were de-identified and data was entered into a database on a password-protected computer.

## Statistical analysis

The two types of HNC were compared using chi-square tests for dichotomous categorical variables or Fishers exact test where appropriate. Wald test was used to compare variables with 3 categories. Continuous variables were compared using the non-parametric Wilcoxon test. The primary outcome was disease-free survival defined as survival free of relapse. Death was treated as a competing risk and reported as relapse-free mortality. Data was censored on date of last known follow-up. Overall survival was analyzed as a secondary outcome. All events were measured from the date of diagnosis. Gray's test for equality of cumulative incidence functions was used to assess differences between types of HNC. The cumulative incidence of mortality in the presence of relapse was also modeled. Cumulative incidence looks at the probability of relapse conditional on relapse free survival and competing risk for survival adjusting for the risk of death.

The proportional hazards model for subdistribution was used to model the cumulative incidence of relapse and relapse-free mortality [25]. Univariate competing risk regression models were performed to look at type of HNC. Multivariate models were used adjusting for COPD, age, overall stage, treatment and previous malignancy. Linearity of continuous variables and proportional hazards assumption of categorical variables was tested. Age violated assumptions of linearity and was therefore modeled as age < 55 vs. age ≥ 55. Overall survival was characterized using Kaplan-Meier plots and the Log-rank test was used to compare type of HNC. Cox-proportional hazards model was used to estimate hazard ratios. Level of significance was set at α = 0.05. SAS STAT software v9.3 (Cary, NC: SAS Institute Inc.) was used for all analyses.

## Results

### Primary subsite distribution

There were 582 charts reviewed with 318 (55 %) patients meeting the inclusion criteria. Of those analyzed,

122 (38 %) had been diagnosed with OPSCC and 196 (62 %) patients had other HNSCC primaries (Table 1). Analysis was performed on all available data. However, there were varying levels of availability in patient charts as demonstrated by the variability in sample sizes for specific comparisons.

### Demographics, risk factors and comorbidities

Patients' demographics, risk factors and comorbidities are reported in Table 2. There were no significant differences in smoking history between patients with OPSCC and other types of HNC (n = 312, never smoked 21(17 %) vs 25(13 %), current smoker 48(39 %) vs 91(46 %) and quit smoking 53(43 %) vs 74(38 %), p = 0.3002). The same was shown when pack year history was analyzed (Current smokers: 41.5 % vs 44.09 % p = 0.9891; Quit smoking: 27.79 % vs 32.18 %, p = 0.2969). Those with OPSCC, however, were significantly less likely to have COPD as a co-morbidity (n = 318, 19(16 %) vs 53(27 %), p = 0.0175). Particularly of note there were no significant differences in patients diagnosed at age <55 years (n = 316, 91(75 %)) compared to those age 55 years and older (147(75 %), p = 0.8123), in patient gender (n = 318, males: 97(80 %) vs. 140(71 %), p = 0.1078), in marijuana use (n = 128, 10(8 %) vs 17(9 %), p = 0.8267) or in drinking status (n = 267, never drank 4(3 %) vs 8(4 %), current drinker 84(69 %) vs 126(64 %) and quit drinking 20(16 %) vs 25(13 %), p = 0.7538). Finally, the Charlson probability for 10 year survival demonstrated no significant difference (n = 318, >50 % 89(28 %) vs 140(44 %), p = 0.7984).

### Treatment and weight loss

Treatment and weight loss data is summarized in Table 3. These comparisons demonstrated that OPSCCs were more likely to be given combination therapy, including "surgery and radiation therapy" (S-RT), "surgery

**Table 1** Anatomical subsite distribution of HNSCC primary tumours

| Site | Frequency (n) | Percent |
| --- | --- | --- |
| Oropharynx | 122 | 38.4 % |
| Lip & Oral Cavity | 86 | 27.0 % |
| Larynx | 72 | 22.6 % |
| Hypopharynx | 15 | 4.7 % |
| Nasopharynx | 10 | 3.1 % |
| Nasal Cavity | 8 | 2.5 % |
| Paranasal Sinuses | 4 | 1.3 % |
| Salivary Glands | 1 | 0.3 % |

**Table 2** Demographics and risk factors

| Demographics/risk factors | | Oropharygneal | Non-oropharyngeal | p-value[*] |
|---|---|---|---|---|
| Age at Diagnosis (n = 316) | <55 | 31(25 %) | 47(24 %) | 0.8123 |
| | ≥55 | 91(75 %) | 147(75 %) | |
| | Unknown | 0(0 %) | 2(1 %) | |
| Sex (n = 318) | Female | 25(20 %) | 56(29 %) | 0.1078 |
| | Male | 97(80 %) | 140(71 %) | |
| | Unknown | 0(0 %) | 0(0 %) | |
| Family Hx of Cancer (n = 245) | No | 27(22 %) | 41(21 %) | 0.4858 |
| | Yes | 79(65 %) | 98(50 %) | |
| | Unknown | 16(13 %) | 57(29 %) | |
| Cancer History (n = 318) | None | 93(76 %) | 143(73 %) | 0.5262[a] |
| | HNC | 4(3 %) | 12(6 %) | |
| | Other | 25(20 %) | 41(21 %) | |
| | Unknown | 0(0 %) | 0(0 %) | |
| Smoking History (n = 312) | Never | 21(17 %) | 25(13 %) | 0.3002[a] |
| | Quit | 53(43 %) | 74(38 %) | |
| | Current | 48(39 %) | 91(46 %) | |
| | Unknown | 0(0 %) | 6(3 %) | |
| Alcohol History (n = 267) | Never | 4(3 %) | 8(4 %) | 0.7538[a] |
| | Quit | 20(16 %) | 25(13 %) | |
| | Current | 84(69 %) | 126(64 %) | |
| | Unknown | 14(11 %) | 37(19 %) | |
| Marijuana Use (n = 128) | No | 41(34 %) | 60(31 %) | 0.8267 |
| | Yes | 10(8 %) | 17(9 %) | |
| | Unknown | 71(58 %) | 119(61 %) | |
| COPD (n = 318) | No | 103(84 %) | 143(73 %) | **0.0175** |
| | Yes | 19(16 %) | 53(27 %) | |
| | Unknown | 0(0 %) | 0(0 %) | |
| Pack-Year History (n = 312) | Never | 0 | 0 | n/a |
| | Current | 41.512 yrs. | 44.089 yrs. | 0.9891[b] |
| | Quit | 27.791 yrs. | 32.175 yrs. | 0.2969[b] |
| Charlson Prob. 10-Yr. Survival (n = 318) | <50 % | 33(10 %) | 56(18 %) | 0.7984 |
| | >50 % | 89(28 %) | 140(44 %) | |
| | Unknown | 0(0 %) | 0(0 %) | |

[*]α = 0.05, significant results in bold using chi-square test; [a]Wald test applied. [b]non-parametric Wilcoxon test applied

and chemotherapy", and "surgery, radiation therapy and chemotherapy" (S-CRT), as initial treatment as compared to other HNSCCs (n = 313, 84(69 %) vs 76(39 %), p = <0.001). OPSCCs were also significantly less likely to have primary surgery as initial treatment than other HNSCCs (n = 313, 14(11 %) vs 93(47 %), p = <0.001). During therapy, patients with OPSCCs also experienced greater weight loss by the end of treatment (n = 280, mean difference −3.0 kg (±5.3 SD), p < 0.001) and at follow-up (n = 251, mean difference −1.9 kg (± 9.0 SD), p = 0.0457).

### Disease characteristics

Disease characteristics are reported in Table 4. In terms of pathology, OPSCC tumours were more likely to be poorly differentiated/undifferentiated (n = 267, 49(40 %) vs 42(21 %), p < 0.001), be non-keratinizing (n = 169, 25(20 %) vs 17(9 %), p < 0.001), greater than 2 cm on presentation (n = 253, 72(59 %) vs 78(40 %), p = 0.0061), have had locoregional nodal spread (n = 315, 103(84 %) vs 55(28 %), p < 0.001) and to be overall stage 4 (n = 313, 55(45 %) vs 64(33 %), p = 0.0315). In the subset of 57 patients that had p16 testing for HPV, OPSCC were

A different entity: a population based study of characteristics and recurrence patterns...

5

**Table 3** Primary treatments and weight loss

| Primary treatment/weight Loss | | Oropharygneal | Non-oropharyngeal | p-value[*] |
|---|---|---|---|---|
| Combination Therapy (n = 313) | No | 35(29 %) | 118(60 %) | **<0.0001** |
| | Yes | 84(69 %) | 76(39 %) | |
| | Unknown | 3(2 %) | 2(1 %) | |
| Primary Surgery (n = 313) | No | 105(86 %) | 101(52 %) | **<0.0001** |
| | Yes | 14(11 %) | 93(47 %) | |
| | Unknown | 3(2 %) | 2(1 %) | |
| Median Weight Loss (kg) by Treatment End (n = 280) | | −5.7(31.4[b]) | −1.3(37.3[b]) | **<0.0001[a]** |
| Median Weight Loss (kg) at Follow-up (n = 251) | | −6.9(48.5[b]) | −4.5(66.45[b]) | **0.0457[a]** |

[*] α = 0.05, significant results in bold using chi-square test; [a]non-parametric Wilcoxon test applied; [b]weight loss range

more likely to be p16(+) (37(30 %) vs 1(1 %), $p < .001$) compared to other HNSCCs.

**Patient prognosis**

Prognostic data by HNSCC primaries are presented in Tables 5, 6 and 7. 26.73 % (85) of patients experienced relapse (median follow-up time 1.4 years, IQR 0.57 to 1.74). During follow-up 11.64 % (37) died without

relapse (median follow-up time 0.7 years, IQR 0.28 to 1.05). The cumulative incidence of relapse at 1-year was 7.03 % (95 % CI 3.26 % to 12.74 %) for OPSCCs compared to 20.61 % (95 % CI 14.93 % to 26.95 %) in other HNSCCs (Table 5). The Gray test indicated a difference in cummulative incidence functions (Fig. 1) for relapse between OPSCC and non-OPSCC tumours ($p = 0.0042$). However there was no evidence of a difference between

**Table 4** Disease characteristics

| Pathological factors | | Oropharygneal | Non-oropharyngeal | p-value[*] |
|---|---|---|---|---|
| Tumour size (n = 253) | ≤2 | 31(25 %) | 72(37 %) | **0.0061** |
| | >2 | 72(59 %) | 78(40 %) | |
| | Unknown | 19(16 %) | 46(23 %) | |
| Node Status (n = 315) | Negative | 19(16 %) | 138(70 %) | **<0.0001** |
| | Positive | 103(84 %) | 55(28 %) | |
| | Unknown | 0(0 %) | 3(2 %) | |
| Metastasis (n = 313) | No | 121(99 %) | 190(97 %) | 0.5242 |
| | Yes | 0(0 %) | 2(1 %) | |
| | Unknown | 1(1 %) | 4(2 %) | |
| Overall TMN Stage (n = 313) | <4 | 66(54 %) | 128(65 %) | **0.0315** |
| | 4 | 55(45 %) | 64(33 %) | |
| | Unknown | 1(1 %) | 4(2 %) | |
| Keratinization (n = 169) | Non-Keratinizing | 25(20 %) | 17(9 %) | **<0.0001** |
| | Keratinizing | 33(27 %) | 94(48 %) | |
| | Unknown | 64(52 %) | 85(43 %) | |
| Grade (n = 267) | ≥3 | 49(40 %) | 42(21 %) | **<0.0001[a]** |
| | 2 | 41(34 %) | 108(55 %) | |
| | 1 | 1(1 %) | 26(13 %) | |
| | Unknown | 31(25 %) | 20(10 %) | |
| p16 Status (n = 57) | Negative | 8(7 %) | 11(6 %) | **<0.0001** |
| | Positive | 37(30 %) | 1(1 %) | |
| | Unknown | 77(63 %) | 184(94 %) | |

[*] α = 0.05, significant results in bold using chi-square test; [a]Wald test applied

**Table 5** Cumulative incidence of relapse and relapse-free mortality at 1 year

| Subsite | Cumulative relapse at 1 year (95 % CI) | p-value[*] | Cumulative relapse-free mortality at 1 year (95 % CI) | p-value[*] |
|---|---|---|---|---|
| Oropharynx | 7.03 % (3.26–12.74 %) | **0.0042** | 9.76 % (5.13–16.16 %) | 0.1167 |
| Non-OPC | 20.61 % (14.93–26.95 %) | | 7.76 % (4.43–12.28 %) | |

[*]α = 0.05, significant results in bold using Gray's test for equality of cumulative incidence

the groups for the cummulative incidence function (Fig. 2) for relapse free mortality ($p = 0.1167$). The cumulative incidence of relapse free mortality at 1-year was 9.76 % (95 % CI 5.13 % to 16.16 %) for OPSCCs compared to 7.76 % (95 % CI 4.43 % to 12.28 %) for non-OPSCC tumours (Table 5).

In univariate analysis, the hazard of relapse was 2.119 times greater for non-OPSCC tumors ($p = 0.0034$) than OPSCCs. After adjusting the risk model for age ≥ 55, overall stage, treatment, COPD and previous malignancy, the hazard of relapse was 1.899 (95 % CI 0.998 to 3.611, $p = 0.0.0505$). The hazard of relapse-free mortality in univariate analysis was 0.636 times less for non-OPSCC tumors ($p = 0.053$) than OPSCCs. In multivariate analysis after adjusting for age ≥ 55, overall stage, treatment, COPD and previous malignancy, the hazard of relapse-free mortality was 0.896 (95 % CI 0.366 to 2.194, $p = 0.809$).

Overall one-year mortality in the non-OPSCC group was 13.70 % (SE 0.26) and 12.87 % (SE 0.32) in the OPSCC group (Fig. 3). The log-rank test showed no evidence of a difference in mortality rate between the two groups ($p = 0.6150$). The unadjusted hazard ratio was 1.13(95 % CI 0.698 to 1.823, $p = 0.6229$) for death for non-OPSCC tumours compared to OPSCCs. On

multivariate analysis however, an overall survival was appreciated. Specfically, after adjusting for age ≥ 55, overall stage, treatment, COPD and previous malignancy the hazard ratio was 1.822(95 % CI 1.025 to 3.238, $p = 0.0408$) for overall mortality in the non-OPSCC group.

## Discussion

In this population based study, it was found that the NS OPSCC population differed from other HNCs in a similar manner to those previously observed in other populations, however, there were some notable differences. Unlike many previous studies there were no significant differences noted when patient age, sex, alcohol history or Charlson Comorbidity Indices were compared between these groups. There was also no significant difference elucidated when smoking history was compared, although OPSCC patients were less commonly diagnosed with COPD. For this reason it may be hypothesized that other HNSCC patients had more exposure to tobacco smoke, although this remains an imperfect metric.

Weight loss comparisons at follow-up and by treatment end demonstrated significantly more weight loss

**Table 6** Univariate and multivariate competing risk regression analysis for relapse and mortality-free relapse

| Variable | Category | Univariate competing risk regression (95 % CI) | p-value[*] | Multivariate competing risk regression (95 % CI) | p-value[*] |
|---|---|---|---|---|---|
| Relapse | | | | | |
| Primary site | Non-oropharyngeal vs Oropharyngeal | 2.119 (1.282–3.501) | **0.0034** | 1.899 (0.998–3.611) | **0.0505** |
| COPD | Yes vs. No | | | 1.298 (0.777–2.170) | 0.3194 |
| Prior Cancer | Yes vs. No | | | 1.083 (0.644–1.819) | 0.7645 |
| Primary Treatment | Surgery vs. Chemotherapy/ Radiation | | | 1.306 (0.734–2.323) | 0.3645 |
| Stage | Stage 4 vs Other | | | 1.506 (0.930–2.438) | 0.0.0960 |
| Age | Age ≥ 55 vs <55 | | | 0.960 (0.587–1.571) | 0.8714 |
| Mortality-free Relapse | | | | | |
| Primary site | Non-oropharyngeal vs Oropharyngeal | 0.636 (0.314–1.288) | 0.053 | 0.896 (0.366–2.194) | 0.8098 |
| COPD | Yes vs. No | | | 1.669 (0.734–3.794) | 0.2218 |
| Prior Cancer | Yes vs. No | | | 2.507 (1.118–5.624) | **0.0258** |
| Primary Treatment | Surgery vs. Chemotherapy/ Radiation | | | 0.319 (0.115–.884) | **0.0280** |
| Stage | Stage 4 vs Other | | | 2.242 (1.084–4.638) | **0.0295** |
| Age | Age ≥ 55 vs <55 | | | 2.975 (0.925-9.568) | 0.0673 |

[*]α = 0.05, significant results in bold using competing risk regression

**Table 7** Univariate and multivariate Cox proportional hazard model analysis of overall mortality

| Variable | Category | Univariate Cox proportional hazards (95 % CI) | p-value[*] | Multivariate Cox proportional hazards (95 % CI) | p-value[*] |
|---|---|---|---|---|---|
| Overall mortality | | | | | |
| Primary site | Non-oropharyngeal vs Oropharyngeal | 1.128 (0.698–1.823) | 0.6229 | 1.822 (1.025–3.238) | **0.0408** |
| COPD | Yes vs. No | | | 2.022 (1.205–3.394) | **0.0077** |
| Prior Cancer | Yes vs. No | | | 1.622 (0.980–2.683) | 0.0599 |
| Primary Treatment | Surgery vs. Chemotherapy/Radiation | | | 0.367 (0.212–0.636) | **0.0004** |
| Stage | Stage 4 vs Other | | | 2.117 (1.306–3.432) | **0.0023** |
| Age | Age ≥ 55 vs <55 | | | 1.721 (0.928–3.193) | 0.0850 |

[*]α = 0.05, significant results in bold using Cox proportional hazard model

in the OPSCC group. This observation may simply be attributed to the differences in initial treatment between these two cohorts. As seen in Table 3, non-OPC HNSCC patients had a 47 % chance of receiving surgery alone compared to 11 % in the OPSCC group with OPSCCs having a greater chance of receiving combination therapy (69 % vs. 39 %). During this possible seven-week course of combination therapy the ability to have adequate oral intake is frequently severely limited due to the impact radiotherapy has on swallowing subsequently resulting in further weight loss.

Mirroring previous populations studied, in terms of disease characteristics, Nova Scotian patients with OPSCCs were significantly more likely to have lesions that were either poorly or undifferentiated, that were non-keratinizing, overall stage 4, have had nodal spread and to be HPV(+) compared to other HNSCCs. Interestingly, in a univariate analysis even with these classic indicators of poor prognosis OPSCCs in our study were also significantly less likely to experience relapse during the follow-up period. This was despite the lack of significance in the comparison of relapse-free mortality or overall mortality during the follow-up period. When these comparisons were adjusted for age ≥ 55, overall stage, treatment, COPD and previous malignancy in a multivariate analysis, significance decreased for relapse although still clinically significant at p=0.0505. However, significance was gained for overall mortality. This might suggest a significant interaction between non-OPSCC HNC and these other prognostic variables. The favorable

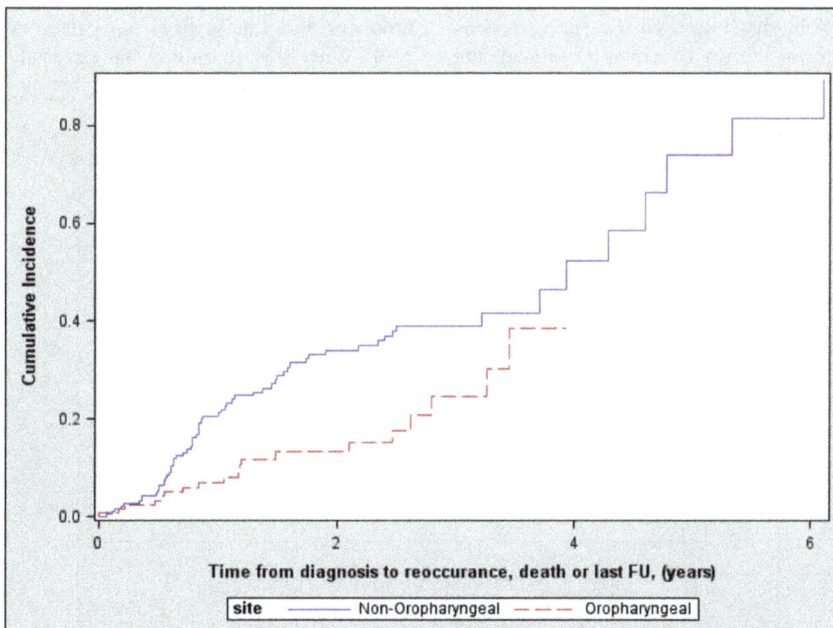

**Fig. 1** Cumulative incidence of relapse between oropharnygeal and non-oropharnygeal tumours (*p* = 0.0042)

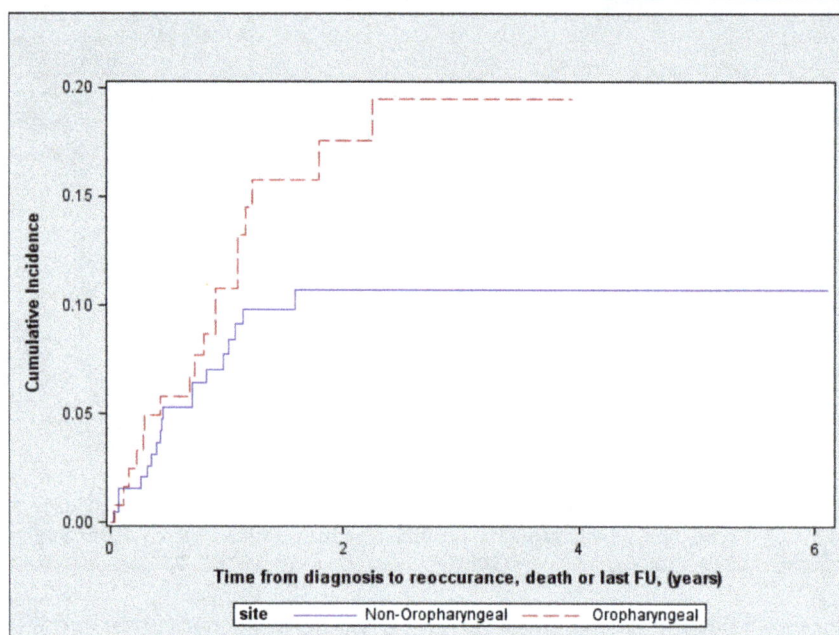

**Fig. 2** Cumulative incidence of relapse free mortality between oropharnygeal and non-oropharnygeal tumours ($p = 0.1167$)

findings in the univarite and multivariate relapse analyses and the multivariate mortality analysis were in keeping with data suggesting better outcomes among HPV related HNSCCs [20–23].

With previous HPV(+) populations demonstrating similar prognostic trends to our OPSCC group these findings may simply be attributed to the high percentage of HPV(+) tumors within the oropharyngeal site. This conclusion must be interpreted with caution, however, as we had such a small proportion of the OPSCC population having data relating to HPV status. Furthermore, OPSCCs have been shown to demonstrate three distinct survival curves in the literature with p16+/non-smokers having the best prognosis, followed by p16+/smokers and finally p16-/non-smokers doing the worst [26]. With this in mind, the survival outcomes of our

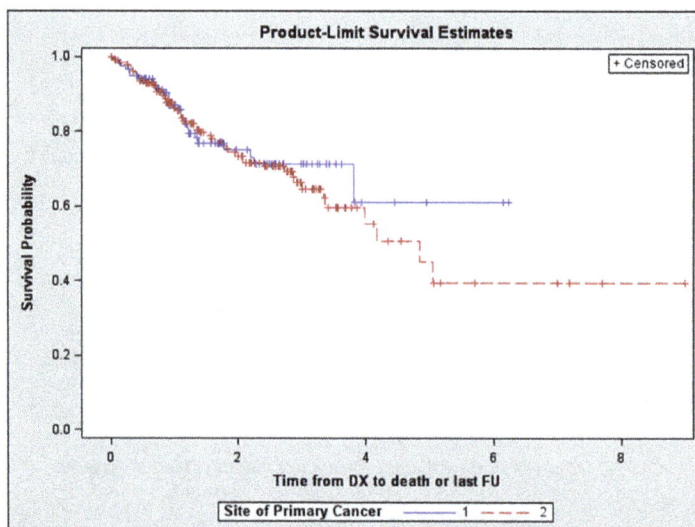

**Fig. 3** Kaplan-Meier curve comparing overall mortality between oropharyngeal (1) and non-oropharyngeal (2) subsites ($p = 0.6150$)

OPSCC group are lower than observed in homogeneous HPV(+) OPSCC populations. This suggests that the HPV(-) OPSCC cohort is influencing these results to some degree and that Nova Scotia's relatively high smoking rate may be placing more patients on the intermediate survival curve described above [26, 27].

The recurrence free survival advantage of OPSCCs has been attributed to the tumours' improved response profiles as compared to other HNSCCs with HPV(+) tumours responding better to chemotherapy and radiation [9, 21, 28, 29]. CRT is, however, associated with increased acute and late toxicities significantly affecting quality of life post-treatment [30]. It has also been shown that combination therapy including surgery for OPSCC has an improved 5-year disease specific survival in stage 3 and 4 disease compared to S-RT and CRT alone [31]. Furthermore, there has been an increase in studies investigating whether we can safely de-escalate treatment for HPV(+) OPSCCs at low risk for distant metastasis, with hopes that treatment related morbidity can be reduced without sacrificing survival outcomes [32–34]. This comes at a time when surgical techniques such as transoral robotic surgery are being developed and tested as possible alternatives to CRT. Recently, these modalities have compared favorably in terms of survival and quality of life in preliminary studies [35].

Evidence is now accumulating suggesting that the classic IUCC/AJCC TNM staging system used to prognosticate HNCs might be inadequate due to the unique presentation and treatment response profile of OPSCCs [36–38]. Most studies show HPV(+) OPSCCs tend to have more nodal spread and higher overall TNM stages than other subsites despite improvements in OS and disease free survival [19–21, 36, 37, 39]. Our research would further support this notion with Nova Scotian OPSCCs presenting at higher overall TNM stages. Despite this, these patients experienced a more favorable prognosis as compared to their HNSCC counterparts in terms of relapse and mortality thus supporting HPV status as a useful prognostic indicator [24, 36, 37].

Our findings would suggest that an alternative staging system might be warranted for this particular subset of SCC. This concept is not new, as the IUCC/AJCC staging system for HNC has been scrutinized for years to further improve its suboptimal prognostic ability [40]. Other staging systems have been developed for HNC in an attempt to mitigate this deficit but there has yet to be an appropriate alternative shown to be effective [40–42]. Notably Huang et al. have shown that an alternative anatomical stage grouping has superior prognostic ability to the classic system and may be further enhanced by the addition of non-anatomic factors [43]. When this new staging system was applied to our patient cohort there were significantly more OPSCCs presenting as stage 1 or 2 disease, which better correlates with their improved prognosis (Table 8). These findings may merit a more in-depth survival analysis in the future.

Our findings suggest that until the advent of a prognostically accurate staging system that takes HPV status into account the presence of an oropharyngeal subsite primary should be considered a positive prognostic indicator regardless of HPV status. This may be of particular importance when HPV status is unknown. More importantly, this highlights the need for universal p16 testing, which is further amplified by recent evidence demonstrating that p16 positive non-OPSCC tumours have similarly improved survival outcomes as compared to p16 negative non-OPSCC tumours [44].

With the disease characteristics of Nova Scotian OPSCC's so closely mirroring those of HPV(+) populations, the oncogenic role of this virus within the oropharynx is further solidified. Although the effect of HPV vaccination on incidence reduction of OPSCCs within the population will take many years to become fully apparent there has been promising research suggesting this is the case [45]. Our findings support established population based vaccination programs shown to be effective in both sexes [46].

This study provided some intriguing findings on OPSCC in NS patients, however, did have some limitations that must be recognized in interpretation. Of course, any retrospective chart review relies on the accuracy of the written record, the presence of important information in the record and the accessibility of that record. For this reason many comparisons have different sample sizes based on the availability of patient data. Further, our interval for follow-up of patients in this study may not have been of adequate length to accurately elucidate OS trends for this population. A

**Table 8** Comparison of Huang et al.'s recursive partitioning analysis (RPA) staging against IUCC/AJCC staging for the oropharyngeal subsite

| Stages at presentation | | RPA staging | IUCC/AJCC staging | p-value[*] |
|---|---|---|---|---|
| Oropharyngeal Subsite | 1 or 2 | 92(75 %) | 12(10 %) | **<0.001** |
| | 3 or 4 | 29(24 %) | 109(89 %) | |
| | Unknown | 1(1 %) | 1(1 %) | |

[*]α = 0.05, significant results in bold using chi-square test

larger sample would also provide increased statistical power to further study the relationships between our subgroups and the prognostic variables analyzed herein.

Finally, HPV status in particular was scarce in patient records during this time period thus making the exact influence of the virus difficult to elucidate. While the population tested for p16 was small, based on trends within the oropharynx and the characteristics demonstrated herein it is likely that many of the trends observed in Nova Scotia's OPSCC cohort could be attributed to HPV infection alone. For this reason we believe that if all patients had been tested the number of HPV associated OPSCCs would be similar to other North American populations. The small number of specimens tested is at least in part due to their date of diagnosis predating routine p16 testing in NS, which was implemented in 2009. Although all patients were treated during 2010 or 2011 only 79 % of them were diagnosed within this time period. Furthermore, among these late diagnoses many would have presented with nodal disease thus limiting the adequacy of p16 testing, as tissue samples would have been limited to fine needle aspirates [47].

## Conclusions
In conclusion, this study demonstrates that Nova Scotian patients diagnosed with OPSCCs treated at the NSCC between 2010 and 2011 did in fact possess disease characteristics distinct from other HNSCC subsites. The disease characteristics observed were in line with previous studies on HPV(+) OPSCCs further supporting the potential that HPV infection is playing an important oncogenic role in NS. Furthermore, despite more advanced presentations, based on IUCC/AJCC staging, these OPSCC tumours tend to have a more favorable prognosis than their other HNSCC counterparts. These findings support the implementation of universal p16 testing for accurate prognostication of HNSCCs and the potential inclusion of p16 into future staging systems for OPSCC. Ultimately, these unique Nova Scotian trends when combined with other studies across Canada should help guide treatment and prevention resource allocation decisions in the future.

### Abbreviations
COPD: Chronic obstructive pulmonary disease; HNC: Head and neck cancer; HNSCC: Head and neck squamous cell carcinoma; HPV: Human papillomavirus; HPV(+): Human papillomavirus positive; HPV(-): Human papillomavirus negative; NS: Nova Scotia; NSCC: Nova Scotia Cancer Centre; OPSCC: Oropharyngeal squamous cell carcinoma; OPC: Oropharyngeal cancer; OS: Overall survival; SCC: Squamous cell carcinoma; S-CRT: Surgery, radiation therapy and chemotherapy; S-RT: Surgery and radiation therapy; US: United States; UK: United Kingdom.

### Competing interests
To all of the authors' knowledge this manuscript adheres to the Journal of Otolaryngology-Head & Neck Surgery's editorial policies and there are no competing interests involved.

### Authors' contributions
SLS, RH and MR conceptualized the study. SM wrote the final manuscript. SM and MH were responsible for maintenance of the database, data acquisition, analysis and manuscript preparation including revision and editing. KT performed statistical analysis along with revision and editing of the manuscript. All authors read and approved the final manuscript.

### Acknowledgements
This project was partially funded by Cancer Care Nova Scotia, by way of a Norah Stephen Oncology Scholars Award through the Beatrice Hunter Cancer Research Institute. Further, the authors acknowledge with gratitude Dr. Geoffrey Liu, University Health Network, University of Toronto, for both financial and infrastructure support for this project. The funding bodies played no role in the design, collection, analysis, or interpretation of data; in the writing of the manuscript; or in the decision to submit the manuscript for publication.

### Author details
[1]Dalhousie University, Faculty of Medicine, Halifax, Nova Scotia, Canada. [2]Dalhousie University, Research Methods Unit, Halifax, Nova Scotia, Canada. [3]Department of Surgery, Division of Otolaryngology, Capital District Health Authority, Halifax, Nova Scotia, Canada. [4]Department of Radiation Oncology, Capital District Health Authority, Halifax, Nova Scotia, Canada. [5]Department of Internal Medicine, Division of Medical Oncology, Capital District Health Authority, Halifax, Nova Scotia, Canada.

### References
1. Jemal A, Bray F, Center MM, Ferlay J, Ward E, Forman D. Global cancer statistics. CA Cancer J Clin. 2011;61:69–90.
2. Warnakulasuriya S. Global epidemiology of oral and oropharyngeal cancer. Oral Oncol. 2009;45:309–16.
3. Canadian Cancer Statistics 2014 [http://www.cancer.ca/~/media/cancer.ca/CW/cancer%20information/cancer%20101/Canadian%20cancer%20statistics/Canadian-Cancer-Statistics-2014-EN.pdf]
4. Johnson-Obaseki S, McDonald JT, Corsten M, Rourke R. Head and neck cancer in Canada: trends 1992 to 2007. Otolaryngol Head Neck Surg. 2012;147:74–8.
5. Attner P, Du J, Nasman A, Hammarstedt L, Ramqvist T, Lindholm J, et al. The role of human papillomavirus in the increased incidence of base of tongue cancer. Int J Cancer. 2010;126:2879–84.
6. Chaturvedi AK, Engels EA, Anderson WF, Gillison ML. Incidence trends for human papillomavirus-related and -unrelated oral squamous cell carcinomas in the United States. J Clin Oncol. 2008;26:612–9.
7. Ryerson AB, Peters ES, Coughlin SS,Chen VW, Gillison ML, Reichman ME, et al. Burden of potentially human papillomavirus-associated cancers of the oropharynx and oral cavity in the US, 1998-2003. Cancer. 2008;113:2901–9.
8. Nasman A, Attner P, Hammarstedt L, Du J, Eriksson M, Giraud G, et al. Incidence of human papillomavirus (HPV) positive tonsillar carcinoma in Stockholm, Sweden: an epidemic of viral-induced carcinoma? Int J Cancer. 2009;125:362–6.
9. Ramqvist T, Dalianis T. An epidemic of oropharyngeal squamous cell carcinoma (OSCC) due to human papillomavirus (HPV) infection and aspects of treatment and prevention. Anticancer Res. 2001;31:1515–20.
10. Chaturvedi AK, Anderson WF, Lortet-Tieulent J, Curado MP, Ferlay J, Franceschi S, et al. Worldwide trends in incidence rates for oral cavity and oropharyngeal cancers. J Clin Oncol. 2013;31:4550–9.
11. Chaturvedi AK, Engels EA, Pfeiffer R, Hernandez BY, Xiao W, Kim E, et al. Human papillomavirus and rising oropharyngeal cancer incidence in the United States. J Clin Oncol. 2011;29:4924–301.
12. Hashibe M, Brennan P, Chuang SC, Boccia S, Castellsague X, Chen C, et al. Interaction between tobacco and alcohol use and the risk of head and neck cancer: pooled analysis in the International Head and Neck Cancer Epidemiology Consortium. Cancer Epidemiol Biomarkers Prev. 2009;18:541–50.
13. Health Canada tobacco use statistics [http://www.hc-sc.gc.ca/hc-ps/tobac-tabac/research-recherche/stat/index-eng.php]

14. Health Canada drug and alcohol use statistics [http://www.hc-sc.gc.ca/hc-ps/drugs-drogues/stat/index-eng.php]
15. Romanitan M, Nasman A, Ramqvist T, Dahlstrand H, Polykretis L, Vogiatzis P, et al. Human papillomavirus frequency in oral and oropharyngeal cancer in Greece. Anticancer Res. 2008;28:2077–80.
16. Herrero R, Castellsague X, Pawlita M, Lissowska J, Kee F, Balaram P, et al. Human papillomavirus and oral cancer: the International Agency for Research on Cancer multicenter study. J Natl Cancer Inst. 2003;95:1772–83.
17. Walboomers JM, Jacobs MV, Manos MM, Bosch FX, Kummer JA, Shah KV, et al. Human papillomavirus is a necessary cause of invasive cervical cancer worldwide. J Pathol. 1999;189:12–9.
18. Gillison M, D'Souza G, Westra W, Sugar E, Xiao W, Begum S, et al. Distinct risk factor profiles for human papillomavirus type 16-positive and human papillomavirus type 16- negative head and neck cancers. J Natl Cancer Inst. 2008;100:407–20.
19. Marur S, D'Souza G, Westra WH, Forastiere AA. HPV-associated head and neck cancer: a virus- related cancer epidemic. Lancet Oncol. 2010;11:781–9.
20. Ragin CC, Taioli E. Survival of squamous cell carcinoma of the head and neck in relation to human papillomavirus infection: review and meta-analysis. Int J Cancer. 2007;121:1813–20.
21. Pfister DG, Fury MG. New Chapter in Our Understanding of Human Papillomavirus-Related Head and Neck Cancer. J Clin Oncol. 2014;32. in press.
22. Fakhry C, Zhang Q, Nguyen-Tan PF, Rosenthal D, El-Naggar A, Garden AS, et al. Human papillomavirus and overall survival after progression of oropharyngeal squamous cell carcinoma. J Clin Oncol. 2014. doi:10.1200/JCO.2014.55.1937.
23. Kreimer AR, Clifford GM, Boyle P, Franceschi S. Human papillomavirus types in head and neck squamous cell carcinomas worldwide: a systematic review. Cancer Epidemiol Biomarkers Prev. 2005;14:467–75.
24. Charlson M, Szatrowski TP, Peterson J, Gold J. Validation of a combined comorbidity index. J Clin Epidemiol. 1994;47:1245–51.
25. Fine JP, Gray RJ. A proportional hazards model for the subdistribution of a competing risk. J Am Stat Assoc. 1999;94:496–509.
26. Ang KK, Harris J, Wheeler R, Weber R, Rosenthal DI, Nguyen-Tân PF, et al. Human papillomavirus and survival of patients with oropharyngeal cancer. N Engl J Med. 2011;363:24–35.
27. Statistics Canada: Smokers, by sex, province and territories (percent) [http://www.statcan.gc.ca/tables-tableaux/sum-som/l01/cst01/health74b-eng.htm]
28. Fakhry C, Westra WH, Li S, Cmelak A, Ridge JA, Pinto H, et al. Improved survival of patients with human papillomavirus- positive head and neck squamous cell carcinoma in a prospective clinical trial. J Natl Cancer Inst. 2008;100:261–9.
29. Lindquist D, Romanitan M, Hammarstedt L, Näsman A, Dahlstrand H, Lindholm J, et al. Human papillomavirus is a favourable prognostic factor in tonsillar cancer and its oncogenic role is supported by the expression of E6 and E7. Mol Oncol. 2007;1:350–5.
30. Machtay M, Moughan J, Trotti A, Garden AS, Weber RS, Cooper JS, et al. Factors associated with severe late toxicity after concurrent chemoradiation for locally advanced head and neck cancer: an RTOG analysis. J Clin Oncol. 2008;26:3582–9.
31. O'Connell D, Seikaly H, Murphy R, Fung C, Cooper T, Knox A, et al. Primary surgery versus chemoradiotherapy for advanced oropharyngeal cancers: a longitudinal population study. J Otolaryngol Head Neck Surg. 2013;42:31.
32. Ferris RL, Harry Q, Panian B. Phase II Randomized Trial of Transoral Surgical Resection followed by Low-dose or Standard-dose IMRT in Resectable p16+ Locally Advanced Oropharynx Cancer. 2013. ClinicalTrials.gov identifier: NCT01898494. https://clinicaltrials.gov/ct2/show/NCT01898494.
33. Haughey BH. Adjuvant De-escalation, Extracapsular spread, P16+, Transoral (A.D.E.P.T) Trial for Oropharynx Malignancy. 2013. ClinicalTrials.gov identifier: NCT01687413. https://clinicaltrials.gov/ct2/show/NCT01687413.
34. O'Sullivan B, Huang SH, Siu LL, Waldron J, Zhao H, Perez-Ordonez B, et al. Deintensification candidate subgroups in human papillomavirus–related oropharyngeal cancer according to minimal risk of distant metastasis. J Clin Oncol. 2013;31:543–50.
35. Nichols AC, Yoo J, Hammond JA, Fung K, Winquist E, Read N, et al. Early-stage squamous cell carcinoma of the oropharynx: radiotherapy vs. trans-oral robotic surgery (ORATOR) — study protocol for a randomized phase II trial. BMC Cancer. 2013;13:133.
36. Klozar J, Koslabova E, Kratochvil V, Salakova, M, Tachezy, R. Nodal status is not a prognostic factor in patients with HPV-positive oral/oropharyngeal tumors. J Surg Oncol. 2013;107:625–33.
37. Hong AM, Martin A, Armstrong BK, Lee CS, Jones D, Chatfield MD, et al. Human papillomavirus modifies the prognostic significance of T stage and possibly N stage in tonsillar cancer. Ann Oncol. 2013;24:215–9.
38. Smith EM, Ritchie JM, Summersgill KF, Klussmann JP, Lee JH, Wang D, et al. Age, sexual behavior and human papillomavirus infection in oral cavity and oropharyngeal cancers. Int J Cancer. 2004;108:766–72.
39. Hong AM, Dobbins TA, Lee CS, Jones D, Harnett GB, Armstrong BK, et al. Human papillomavirus predicts outcome in oropharyngeal cancer in patients treated primarily with surgery or radiation therapy. Br J Cancer. 2010;103:1510–7.
40. Groome PA, Schulze KM, Mackillop WJ, Grice B, Goh C, Cummings BJ, et al. A comparison of published head and neck stage groupings in carcinomas of the tonsillar region. Cancer. 2001;92:1484–94.
41. Jones GW, Browman G, Goodyear M, Marcellus D, Hodson DI. Comparison of the additions of T and N integer scores with TNM stage groups in head and neck cancer. Head Neck. 1993;15:497–503.
42. Hart AA, Hilgers FJ, Manni JJ. The importance of correct stage grouping in oncology. Cancer. 1995;11:2656–62.
43. Huang SH, Xu W, Waldron J, Siu L, Shen X, Tong L, et al. Refining American Joint Committee on Cancer/Union for International Cancer Control TNM stage and prognostic groups for human papillomavirus–related oropharyngeal carcinomas. J Clin Oncol. 2015;33:836–45.
44. Chung CH, Zhang Q, Kong CS, Harris J, Fertig EJ, Harari PM, et al. p16 protein expression and human papillomavirus status as prognostic biomarkers of nonoropharyngeal head and neck squamous cell carcinoma. J Clin Oncol. 2014. doi:10.1200/JCO.2013.54.5228.
45. Herrero R, Quint W, Hildesheim A, Gonzalez P, Struijk L, Katki HA, et al. Reduced prevalence of oral human papillomavirus (HPV) 4 years after bivalent HPV vaccination in a randomized clinical trial in Costa Rica. PLoS One. 2013;8:e68329.
46. Giuliano AR, Palefsky JM, Goldstone S, Moreira ED Jr, Penny ME, Aranda C, et al. Efficacy of quadrivalent HPV vaccine against HPV infection and disease in males. N Engl J Med. 2011;364:401–11.
47. Lastra RR, Pramick MR, Nakashima MO, Weinstein GS, Montone KT, Livolsi VA, et al. Adequacy of fine-needle aspiration specimens for human papillomavirus infection molecular testing in head and neck squamous cell carcinoma. Cytojournal. 2013;10:21.

# 2

# Identification of altered protein abundances in cholesteatoma matrix via mass spectrometry-based proteomic analysis

Derrick R. Randall, Phillip S. Park and Justin K. Chau[*]

## Abstract

**Background:** Cholesteatoma are cyst-like structures lined with a matrix of differentiated squamous epithelium overlying connective tissue. Although epithelium normally exhibits self-limited growth, cholesteatoma matrix erodes mucosa and bone suggesting changes in matrix protein constituents that permit destructive behaviour. Differential proteomic studies can measure and compare the cholesteatoma proteome to normal tissues, revealing protein alterations that may propagate the destructive process.

**Methods:** Human cholesteatoma matrix, cholesteatoma-involved ossicles, and normal middle ear mucosa, post-auricular skin, and non-involved ossicles were harvested. These tissues were subjected to multiplex peptide labeling followed by liquid chromatography and tandem mass spectrometry analysis. Relative protein abundances were compared and evaluated for ontologic function and putative involvement in cholesteatoma.

**Results:** Our methodology detected 10 764 peptides constituting 1662 unique proteins at 95 % confidence or greater. Twenty-nine candidate proteins were identified in soft tissue analysis, with 29 additional proteins showing altered abundances in bone samples. Ontologic functions and known relevance to cholesteatoma are discussed, with several candidates highlighted for their roles in epithelial integrity, evasion of apoptosis, and immunologic function.

**Conclusion:** This study produced an extensive cholesteatoma proteome and identified 58 proteins with altered abundances contributing to disease pathopathysiology. As well, potential biomarkers of residual disease were highlighted. Further investigation into these proteins may provide useful options for novel therapeutics or monitoring disease status.

## Background

Cholesteatoma is a benign epidermal inclusion cyst that develops within the temporal bone and exhibits locally destructive behavior. Without treatment, cholesteatomas can progressively expand and destroy middle ear and temporal bone structures. This process can lead to secondary infections, which can result in complications such as tympanic membrane perforation, chronic otorrhea, hearing loss, vestibular dysfunction, facial nerve

* Correspondence: justin.chau@gmail.com
This article was presented at the Canadian Society of Otolaryngology – Head & Neck Surgery Poliquin Competition, Winnipeg, MB, June 8, 2015
Section of Otolaryngology – Head & Neck Surgery, Department of Surgery, University of Calgary, Calgary, Foothills Medical Centre, 1403 - 29 Street NW, Calgary, AB T2N 2T9, Canada

paresis, and intracranial extension [1]. Regardless of surgical technique, cholesteatoma have propensity to recur [2], requiring exteriorization of the middle ear through canal wall down procedures or "second look" tympano-mastoidectomy for surveillance of disease in intact canal wall procedures.

Increased understanding of molecular changes in bone through orthopedic and otitis media literature led to theories of cholesteatoma-related bone destruction through cellular resorption, mechanical compression, and second mediator effects [2–7]. Bone erosion involved in the progression of disease may be intrinsic to the cholesteatoma—increased matrix growth factor and cytokine expression, pressure effect of outward growth, and host granulation enzymes. Extrinsic factors include bacterial superinfection, altered osteoclast activity in response to invasion, and changes in bone architecture and cell population [3, 7, 8]. Numerous targeted molecular and genome wide studies on cholesteatoma specimens support some of these hypotheses but fail to appreciate the complex interplay between multiple changes at the cellular level.

Differential proteomic analysis evaluates the active protein constellation between normal and pathologic states [9]. Initiated as two-dimensional gel electrophoresis (2DGE) with densitometry or visual evaluation, modern proteomic analysis evolved to incorporate mass-spectrometry in protein identification from individual 2DGE studies to current chromatographic separation and tandem mass spectrometry techniques capable of analyzing multiple tissue conditions simultaneously. Modern mass spectrometry-based techniques have improved the ability to recognize novel, replicable protein derangements in various diseases and tissues by comparing disease to normal states [10]. These changes can be detected among proteins expressed at very low levels and several orders of magnitude below that of the most abundant proteins.

Previous proteomic approaches to cholesteatoma identified several proteins with altered presence in comparison to post-auricular skin through 2DGE [11]. In this study, we employed a multiplex differential mass spectrometry-based approach termed isotope-tagged relative abundance quantification (iTRAQ) to characterize simultaneously the cholesteatoma matrix proteome in reference to native middle ear mucosa and post-auricular skin as well as to evaluate the bone proteome of ossicles involved by cholesteatoma compared to normal ossicles. With this design we were able to detect agents underlying the pathophysiologic process and destructive behavior demonstrated by cholesteatoma as well as identify and quantify potential biomarkers of disease.

## Methods
### Sample collection
This study received ethical approval from the University of Calgary Conjoint Health Research Ethics Board (REB-14-0883). Patient tissue samples were obtained during primary tympanomastoidectomy from patients with acquired cholesteatoma, whereby cholesteatoma matrix was excised and cleaned of keratin debris; middle ear mucosa was collected from uninvolved regions of the mastoid cavity; post-auricular skin was taken as a 1 mm wide strip of skin along the margin of the skin incision with subcutaneous tissue removed by sharp dissection under an operating microscope. Cholesteatoma-involved ossicles were harvested during tympanomastoidectomy from patients with evidence of ossicular destruction. Control ossicles were obtained from patients undergoing

labyrinthectomy for vestibular schwannoma or ossicular reconstruction for traumatic ossicular discontinuity. Tissue samples were immediately placed on ice then stored at −80 °C until sample processing.

### Protein extraction
Samples were thawed on ice then washed three times in 4 °C phosphate-buffered saline containing complete protease inhibitor (Roche, Mississauga, ON). Sample processing was performed by the following methods for either soft tissue or bone, in an identical fashion for each tissue sample, with all buffers containing cOmplete protease inhibitor (Roche, Mississauga, ON).

Soft tissue samples were pooled as mucosa, matrix, or skin samples. Each pool was incubated at 4 °C for 16 h in modified RIPA buffer with protease inhibitor. Samples were then sonicated on ice for 7 s at 20 % power for 5 cycles with 30 s cooling periods. The resultant lysates were centrifuged for 60 min at 12 000 g at 4 °C in an Allegra X-15R centrifuge (Beckman-Coulter, Mississauga, ON) and the supernatant preserved. Equivalent total protein concentrations from each pool were precipitated in 100 % chilled ethanol (Sigma, Oakville, ON) by incubating 24 h at −20 °C followed by 20 min centrifugation at $2500\,g$ (4 °C). The pellet was preserved, washed once with 80 % ethanol (v/v), centrifuged at $2500\,g$ (4 °C), decanted, and air dried for 5 min. The precipitated samples were stored at −80 °C until iTRAQ analysis.

Individual bone samples were incubated at room temperature in 0.06 M hydrocholoric acid (HCl) for 16 h. The diluent (D1) was removed and the bone samples incubated in 1.2 M HCl at 4 °C for 16 h to decalcify the bone. After decalcification, the diluent (D2) was removed, and bone samples were pooled into two groups (control ossicles or cholesteatoma-involved ossicles) then washed with extraction buffer 1 (E1: 6 M guanidine-HCl and 100 mM Tris–HCl with protease inhibitor). Buffer E1 was added to the pooled samples, which were sonicated on ice for 7 s at 20 % power for 5 cycles with 30 s cooling periods. Samples were incubated for 72 h at 4 °C then centrifuged for 20 min at 12 000 g (4 °C). Supernatant E1 was removed and stored at −80 °C. Samples were washed with extraction buffer 1.5 (E1.5: 6 M guanidine-HCl, 100 mM HEPES, 0.5 M $Na_4EDTA$, protease inhibitor), then buffer E1.5 was added to the pellet, agitated, and incubated 72 h at 4 °C. Samples were centrifuged for 20 min at 12 000 g at 4 °C, and supernatant E1.5 removed and stored at −80 °C. Samples were washed with extraction buffer 2 (E2: 6 M HCl, 6 M guanidine-HCl, 100 mM 100 mM Tris, protease inhibitor), then buffer E2 was added to the pellet, fragmented, and incubated 20 h at 4 °C. Samples D2, E1, E1.5, and E2 were combined in their respective pooled samples and precipitated by the same method as the soft tissue samples and stored at −80 °C until iTRAQ analysis.

## iTRAQ reagent preparation

Two LC-MS/MS tracts were defined and run on separate days in order to minimize the impact of high abundance proteins from each tissue type limiting the ability to detect low abundance proteins: one for soft tissue and one for bone samples. Soft tissue and bone lysates were labelled with iTRAQ reagent according to the University of Victoria Protein Centre protocols. 100 µg of total protein from each sample underwent acetone precipitation followed by resuspension in iTRAQ buffer and trypsin digestion. Each protein lysate was labeled with a distinct isotopic iTRAQ reagent: control ossicles (113 Da), cholesteatoma-involved ossicles (115 Da); cholesteatoma matrix 1 (113 Da), cholesteatoma matrix 2 (114 Da), mucosa (115 Da), post-auricular skin (116 Da). These samples were combined and subjected to alkaline (pH 10) reversed phase high performance liquid chromatography on an XBridge C18 BEH300 250 mm X 4.6 mm, 5 µm, 300A HPLC column (Waters, MA, USA), with fractions collected every minute for 96 min.

## LC-MS/MS analysis

Fractions were separated by on-line reversed phase liquid chromatography using a Thermo Scientific EASY-nanoLC II system with a reversed-phase pre-column Magic C-18AQ (100 µm I.D., 2 cm length, and an in-house prepared reversed-phase nano-analytical column packed with Magic C-18AQ (75 µm I.D., 15 cm length, 5 µm, 100 Å; Michrom BioResources Inc, Auburn, CA). The chromatography system was coupled on-line to an LTQ Orbitrap Velos Pro mass spectrometer equipped with a Nanospray Flex source (Thermo Fisher Scientific, Bremen, Germany) and run over a 120 min gradient from 95 % solvent A (2 % Acetonitrile, 0.1 % Formic acid):5 % solvent B (90 % Acetonitrile, 0.1 % Formic acid) to 100 % solvent B. Mass spectrometry data were acquired with a time of flight survey scan of mass range 400–1800 amu where the most abundant ions exceeding 5000 counts and charge state 2–4 selected for fragmentation.

## Data acquisition and analysis

The resulting data were analyzed by Proteome Discoverer 1.4 software suite (Thermo Scientific) using stringency criteria: s/n cut-off: 1.5; total intensity threshold: 0; minimum peak count: 1; precursor mass: 350–5000 Da. The peak lists were submitted to an in-house database search using Mascot 2.4 (Matrix Science), and were searched against the Uniprot-Swissprot database (May 30, 2015 update; 540,261 sequences; 191,876,607 residues) assuming 2 or less missed trypsin cut sites as well as fixed methylthio and variable oxidation and deamidation modifications.

Target false discovery rate was set a 0.01. All identified proteins were assessed for gene ontology functions with an additional function set for structural components and those proteins with bone-related functions. Candidate proteins were selected if their relative abundances were greater than 1.5-fold ($\log_2$ scale) increased or decreased in cholesteatoma matrix compared to either middle ear mucosa or post-auricular skin for soft tissue analysis, or if proteins in cholesteatoma-involved bone were greater than 1.5-fold ($\log_2$ scale) increased or decreased relative to control ossicles and found to have ontologic functions corresponding to cellular metabolism, bone structure, bone metabolism, or epithelial content.

## Results

The soft tissue arm of our study included representative samples from 12 cholesteatoma matrices, eight non-diseased middle ear mucosa fragments, and nine post-auricular skin samples. Healthy mucosa not involved with cholesteatoma could not be identified in four patients and was not collected; three post-auricular skin samples were suboptimal samples and not included. iTRAQ analysis of the included samples detected 10 720 spectra representing 8372 unique peptides. Setting stringency at 95 % probability of protein recognition and at least two peptides per protein identified 1490 proteins from 8315 of these peptides, corresponding to an average of 5.58 peptides per protein. The ontologic functions of these proteins are displayed in Fig. 1a. Cellular metabolism, signal transduction, and DNA replication/transcription/repair functions comprise more than 50 % of the identified proteins.

With respect to the bone lysate analysis, which included eight cholesteatoma-involved ossicles and eight control ossicles, 3159 spectra and 2392 unique peptides produced 480 proteins with at least two peptides and 95 % confidence of identification (4.96 peptides per protein). After subtracting protein clusters representing homologous protein family members, 428 were recognized with greater than 95 % confidence and further scrutinized. Gene ontology functions for the identified proteins are shown in Fig. 1b. The most common functions identified were metabolism, signal transduction, and bone structure, which accounted for 50 % of all proteins; 10 % of proteins played a role in bone structure and another 7 % in bone metabolism. In comparison to the soft tissue analysis there were 256 common proteins, indicating our study identified 1662 proteins from cholesteatoma and involved middle ear structures.

Figures 2 and 3 display the proteins identified in the soft tissue analysis with relative abundances of proteins in mucosa and skin, respectively, compared to cholesteatoma matrix. Proteins exceeding the relative abundance threshold are highlighted in red and represent potential

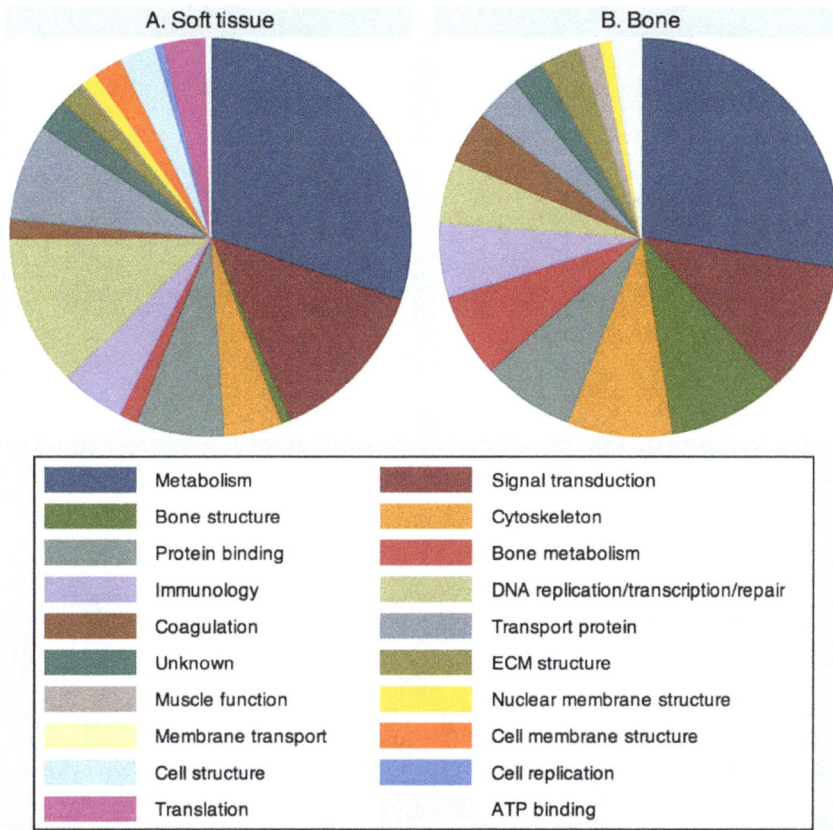

**Fig. 1** Ontologic functions of proteins identified in (**a**). Soft tissue analysis and (**b**). Bone analysis. General metabolic function and signal transduction properties represent the most common ontologic functions in both tissue sets, but wide variation exists among the remaining categories

candidates in cholesteatoma pathophysiology or biomarkers of disease. These 29 proteins are listed in Table 1 with their relative abundances in cholesteatoma matrix in reference to both uninvolved mucosa and post-auricular skin. Positive numbers indicate increased abundance in cholesteatoma while negative values indicate a higher relative abundance in normal tissue. Similarly, Fig. 4 shows all proteins identified in the bone analysis with potential candidates based on relative abundance alterations marked; Table 2 contains the 33 proteins marked in Fig. 4 sorted by relative abundance in cholesteatoma-involved ossicles to uninvolved ossicles. Four proteins were present in altered abundances in both the soft tissue and bone tissue analyses: creatine kinase B-type (CKB), tenascin-X (TNXB), serum amyloid P-component (APCS), and keratin type 2 cytoskeletal 8 (KRT8).

## Discussion

Our study used a mass spectrometry-based proteomic approach to evaluate the relative abundance changes between proteins found within middle ear mucosa and post-auricular skin relative to cholesteatoma matrix. A second arm of the study investigated the protein changes occurring in bone involved with cholesteatoma relative to healthy ossicles. We identified a number of potential candidates in the molecular changes among the functional components of the cholesteatoma matrix leading to uncontrolled growth and bony destruction.

Recognizing proteins with either increased or decreased abundance in both skin and mucosa reflect deviations from normal, particularly when they are functional rather than primarily structural in nature. Proteins fitting this description include members of the S100 family (A7, A8, and A9) and SERPINB3. S100 proteins are elevated in hyperproliferative skin disorders with primary roles in cell cycle regulation and cell differentiation [12, 13]. S100A7 also functions in an antibacterial capacity through the Toll-like receptor pathway in response to the bacterial protein flagellin [14], which is found in *P. aeruginosa* and *E. coli*, among other bacteria. SERPINB3 is a serine

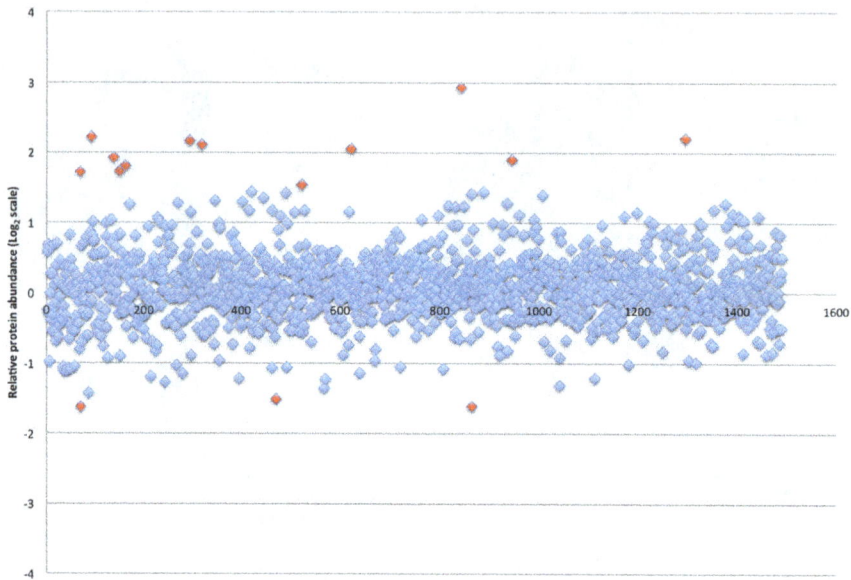

**Fig. 2** Logarithm (base 2) plot of relative abundances of all proteins identified in cholesteatoma matrix in reference to control mucosa. Positive values indicate greater protein content in cholesteatoma. The 15 proteins exceeding threshold abundances are indicated in red

protease inhibitor associated with cellular atypia, evasion of apoptosis, and cholesteatoma proliferation [15–17]. Our identification of SERPINB3 and the three S100 proteins in cholesteatoma matrix agrees with existing literature noting increased levels in cholesteatoma relative to post-auricular skin [11, 18], but it is a potentially novel finding to find increased abundance relative to middle ear mucosa. Though adult cholesteatoma is a disease of keratinizing epithelium that likely originates from the lateral surface of the tympanic membrane or external auditory canal, its destructive properties occur primarily within the middle ear; as such, finding difference between the

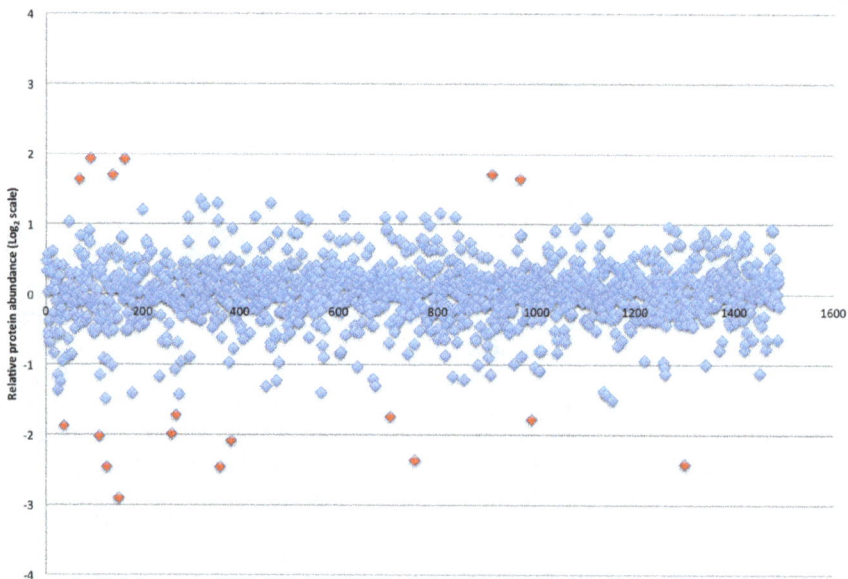

**Fig. 3** Logarithm (base 2) plot of relative abundances of all proteins identified in cholesteatoma matrix in reference to post-auricular skin. Positive values indicate greater protein content in cholesteatoma. The 18 proteins exceeding threshold abundances are indicated in red

**Table 1** Altered soft tissue protein abundances in cholesteatoma matrix relative to normal mucosa and post-auricular skin. Positive values indicate a greater abundance of a protein in cholesteatoma than the reference tissue. Italicized relative abundances indicate values below the detection threshold for one tissue but above detection threshold in the other. Study ID numbers correlate to Figs. 2 and 3

| Protein name (study ID number) | NCBI gene ID | Number of unique peptides | Percent protein coverage (%) | Relative protein abundance | |
|---|---|---|---|---|---|
| | | | | Mucosa | Skin |
| Bleomycin hydrolase (842) | BLMH | 4 | 13.8 | 7.66 | *1.14* |
| Protein S100-A9 (92) | S100A9 | 5 | 55.3 | 4.66 | 3.83 |
| Acyl-coenzyme A thioesterase 1 (1295) | ACOT1 | 2 | 5.7 | 4.62 | *−1.26* |
| Filaggrin (294) | FLG | 10 | 3.7 | 4.50 | *2.14* |
| FA binding protein, epidermal (319) | FABP5 | 7 | 65.2 | 4.32 | *2.55* |
| Filaggrin-2 (621) | FLG2 | 3 | 1.0 | 4.15 | *1.35* |
| Protein S100-A7 (138) | S100A7 | 7 | 54.5 | 3.81 | 3.25 |
| Creatine kinase B-type (944) | CKB | 2 | 7.9 | 3.74 | *1.47* |
| Protein S100-A8 (162) | S100A8 | 5 | 64.5 | 3.50 | 3.80 |
| Thymidine phosphorylase (150) | TYMP | 10 | 35.1 | 3.32 | *1.52* |
| Serine protease inhibitor B3 (69) | SERPINB3 | 22 | 50.3 | 3.30 | 3.12 |
| Myelin protein P0 (523) | MPZ | 6 | 25.0 | 2.92 | *1.06* |
| Desmocollin-3 (989) | DSC3 | 3 | 4.2 | *2.07* | −3.42 |
| Ferritin light chain (965) | FTL | 3 | 19.4 | *1.42* | 3.13 |
| Fatty acid desaturase 2 (1301) | FADS2 | 2 | 3.6 | *1.32* | −5.34 |
| Hydroxymethylglutaryl-CoA synthase, cytoplasmic (705) | HMGCS1 | 2 | 6.0 | *1.30* | −3.32 |
| Fatty acid synthase (37) | FASN | 38 | 23.7 | *1.29* | −3.65 |
| Collagen alpha-1(III) chain (754) | COL3A1 | 3 | 2.7 | *1.26* | −5.15 |
| Collagen alpha-6(VI) chain (260) | COL6A6 | 10 | 7.0 | *1.18* | −3.95 |
| Integrin alpha-M (909) | ITGAM | 4 | 3.9 | *1.16* | 3.28 |
| Keratin, type II cytoskeletal 79 (359) | KRT79 | 15 | 27.7 | *−1.03* | −5.48 |
| Tenascin-X (111) | TNXB | 23 | 8.2 | *−1.18* | −4.05 |
| Serum amyloid P-component (269) | APCS | 5 | 23.3 | *−1.23* | −3.27 |
| Tryptase alpha/beta-1 (382) | TPSAB1 | 4 | 14.5 | *−1.65* | −4.23 |
| Collagen alpha-2(I) chain (151) | COL1A2 | 7 | 54.5 | *−1.86* | −7.48 |
| Mimecan/osteoglycin (126) | OGN | 7 | 24.8 | *−1.89* | −5.49 |
| Keratin type 2 cytoskeletal 8 (471) | KRT8 | 13 | 21.7 | −2.85 | *−1.55* |
| BPI fold containing family member B (865) | BPIFB1 | 3 | 8.5 | −3.06 | *1.68* |
| Fibrillin-1 (70) | FBN1 | 27 | 11.3 | −3.08 | *−1.23* |

cholesteatoma matrix that allows it to overgrow mucosa and destroy neighbouring tissue may be more appreciable by analyzing the mucosa of presumably unaffected middle ear tissue.

A biomarker that is able to distinguish normal mucosa from cholesteatoma could prove useful for intra-operative tissue labeling or frozen section pathologic analysis, aiding the surgeon in removing all diseased tissue. Therefore another objective of this study was to recognize proteins that may function as indicators of residual or recurrent disease. As expected, the landscape of the cholesteatoma matrix proteome resembles that of normal skin, with multiple low-level abundance changes that likely reflect a complex interplay between various proteins and gene expression levels. The ideal candidate protein profile for this would have increased relative abundance in cholesteatoma compared to mucosa. Of the novel protein alterations we identified, some of the most intriguing changes involve BLMH, TYMP, FLBP5, and FLG/FLG2. BLMH represents a good candidate since it is located in superficial epidermis and maintains epithelial integrity [19]. Increased BLMH levels in cholesteatoma relative to mucosa, but unchanged in skin, is logical given that it is found primarily in the superficial and corneal layers of epidermis which are largely deficient in the non-keratinizing middle ear epithelium. This makes it an excellent potential biomarker

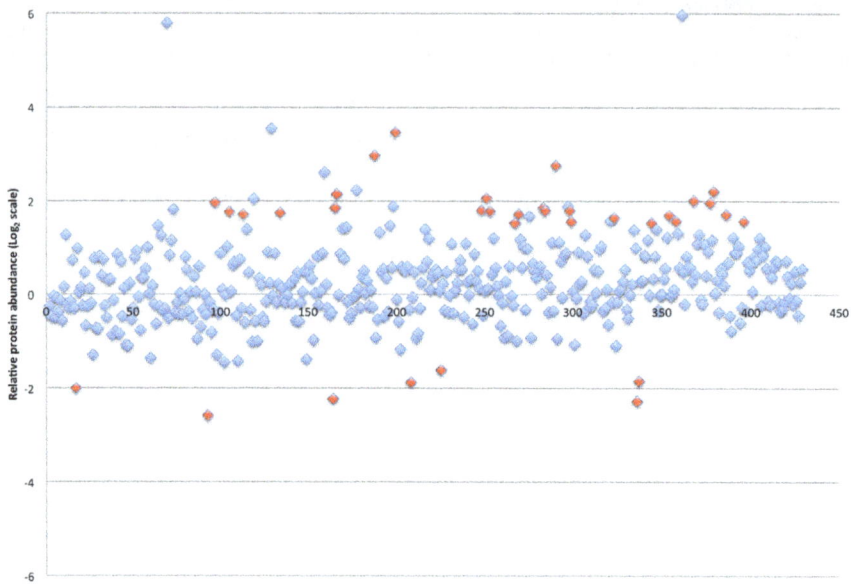

**Fig. 4** Logarithm (base 2) plot of relative abundances of all proteins identified in cholesteatoma-involved ossicles in reference to control ossicles. Positive values indicate greater protein content in cholesteatoma-involved bone. The 34 proteins exceeding threshold abundances and meeting inclusion criteria are highlighted in red

since presence in the middle ear following cholesteatoma excision may represent residual disease. Likewise, FLG is long recognized as elevated in cholesteatoma by histopathologic studies relative to post-auricular skin [20, 21], and we note considerably greater degree of elevation in cholesteatoma compared to mucosa with similar change noted in FLG2, which is co-expressed with FLG during keratinocyte differentiation [22]. Previous data suggests an interaction between FLG and involucrin (IVL), a protein that creates a protective envelope around corneocytes, and increased IVL in cholesteatoma [21, 23]; we identified increased IVL in cholesteatoma matrix, but not at levels meeting detection threshold (1.97-fold increase).

TYMP abundance was elevated in cholesteatoma 3.25-fold in our study compared to mucosa, though less so compared to post-auricular skin. TYMP is an angiogenesis factor involved in avoiding hypoxia-induced apoptosis, though most research focuses on malignant disease [24]. The role of hypoxia in cholesteatoma is poorly understood and thought to stimulate matrix metalloprotease release and subsequent perimatrix degeneration [25]. Elevated TYMP may contribute to the independent growth capability of cholesteatoma particularly when oxygen requirements exceed that available from direct diffusion in aerated portions of the middle ear. In addition to oxygen supply, energy demand is another hurdle cholesteatoma must overcome to continue growth and local destructive potential. Fatty acid metabolism is gaining attention in

cholesteatoma pathophysiology as an available energy source to propagate self-sufficient growth [25]. We found epidermal fatty acid binding protein (FABP5) is highly overabundant in cholesteatoma compared to normal mucosa (4.3-fold), with a lesser increase compared to skin. Initially identified in psoriasis, FABP5 is unique to keratinocytes, is a key factor in keratinocyte differentiation, and interacts with other proteins found at altered abundances in our study [26]. Of note, increased FABP5 stimulates increased IVL and is stabilized by S100A7 [27, 28]. FABP5 also appears to have a role in inflammatory change and tissue injury involving keratinocytes [29].

Other notable observations are the reduction of several structural proteins in cholesteatoma compared to post-auricular skin. These proteins provide insight into the molecular changes occurring that cause the well-recognized fragility of matrix intra-operatively. Desmocollin-3 (DSC3) likely contributes to this friability, as loss of function is found in skin fragility disorders [30], which matches the abundance profile we observed with decreased levels (3.42-fold) in cholesteatoma compared to skin, but above that seen in mucosa. Intercellular tight junction loss in cholesteatoma compared to normal skin has been shown by electrical impedence studies, agreeing with the impaired intercellular connections we found [31]. As shown in Table 1, a large proportion of the proteins reduced in cholesteatoma relative to skin are structural components.

With respect to the bone proteome of cholesteatoma-involved ossicles, the extensive number of changes

**Table 2** Altered abundances of proteins found in the cholesteatoma matrix proteome relative to healthy ossicles. Positive values indicate increased protein abundance in cholesteatoma. Study ID numbers correlate to Fig. 4

| Protein name (study ID number) | NCBI gene ID | Number of unique peptides | Percent protein coverage (%) | Relative protein abundance<br>Normal ossicles |
|---|---|---|---|---|
| Isocitrate dehydrogenase 2 (199) | IDH2 | 3 | 4.6 | 11.02 |
| Creatine kinase B type (187) | CKB | 3 | 9.7 | 7.81 |
| Thioredoxin domain-co8ntaining protein 5 (290) | TXNDC5 | 3 | 12.0 | 6.76 |
| Cytoskeleton-associated protein 4 (379) | CKAP4 | 2 | 4.8 | 4.64 |
| Protein disulfide-isomerase A6 (166) | PDIA6 | 5 | 15.2 | 4.45 |
| Ribosome binding protein 1 (251) | RRBP1 | 3 | 2.4 | 4.19 |
| Peptidyl-prolyl cis-trans isomerase (368) | FKBP10 | 2 | 4.5 | 4.06 |
| ATP synthase subunit α, mitochondrial (97) | ATP5A1 | 9 | 21.2 | 3.92 |
| Superoxide dismutase, mitochondrial (377) | SOD2 | 2 | 17.2 | 3.92 |
| 60S ribosome L14 (298) | RPL14 | 2 | 10.7 | 3.73 |
| Stress-10 protein, mitochondrial (290) | HSPA9 | 3 | 12.0 | 3.73 |
| Guanine nucleotide binding protein subunit β-2 (283) | GNB2L1 | 4 | 18.3 | 3.63 |
| Malate dehydrogenase 2 (165) | MDH2 | 6 | 25.4 | 3.62 |
| Serine protease inhibitor H1 (248) | SERPINH1 | 4 | 14.6 | 3.50 |
| Dolichyl-diphosphooligosaccharide–protein glycosyltransferase (284) | DDOST | 3 | 7.7 | 3.48 |
| Elongation factor Tu (253) | TUFM | 3 | 10.6 | 3.45 |
| ATP synthase subunit β, mitochondrial (105) | ATP5B | 6 | 14.6 | 3.41 |
| ADP/ATP translocase 2 (134) | SLC25A5 | 8 | 24.8 | 3.37 |
| Neutrophil elastase (269) | ELANE | 2 | 6.7 | 3.31 |
| Cathepsin G (113) | CTSG | 5 | 22.4 | 3.29 |
| Staphylococcal nuclease domain-containing protein 1 (386) | SND1 | 2 | 2.5 | 3.28 |
| Very long chain specific acyl-CoA dehydrogenase (354) | ACADVL | 2 | 3.5 | 3.26 |
| Coatamer subunit gamma-1 (323) | COPG1 | 2 | 2.6 | 3.13 |
| Prohibitin-2 (358) | PHB2 | 2 | 9.7 | 2.99 |
| Lamin-B1 (396) | LMNB1 | 2 | 3.4 | 2.98 |
| Valine—tRNA ligase (299) | VARS | 2 | 2.1 | 2.97 |
| Aspartate aminotransferase, mitochondrial (344) | GOT2 | 2 | 5.1 | 2.91 |
| 3-Hydroxyacyl-coA dehydrogenase type 2 (267) | HSD17B10 | 2 | 12.3 | 2.89 |
| Membrane primary amine oxidase (225) | AOC3 | 4 | 3.7 | −3.04 |
| Keratin type II cytoskeletal 8 (337) | KRT8 | 3 | 6.2 | −3.59 |
| Collagen VIII, α-1 chain (208) | COL8A | 3 | 5.0 | −3.66 |
| Cochlin (17) | COCH | 11 | 20.4 | −4.00 |
| Keratin type II cytoskeletal 7 (164) | KRT7 | 6 | 13.4 | −4.70 |
| Tenascin-X (336) | TNXB | 3 | 0.8 | −4.84 |
| Serum amyloid P-component (93) | APCS | 5 | 21.5 | −5.96 |

mirrors the complexity of bone as an organ. Many of these changes relate to increased metabolic function, protein degradation, and inflammatory response and less so with structural components. A number of the proteins are constituents of the endoplasmic reticulum, which is abundant in osteoblasts for their synthetic function. Among the proteins with functional ontologic duties, Tenascin-X (TNXB), Serine protease inhibitor H1

(SERPINH1), and Neutrophil elastase (ELANE), are known factors in bone remodeling. TNXB, decreased in cholesteatoma-involved bone relative to normal ossicles and one of the proteins common to bone and soft tissue analyses, stabilizes extracellular matrix and collagen fibril formation; reduced TNXB is associated with abnormal collagen and elastin deposition and extracellular maturation [32–34]. Whether altered TNXB levels in our study reflect a pathologic or reactive change to cholesteatoma remains to be seen. SERPINH1 is a serine protease inhibitor molecular chaperone with critical function in endochondral bone and cartilage formation [35]. Elevated SERPINH1 in cholesteatoma-involved ossicles suggests either increased bone remodeling or repair of the affected bones. This is also likely the scenario for our observation of increased ELANE in cholesteatoma-involved bone. Involved in innate cellular immune processes, ELANE also functions in Collagen VI breakdown and matrix metalloprotease activation [36]. As noted in the soft tissue analysis, proteins present at increased abundances in cholesteatoma-involved bone may also represent markers of residual disease. Cytoskeleton-associated protein 4 (CKAP4) primarily functions in skin development and maintenance [37], implying its presence in cholesteatoma-involved bone correlates with presence of invasive disease.

Limitations of our study center on the use of a large-scale proteomic approach to the identification of these altered protein abundances. We found several abundance differences between cholesteatoma matrix and skin compared to the difference between matrix and mucosa. This is challenging to explain but may represent an alteration in protein composition in epidermis as cholesteatoma matures. One possible reason for this is that the local environment in the middle ear is different from that of the exposed post-auricular region. Alternatively, dermal elements could be underrepresented or absent in cholesteatoma while they would not be present in mucosa since there is no appreciable submucosa in the middle ear. Yet another consideration is the inability to measure proteins present in very low abundances, since the peptide fragments from these proteins fail to reach detection thresholds due to the presence of peptides from highly expressed proteins. This remains a challenge to all proteomic studies, although mass spectrometry-based techniques have a wider dynamic range than traditional 2DGE [10, 38].

Additional limitations specific to biomarker discovery studies warrant mention. Identification of disease biomarkers represents a chief objective of proteomics, though to date it as been difficult to carry putative biomarkers through to clinical practice, mainly due to variation between populations and study validity [39]. Discovery phase studies generally use samples containing well-defined and discrete disease states that do not necessarily reflect early, subclinical disease, which would be the ideal target for disease prevention. Similarly, patients with advanced disease often present in a condition that does not match the disease state used to identify the biomarker. Current candidates discovered with large scale proteomic approaches currently under inquiry for roles in clinical diagnostics and disease management include proteins altered in COPD [40], lung cancer [40, 41], gastrointestinal malignancy [42],

transplant rejection [43], metabolic diseases [44]. Nonetheless, at present no single protein biomarker discovered through proteomics demonstrates sufficient accuracy to predict disease in a subclinical state [45]. Multiplex approaches to biomarker development present promise to increase understanding of diseases by simultaneously testing multiple proteins and observing abundance changes in concert, and to provide biomarker panels with increased accuracy [45].

## Conclusions

In conclusion, we used a large-scale, two armed proteomic approach to identify and quantify the changes in protein abundance levels in cholesteatoma matrix relative to normal middle ear mucosa and post-auricular skin, as well as in ossicles invaded by cholesteatoma compared to normal ossicles. Given the quantity of proteins involved in epithelial integrity and metabolism, our results provide several avenues for future research into cholesteatoma pathophysiology. Moreover, our inclusion of middle ear mucosa noted novel protein increases in matrix compared to post-auricular skin. One of the exciting findings in our study is the large number of potential biomarkers to use for evaluating residual or recurrent disease, in particular BLMH, TYMP, FLBP5, FLG/FLG2, and CKAP4. Our results describe several accessible proteins that could be used, if future validation demonstrates they are present in altered abundances in cholesteatoma compared to nascent mucosa, as potential therapeutic or diagnostic targets with the aim of reducing recurrent or residual disease and the need for second look tympanomastoidectomy. The greatest challenge with cholesteatoma surgery is eradicating disease without compromising function. Ideally, future cholesteatoma surgery could incorporate intraoperative or postoperative histopathologic margin evaluation using these biomarkers to reduce residual disease and determine timing of second look surgery.

**Competing interests**
The authors declare that they have no competing interests.

**Authors' contributions**
DRR developed the study protocol, prepared ethics approval, performed molecular analysis, analyzed data, and drafted the manuscript. PSP assisted with study design, data analysis, sample collection, and manuscript development. JKC contributed to study design, ethics application preparation, sample collection, data analysis, and manuscript preparation. All authors read and approved the final manuscript.

**Acknowledgments**
The authors thank the University of Calgary Office of Surgical Research (Calgary Surgical Research Development Fund) and the Campbell MacLaurin Foundation for Hearing Research for providing funding to support this study. We also thank Dr. Karl Riabowol for providing laboratory facilities to prepare tissue lysates, Dr. Lorne Clarke for technical advice on bone proteome isolation, and the University of Victoria Genome BC Protein Centre for their expertise in proteomic analysis.

**Funding**

University of Calgary Surgical Research Development Fund, Campbell McLaurin Foundation for Hearing Research.

**References**

1. Prasad SC, Shin SH, Russo A, Di Trapani G, Sanna M. Current trends in the management of the complications of chronic otitis media with cholesteatoma. Curr Opin Otolaryngol Head Neck Surg. 2013;21(5):446–54.

2. Mishiro Y, Sakagami M, Kitahara T, Kondoh K, Okumura S. The investigation of the recurrence rate of cholesteatoma using Kaplan-Meier survival analysis. Otol Neurotol. 2008;29(6):803–6.

3. Jung JY, Chole RA. Bone resorption in chronic otitis media: the role of the osteoclast. ORL J Otorhinolaryngol Relat Spec. 2002;64:95–107.

4. Olszewska E, Wagner M, Bernal-Sprekelsen M, Ebmeyer J, Dazert S, Hildmann H, et al. Etiopathogenesis of cholesteatoma. Eur Arch Otorhinolaryngol. 2004;261(1):6–24.

5. Morales SD, Penido N de O, da Silva NID, Stavale JN, Guilherme A, Fukuda Y. Matrix metalloproteinase 2: an important genetic marker for cholesteatomas. Braz J Otorhinolaryngol. 2007;73:51–7.

6. Nason R, Jung JY, Chole RA. Lipopolysaccharide-induced osteoclastogenesis from mononuclear precursors: a mechanism for osteolysis in chronic otitis. J Assoc Res Otolaryngol. 2009;10:151–60.

7. Louw L. Acquired cholesteatoma pathogenesis: stepwise explanations. J Laryngol Otol. 2010;124(6):587–93.

8. Kuo CL. Etiopathogenesis of acquired cholesteatoma: prominent theories and recent advances in biomolecular research. Laryngoscope. 2015;125(1):234–40.

9. Aggarwal K, Choe LH, Lee KH. Shotgun proteomics using the iTRAQ isobaric tags. Brief Funct Genomic Proteomic. 2006;5(2):112–20.

10. Feist P, Hummon AB. Proteomic challenges: sample preparation techniques for microgram-quantity protein analysis from biological samples. Int J Mol Sci. 2015;16(2):3537–63.

11. Kim JL, Jung HH. Proteomic analysis of cholesteatoma. Acta Otolaryngol. 2004;124(7):783–8.

12. Lee Y, Jang S, Min JK, Lee K, Sohn KC, Lim JS, et al. S100A8 and S100A9 are messengers in the crosstalk between epidermis and dermis modulating a psoriatic milieu in human skin. Biochem Biophys Res Commun. 2012;423(4):647–53.

13. Hattori F, Kiatsurayanon C, Okumura K, Ogawa H, Ikeda S, Okamoto K, et al. The antimicrobial protein S100A7/psoriasin enhances the expression of keratinocyte differentiation markers and strengthens the skin's tight junction barrier. Br J Dermatol. 2014;171(4):742–53.

14. Abtin A, Eckhart L, Mildner M, Gruber F, Schröder JM, Tschachler E. Flagellin is the principal inducer of the antimicrobial peptide S100A7c (psoriasin) in human epidermal keratinocytes exposed to Escherichia coli. FASEB J. 2008;22(7):2168–76.

15. Suminami Y, Kishi F, Sekiguchi K, Kato H. Squamous cell carcinoma antigen is a new member of the serine protease inhibitors. Biochem Biophys Res Commun. 1991;181(1):51–8.

16. Vidalino L, Doria A, Quarta S, Zen M, Gatta A, Pontisso P. SERPINB3, apoptosis and autoimmunity. Autoimmun Rev. 2009;9(2):108–12.

17. Quarta S, Vidalino L, Turato C, Ruvoletto M, Calabrese F, Valente M, et al. SERPINB3 induces epithelial-mesenchymal transition. J Pathol. 2010;221(3):343–56.

18. Ho KY, Huang HH, Hung KF, Chen JC, Chai CY, Chen WT, et al. Cholesteatoma growth and proliferation: relevance with serpin B3. Laryngoscope. 2012;122(12):2818–23.

19. Schwartz DR, Homanics GE, Hoyt DG, Klein E, Abernethy J, Lazo JS. The neutral cysteine protease bleomycin hydrolase is essential for epidermal integrity and bleomycin resistance. Proc Natl Acad Sci USA. 1999;96(8):4680–5.

20. Stammberger M, Bujía J, Kastenbauer E. Alteration of epidermal differentiation in middle ear cholesteatoma. Am J Otol. 1995;16(4):527–31.

21. Min HJ, Park CW, Jeong JH, Cho SH, Kim KR, SH L. Comparative analysis of the expression of involucrin, filaggrin and cytokeratin 4, 10, 16 in cholesteatoma. Korean J Audiol. 2012;16(3):124–9.

22. Makino T, Mizawa M, Yamakoshi T, Takaishi M, Shimizu T. Expression of filaggrin-2 protein in the epidermis of human skin diseases: a comparative analysis with filaggrin. Biochem Biophys Res Commun. 2014;449(1):100–6.

23. Huisman MA, De Heer E, Grote JJ. Survival signaling and terminal differentiation in cholesteatoma epithelium. Acta Otolaryngol. 2007;127(4):424–9.

24. Ikeda R, Tajitsu Y, Iwashita K, Che XF, Yoshida K, Ushiyama M, et al. Thymidine phosphorylase inhibits the expression of proapoptotic protein BNIP3. Biochem Biophys Res Commun. 2008;370(2):220–4.

25. Louw L. Acquired cholesteatoma: summary of the cascade of molecular events. J Laryngol Otol. 2013;127(6):542–9.

26. Dallaglio K, Marconi A, Truzzi F, Lotti R, Palazzo E, Petrachi T, et al. E-FABP induces differentiation in normal human keratinocytes and modulates the differentiation process in psoriatic keratinocytes in vitro. Exp Dermatol. 2013;22(4):255–61.

27. Hagens G, Roulin K, Hotz R, Saurat JH, Hellman U, Siegenthaler G. Probable interaction between S100A7 and E-FABP in the cytosol of human keratinocytes from psoriatic scales. Mol Cell Biochem. 1999;192(1–2):123–8.

28. Ruse M, Broome AM, Eckert RL. S100A7 (psoriasin) interacts with epidermal fatty acid binding protein and localizes in focal adhesion-like structures in cultured keratinocytes. J Invest Dermatol. 2003;121(1):132–41.

29. Kusakari Y, Ogawa E, Owada Y, Kitanaka N, Watanabe H, Kimura M, et al. Decreased keratinocyte motility in skin wound on mice lacking the epidermal fatty acid binding protein gene. Mol Cell Biochem. 2006;284(1–2):183–8.

30. Hartlieb E, Kempf B, Partilla M, Vigh B, Spindler V, Waschke J. Desmoglein 2 is less important than desmoglein 3 for keratinocyte cohesion. PLoS One. 2013;8(1), e53739.

31. Koizumi H, Suzuki H, Ohbuchi T, Kitamura T, Hashida K, Nakamura M. Increased permeability of the epithelium of middle ear cholesteatoma. Clin Otolaryngol. 2015;40(2):106–14.

32. Zweers MC, van Vlijmen-Willems IM, van Kuppevelt TH, Mecham RP, Steijlen PM, Bristow J, et al. Deficiency of tenascin-X causes abnormalities in dermal elastic fiber morphology. J Invest Dermatol. 2004;122(4):885–91.

33. Egging D, van den Berkmortel F, Taylor G, Bristow J, Schalkwijk J. Interactions of human tenascin-X domains with dermal extracellular matrix molecules. Arch Dermatol Res. 2007;298(8):389–96.

34. Egging D, van Vlijmen-Willems I, van Tongeren T, Schalkwijk J, Peeters A. Wound healing in tenascin-X deficient mice suggests that tenascin-X is involved in matrix maturation rather than matrix deposition. Connect Tissue Res. 2007;48(2):93–8.

35. Masago Y, Hosoya A, Kawasaki K, Kawano S, Nasu A, Toguchida J, et al. The molecular chaperone Hsp47 is essential for cartilage and endochondral bone formation. J Cell Sci. 2012;125(Pt 5):1118–28.

36. Kielty CM, Lees M, Shuttleworth CA, Woolley D. Catabolism of intact type VI collagen microfibrils: susceptibility to degradation by serine proteinases. Biochem Biophys Res Commun. 1993;191(3):1230–6.

37. Koster MI. p63 in skin development and ectodermal dysplasias. J Invest Dermatol. 2010;130(10):2352–8.

38. Choe LH, Aggarwal K, Franck Z, Lee KH. A comparison of the consistency of proteome quantitation using two-dimensional electrophoresis and shotgun isobaric tagging in Escherichia coli cells. Electrophoresis. 2005;26(12):2437–49.

39. Lin JL, Bonnichsen MH, Nogeh EU, Raftery MJ, Thomas PS. Proteomics in detection and monitoring of asthma and smoking-related lung diseases. Expert Rev Proteomics. 2010;7(3):361–72.

40. Ohlmeier S, Vuolanto M, Toljamo T, Vuopala K, Salmenkivi K, Myllärniemi M, et al. Proteomics of human lung tissue identifies surfactant protein A as a marker of chronic obstructive pulmonary disease. J Proteome Res. 2008;7(12):5125–32.

41. Bajtarevic A, Ager C, Pienz M, Klieber M, Schwarz K, Ligor M, et al. Noninvasive detection of lung cancer by analysis of exhaled breath. BMC Cancer. 2009;9:348.

42. Kuramitsu Y, Nakamura K. Proteomic analysis of cancer tissues: shedding light on carcinogenesis and possible biomarkers. Proteomics. 2006;6(20):5650–61.

43. Cohen Freue GV, Meredith A, Smith D, Bergman A, Sasaki M, Lam KK, et al. Biomarkers in Transplantation and the NCE CECR Prevention of Organ Failure Centre of Excellence Teams. Computational biomarker pipeline from discovery to clinical implementation: plasma proteomic biomarkers for cardiac transplantation. PLoS Comput Biol. 2013;9(4), e1002963.

44. Randall DR, Sinclair GB, Colobong KE, Hetty E, Clarke LA. Heparin cofactor II-thrombin complex in MPS I: a biomarker of MPS disease. Mol Genet Metab. 2006;88(3):235–43.

45. Schiess R, Wollscheid B, Aebersold R. Targeted proteomic strategy for clinical biomarker discovery. Mol Oncol. 2009;3(1):33–44.

# 3

# Depression as a predictor of postoperative functional performance status (PFPS) and treatment adherence in head and neck cancer patients: a prospective study

Brittany Barber[1*], Jace Dergousoff[2], Margaret Nesbitt[1], Nicholas Mitchell[2], Jeffrey Harris[1], Daniel O'Connell[1], David Côté[1], Vincent Biron[1] and Hadi Seikaly[1]

## Abstract

**Background:** Head and neck cancer (HNC) is a debilitating disease due in part to its effects on function, including speech, swallowing, and cosmesis. Previous studies regarding depression in HNC have focused on demographic predictors, incidence, and quality of life studies. There is, however, a paucity of studies that objectively address depressive symptoms in HNC patients and the resultant effects on post-treatment functional performance status. The aim of this study was to assess the relationship between preoperative depressive symptoms (PDS) and postoperative functional performance status (PFPS), in addition to other predictors of rehabilitation and survival.

**Methods:** A prospective cohort study was undertaken at the University of Alberta, including all new adult HNC patients undergoing surgery as primary therapy for HNC from May 2013 to January 2014. Baseline depressive symptoms were measured on the Quick Inventory of Depressive Symptoms (QIDS) questionnaire 2 weeks preoperatively and PFPS was assessed 12 months postoperatively on the Functional Assessment of Cancer Therapy-Head & Neck (FACT-HN) scale. Secondary outcomes included completion of adjuvant therapy, narcotic dependence, return to detrimental habits, loss of follow-up, and length of hospital stay (LOHS). Differences between the Normal-Mild and Moderate-Severe QIDS groups were assessed using Mann–Whitney and Fischer Exact statistical analyses.

**Results:** Seventy-one patients were included in the study. Mild and Moderate-Severe PDS were 35.2 % and 18.3 %, respectively. Significantly lower FACT-HN scores were noted in the Moderate-Severe group at 12 months (p = 0.03). The risk ratio (RR) for FACT-HN score < 50 % at 12 months in the Moderate-Severe group was 5.66. In addition, significantly lower completion of adjuvant treatment (p = 0.03), significantly higher incidence of narcotic dependence (p = 0.004), and significantly higher LOHS (24 days vs. 18 days; p = 0.02) was observed in the Moderate-Severe group. There was no significant difference in loss of follow-up between the 2 groups (p = 0.64).

**Conclusions:** The incidence and severity of PDS in HNC patients treated with surgery is high (53.5 %). Patients with Moderate-Severe PDS have significantly decreased PFPS, increased narcotic use, decreased completion of adjuvant therapy, and a longer LOHS. HNC patients should be monitored closely for depressive symptoms.

**Keywords:** Depression, Head neck cancer, Postoperative functional performance

---

* Correspondence: brittanybarber0@gmail.com
[1]Division of Otolaryngology-Head & Neck Surgery, University of Alberta Hospital, 1E4, Walter Mackenzie Centre, 8440-112 St, Edmonton, AB T6G 2B7, Canada
Full list of author information is available at the end of the article

## Introduction

Head and neck cancer (HNC) is a debilitating disease due in part to its effects on daily patient function including speech, swallowing, and cosmesis. Previous studies have demonstrated that approximately 40 % of patients become depressed in the first year after their diagnosis and treatment for head and neck cancer, and more importantly, this goes unrecognized and untreated [1]. Misono et al. [2] revealed that oral cavity and laryngeal cancer make up 2 of the 4 highest suicide populations amongst cancer patients. These finding may be attributed to the devastating combination of predisposing factors for HNC, incapacitating symptoms, and the sequelae of treatment.

Depression is also a devastating disease robbing patients of function and quality of life. Previous studies regarding depression in HNC have focused on demographic predictors, incidence, and quality of life studies. There is, however a paucity of studies that objectively address depressive symptoms in the HNC patients and their effect on posttreatment functional performance status. Limited literature exists regarding the effect of depression on other factors that may affect rehabilitation and survival, such as completion of adjuvant treatment and return to detrimental habits.

The aim of this study was to assess the relationship between preoperative depressive symptoms (PDS) and postoperative functional performance status (PFPS), in addition to other predictors of rehabilitation and survival.

## Methods

Institutional ethical approval was obtained from the Human Research Ethics Board (HREB) at the University of Alberta. Informed consent was obtained from all participating subjects.

A prospective cohort study of HNC patients presenting to a tertiary cancer care practice at the University of Alberta Hospital was undertaken. The study population consisted of adult patients undergoing major head and neck ablative and reconstructive surgery and adjuvant therapy for a new HNC. HNCs considered eligible for inclusion were mucosal squamous cell carcinoma (SCC), salivary gland tumors, and skin cancers. Thyroid and ocular cancers were excluded from the study given differences in the extent of surgical management for each group. Patients were recruited at the time of preoperative surgical education sessions approximately 2 weeks prior to surgery from September 1, 2013 to March 1, 2014.

## Demographic assessment

Adult patients undergoing surgery and adjuvant radiotherapy for a new HNC were included. Patients with a pre-existing psychiatric history, those who were unable to read or comprehend the questionnaires or lacked capacity to consent, and those unwilling to present for follow-up questionnaires or assessment were excluded. Demographic data regarding age, gender, comorbidities, primary tumor site and stage, pre-treatment substance abuse, and presence of supportive caregivers was collected. Advanced-stage cancers were defined as those tumors with a clinical T-stage greater than 2 or N-stage greater than 0. Patient comorbidities were identified and Charlson Comorbidity Index was calculated for each patient.

## Preoperative depressive symptom (PDS) assessment

Once determined eligible, patients underwent baseline evaluation with the Quick Inventory of Depressive Symptomatology Self-Report (QIDS-SR) questionnaire [3]. This is a self-report, validated questionnaire involving 16 items under the typical 9 domains assessed with regard to depressed mood. This was not utilized as a diagnostic test for depression, but as a screening tool for examining the severity of depressive symptoms. The QIDS-SR is scored from 0 to 27, and patients were classified as normal, mild, moderate, severe (Table 1), with higher scores indicative of more severe depressive symptoms. Previous studies have demonstrated an internal consistency between physician-rated QIDS-SR score and self-report scores as high as 0.94 [4].

The Functional Assessment of Cancer Therapy for Head and Neck patients (FACT-HN) is a multidimensional, self-reported assessment of post-treatment functional performance status that was specifically designed for head and neck cancer patients, and has been used extensively in Radiation Therapy Oncology Group (RTOG) trials [5–7]. Social, emotional, physical, family, and well-being domains are addressed, and questions related to these domains are answered on a 5-point Likert scale by the patients. Questionnaires are scored from 0 to 144 with higher scores representative of better functioning. Scores of less than 50 % on the FACT-HN correlate with clinical functional decline [5]. A previous analysis of test-retest reliability regarding the stability of the stand-alone FACT-HN questionnaire has demonstrated an intraclass correlation of 0.89 [8].

**Table 1** Scoring rubric for QIDS-SR questionnaire as previously published by Rush et al. [3]

| QIDS-SR | |
| --- | --- |
| Normal | 0–5 |
| Mild | 6–10 |
| Moderate | 11–15 |
| Severe | 16–20 |
| Very Severe | >20 |

QIDS-SR Quick Inventory of Depressive Symptomatology-Self Report

## Outcome measures

The primary outcome assessed was the FACT-HN score 12 months postoperatively. Secondary outcomes were those not evaluated in previous literature, including completion of adjuvant therapy (defined as completion of all adjuvant treatments including chemotherapy and radiotherapy), narcotic dependence (defined as persistent use greater than 3 months postoperatively), and loss of follow-up (defined as patients not presenting for 2 consecutive scheduled follow-up appointments with no attempts to reschedule). Return-to-habit status was defined as a postoperative return to detrimental habits, such as tobacco, alcohol, or illicit drug abuse. Length of hospital stay (LOHS) was also calculated for each patient and compared between groups.

After patients were determined eligible for the study, they underwent a baseline QIDS-SR assessment approximately 2–3 weeks prior to surgery during routine preoperative surgical education sessions. Patients were then classified into the Normal-Mild group (0–10) or the Moderate-Severe group (11–27) based on the scores demonstrated in Table 1. Subsequently, the patients underwent resection and reconstructive surgery with routine postoperative care including adjuvant therapy. Follow-up appointments were arranged for 2 weeks, 3, 6, and 12 months postoperatively, as is standard protocol. Patients were reassessed at 12 months postoperatively with both a QIDS and FACT-HN assessment. Secondary outcomes were also assessed at 12 months.

Treatment for depressive symptoms was initiated in the standard clinical fashion, but was not considered part of this observational study. If patients scored in the Mild category, a discussion regarding depressive symptoms was initiated and patients were referred to Psychiatry for assessment upon request. If patients scored in the Moderate or Severe groups, they were referred to Psychiatry for assessment and options for treatment were discussed with the patient. Outcomes of treatment discussion with Psychiatry were recorded and followed for the Moderate-Severe group.

## Statistical analysis

The Normal-Mild group was compared to the Moderate-Severe group regarding FACT-HN scores using a Mann–Whitney analysis. A multiple regression analysis was additionally performed using other known predictors of postoperative functional performance status to assess the predictive value of PDS on PFPS. A risk ratio (RR) was also calculated for a score less than 50 % on the FACT-HN for those patients with Moderate-Severe PDS [5]. Secondary outcomes were assessed using a Fischer Exact analysis as well as a Spearman Correlation analysis to confirm statistically significant findings. LOHS was compared between groups using a Mann–Whitney analysis. Normal-Mild and Moderate-Severe groups were also compared regarding demographic variables, comorbidities, pre-treatment ETOH or illicit drug use, supportive care-givers, and tumor sites, and TNM-staging using Mann–Whitney and Fisher exact analyses. Statistical analysis was performed using SPSS software (SPSS, Version 21.0, Chicago, IL).

## Results

Seventy-five patients were approached for recruitment to the study; 1 refused participation, 2 did not fully complete the baseline QIDS questionnaire, and 1 did not undergo adjuvant therapy. The compliance rate for baseline PDS assessment was thus 96 % (72 of 75 patients). Of the 71 patients eligible for participation, 58 patients (81.7 %) scored in the Normal-Mild range upon baseline assessment, with the remaining 13 (18.3 %) scoring in the Moderate-Severe group.

Initial examination of demographic data for the entire cohort revealed findings typical of the HNC population, with a mean age of 59.7, a male gender predominance (70.4 %), and primarily advanced-stage disease (90.1 %). The Charlson Comorbidity Index (CCI) for the entire cohort was 70.2 %. Further examination of each study group revealed no differences in mean age, gender, TNM staging, cancer site, reconstruction, adjuvant therapy, pre-treatment substance abuse, presence of supportive care-givers, or Charlson Comorbidity Index between the Normal-Mild and Moderate-Severe groups (Table 2).

At baseline 35.2 % of patients displayed Mild-only depressive symptoms and 18.3 % of patients displayed Moderate-Severe depressive symptoms. None of the patients expressed or recorded thoughts of suicidal ideation. More extensive evaluation of the domains of the QIDS questionnaire revealed significantly higher scores in the sleep, mood, appetite, concentration, energy level, and psychomotor domains for the Moderate-Severe group, indicating dysfunction in these specific areas (Table 3).

There were no statistically significant differences between baseline and 12-month QIDS scores in the Normal-Mild ($p = 0.67$), or Moderate-Severe groups ($p = 0.58$) (Table 4). FACT-HN scores at the 12th postoperative month demonstrated a statistically significant difference between subjects in the Normal-Mild and Moderate-Severe groups ($p = 0.03$). A multiple regression analysis was performed including other known and collected predictors of PFPS, which demonstrated Moderate-Severe PDS as a statistically significant predictor of postoperative FACT-HN scores (Table 5). The risk ratio for FACT-HN score less than 50 % with Moderate-Severe PDS was calculated to be 5.66.

**Table 2** Demographic and disease-specific findings for entire cohort and individual study groups

| Variable | Entire cohort (n = 71) | Normal-Mild (n = 58) | Moderate-Severe (n = 13) | P-value |
|---|---|---|---|---|
| Average age | 59.7 | 60.4 | 59.7 | 0.79 |
| Gender | | | | |
| Males | 50 (70.4 %) | 46 (79.3 %) | 8 (61.5 %) | 0.65 |
| Females | 21 (29.6 %) | 12 (20.7 %) | 5 (38.5 %) | 0.51 |
| TNM staging | | | | |
| Early | 7 (9.9 %) | 12 (20.7 %) | 3 (23.1 %) | 0.35 |
| Advanced | 64 (90.1 %) | 46 (79.3 %) | 10 (76.9 %) | 0.32 |
| Site | | | | |
| Oral Cavity/Oropharynx | 39 (54.9 %) | 29 (50.0 %) | 10 (76.9 %) | 0.07 |
| Larynx | 9 (12.7 %) | 9 (15.5 %) | 0 (0.0 %) | 0.11 |
| Other | 23 (32.4 %) | 20 (34.5 %) | 3 (23.1 %) | 0.32 |
| Reconstruction | | | | |
| Osseocutaneous FF | 11 (15.5 %) | 9 (15.5 %) | 2 (15.4 %) | 1.00 |
| Fasciocutaneous FF | 58 (81.7 %) | 48 (82.8 %) | 10 (76.9 %) | 0.24 |
| Pedicled/Rotational | 2 (2.8 %) | 1 (1.7 %) | 1 (7.7 %) | 0.35 |
| Adjuvant therapy | | | | |
| Radiation therapy (RT) | 57 (80.3 %) | 46 (79.3 %) | 11 (84.6 %) | 0.56 |
| Chemotherapy (C) | 32 (45.1 %) | 26 (44.8 %) | 6 (46.2 %) | 0.22 |
| Chemoradiation Therapy (CRT) | 32 (45.1 %) | 26 (44.8 %) | 6 (46.2 %) | 0.22 |
| Pre-treatment substance abuse | 16 (22.5 %) | 15 (25.9 %) | 1 (7.7 %) | 0.82 |
| Supports/Caregivers available | 61 (85.9 %) | 48 (82.8 %) | 11 (84.6 %) | 0.81 |
| Charlson comorbidity index | Mean 70.2 %, Median 77 % | Mean 70.2 %, Median 77 % | Mean 70.2 %, Median 90 % | 0.65 |

FF free flap, RT radiation therapy, CRT chemoradiation therapy, C chemotherapy

Analysis of the secondary outcomes revealed a significantly lower rate of completion of adjuvant therapy in the Moderate-Severe group when compared to the Normal-Mild group ($\chi2 = 6.1$, $p = 0.03$). A statistically higher rate of narcotic dependence was found in the Moderate-Severe group ($\chi2 = 8.8$, $p < 0.01$). Higher rates of return-to-habit status were identified in the Moderate-Severe group (50 %) as compared to the Normal-Mild group (10.7 %). These results were not significant using a Fisher Exact analysis, though a trend was evident ($\chi2 = 3.7$, $p = 0.05$). No statistically significant difference was noted between groups regarding loss of follow-up ($\chi2 = 0.67$, $p = 0.64$) (Table 6). The mean LOHS for patients in the Moderate-Severe group was significantly longer than the Normal-Mild group Normal-Mild group (18 vs 24 days, $p = 0.02$).

Interventions for patients with Moderate-Severe symptoms are summated in Table 7. Of the patients in the Moderate-Severe group, 5 (38.5 %) were deceased at 12 months, and 4 (30.8 %) were living with recurrence. In the Normal-Mild group, 21 patients (30.0 %) were living with recurrence at 12 months, thus no difference in recurrence was detected between groups at 12 months ($\chi2 = 2.1$, $p = 0.22$). However, both disease-specific (DSS)

**Table 3** Mean QIDS-SR scores at baseline and 12 months postoperatively for Normal-Mild and Moderate-Severe groups

| | Mean baseline QIDS-SR | Mean 12-Month QIDS-SR | P-value |
|---|---|---|---|
| Normal-Mild | 5.35 | 8.13 | 0.67 |
| Moderate-Severe | 14.8 | 17.1 | 0.58 |

QIDS-SR Quick Inventory of Depressive Symptomatology-Self Report

**Table 4** Baseline preoperative depressive symptoms (PDS) demonstrating significant differences between Normal-Mild and Moderate-Severe groups in 6 of 9 domains on the QIDS-SR

| Preoperative Depressive Symptom (PDS) | P-value |
|---|---|
| Sleep | 0.03* |
| Mood | 0.01* |
| Appetite | 0.01* |
| Concentration | 0.01* |
| Self-Worth | 0.61 |
| Death-Suicide | 0.61 |
| Interest | 0.10 |
| Energy level | <0.01* |
| Psychomotor | <0.01* |

*denotes statistical significance

**Table 5** Multiple regression analysis including other known predictors of PFPS as measured on the FACT-HN, demonstrating severity of PDS as a predictor of PFPS

| Variable | P-value |
|---|---|
| Age | 0.37 |
| Gender | 0.38 |
| Social Supports | 0.77 |
| Advanced Stage | 0.76 |
| Charlson Comorbidity Index | 0.73 |
| Moderate-Severe Preoperative Depressive Symptoms (PDS) | 0.03* |

*denotes statistical significance

and overall survival (OS) were statistically significantly worse in the Moderate-Severe group at 12 months ($p = 0.00$, $p = 0.00$) (Table 8, Fig. 1). No non-cancer-related deaths occurred within 12 months of follow-up.

## Discussion

This study demonstrates that the baseline prevalence and severity of preoperative depressive symptoms is high (53.5 %) in HNC patients, and that moderate or severe preoperative depressive symptoms is associated with lower overall postoperative functional performance status, higher rates of narcotic dependence, decreased treatment adherence, and a longer length of hospital stay. This relationship is independent of demographic factors, tumor site, TNM staging, surgical reconstruction, type or presence of adjuvant treatment, and medical comorbidities. These preliminary findings suggest that depressive symptoms in HNC patients impart significant effects on post-treatment rehabilitation and potentially overall survival.

Postoperative functional performance status (PFPS) has broad implications for postoperative course in HNC patients, given the extensive rehabilitation required for swallowing, speech, wound/stoma maintenance, and upper extremity physiotherapy. Moreover, functional status can impact ability to physically attend adjuvant treatments, and this can be compounded by depressive symptoms. As such, PFPS and depressive symptoms alike should be examined as contributors to survival, given their association with low treatment adherence in other types of cancer [9, 10]. This study demonstrates a significantly lower post-treatment

**Table 6** Relationship between PDS and secondary outcomes using Fisher Exact analysis

| Variable | P-value |
|---|---|
| Completion of adjuvant therapy | 0.01* |
| Narcotic dependence | <0.01* |
| Return-to-habit | 0.05 |
| Loss of Follow-up | 0.64 |

*denotes statistical significance

**Table 7** Outcomes and interventions of Moderate-Severe HNC group

| Patient | Intervention | Status |
|---|---|---|
| 1 | Antidepressant | Deceased |
| 2 | Antidepressant | Living |
| 3 | Antidepressant | Deceased |
| 4 | Refused antidepressant; anxiolytic | Deceased |
| 5 | Antidepressant + anxiolytic | Deceased |
| 6 | Antidepressant + anxiolytic | Living; recurrence |
| 7 | Antidepressant + anxiolytic | Living |
| 8 | Refused antidepressant; anxiolytic | Living; recurrence |
| 9 | Antidepressant | Living |
| 10 | Antidepressant | Living |
| 11 | Refused antidepressant; anxiolytic | Deceased |
| 12 | Antidepressant + anxiolytic | Living; recurrence |
| 13 | Antidepressant + anxiolytic | Living; recurrence |

functional status in patients displaying Moderate-Severe PDS, with a RR of 5.66 in obtaining a score less than 50 % on the FACT-HN questionnaire 12 months postoperatively. A similar study by Lin et al. [11] examined the relationship between severe depressive symptoms and specific swallowing and speech outcomes using the MD Anderson Dysphagia Inventory (MDADI) and Beck Depression Inventory Fast Screen (BDI-FS), and found significantly lower MDADI scores for depressed patients 1 year post-treatment. This study also demonstrated a lower overall quality of life (QOL) in patients with lower BDI –FS scores at this time interval. Although it was not our express intention to examine QOL with increasing severity of PDS, previous studies have correlated decreasing FACT-HN scores with decreasing QOL, which in turn has been shown to be a significant prognostic factor in HNC survival [12].

Narcotic dependence was found to be significantly associated with PDS ($p = 0.004$). In the Moderate-Severe group, 4 of the 8 patients remaining alive had recurrence, which may have contributed to the increased incidence of narcotic dependence. However, there was no significant difference between the Normal-Mild and Moderate-Severe groups regarding recurrence at 12 months, thus this confounder should be eliminated. The relationship between narcotic dependence, pain, PDS, and PFPS is not clear. It is possible that patients with more severe PDS have chronic pain throughout the treatment process that contributes to a decreased PFPS. A previous study by Shuman et al. [13] showed that severe depressive symptoms were a significant predictor of pain in head and neck cancer patients 1-year post-treatment. Conversely, other authors [14] have demonstrated an inverse relationship wherein pain is a predictor of depression in post-

**Table 8** Locoregional recurrence, disease-specific survival, and overall survival in Normal-Mild and Moderate-Severe groups 12 months post-treatment

| Variable | Entire cohort (n = 71) | Normal-Mild (n = 58) | Moderate-Severe (n = 13) | p-value |
|---|---|---|---|---|
| Recurrence | 25 (35.2 %) | 21 (36.2 %) | 4 (30.8 %) | 0.22 |
| Disease-Specific Survival (DSS) | 59 (83.1 %) | 51 (87.9 %) | 8 (61.5 %) | <0.01 |
| Overall Survival (OSS) | 51 (87.9 %) | 51 (87.9 %) | 8 (61.5 %) | <0.01 |

*DSS* disease-specific survival, *OS* overall survival

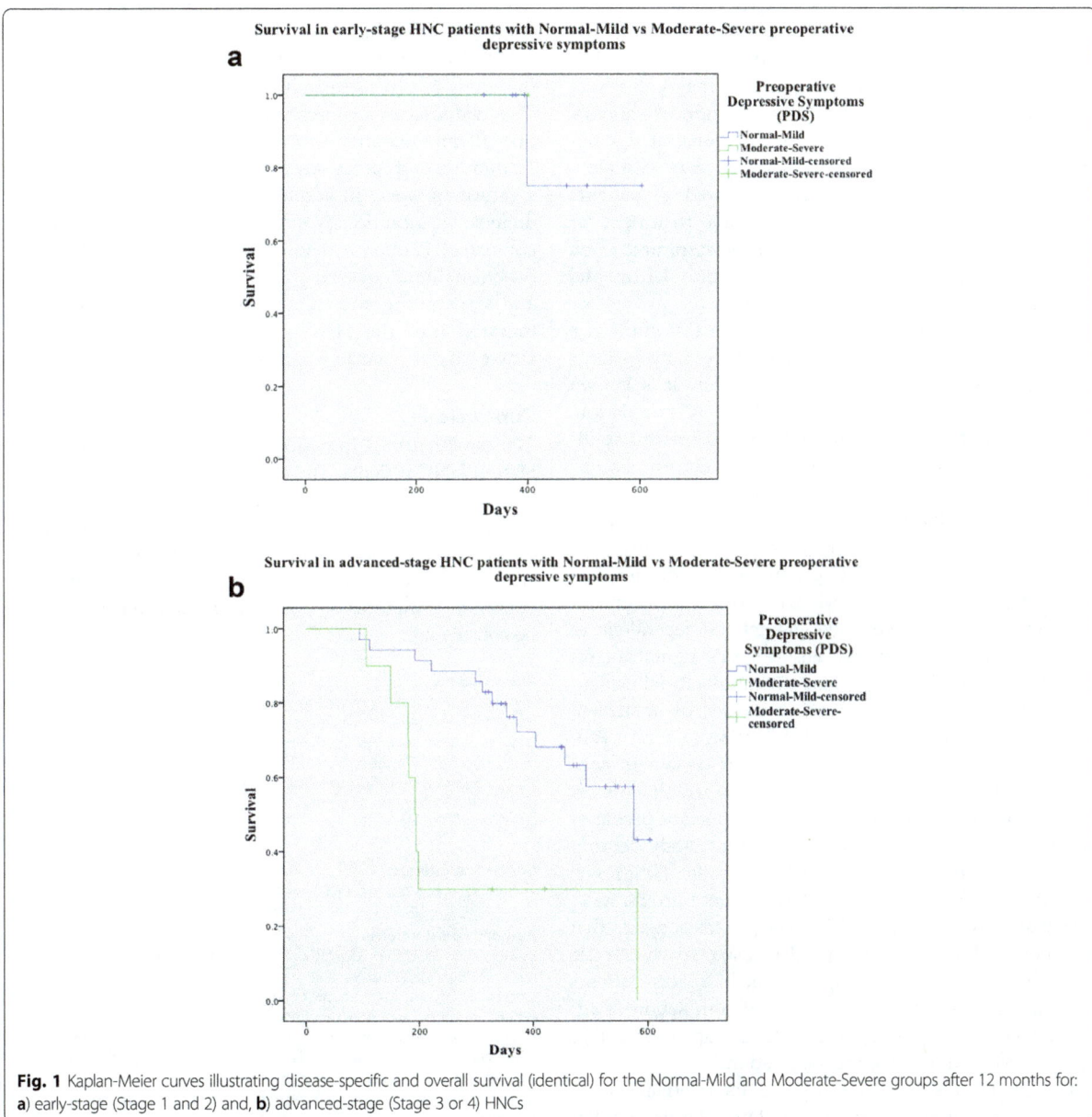

**Fig. 1** Kaplan-Meier curves illustrating disease-specific and overall survival (identical) for the Normal-Mild and Moderate-Severe groups after 12 months for: **a**) early-stage (Stage 1 and 2) and, **b**) advanced-stage (Stage 3 or 4) HNCs

treatment cancer survivors. Therefore, it can be inferred that these symptoms can occur in parallel, and should be monitored throughout diagnosis and treatment.

There was a near-significant relationship between PDS and a return to detrimental habits in our HNC population ($p = 0.05$). There is a well-established relationship between addictions and mental illness, and thus, this relationship, although marginal in this study, is not unexpected. No significant difference in pre-treatment substance abuse was detected between groups that could have been considered to contribute to QIDS scores or even treatment adherence. A recent study by Berg et al. [15] demonstrated that, among survivors of all smoking-related cancers, severe depressive symptoms were a significant risk factor for continued tobacco use, yet it is not known how much this relationship may contribute to survival and recurrence in this population of patients. A previous study by Jerjes et al. [16] demonstrated a significant reduction in mortality at 3 and 5 years with alcohol and tobacco cessation when compared to patients engaging in persistent use. Surveillance and treatment for severe depressive symptoms is potentially warranted, given the tendency of HNC patients for relapse into detrimental habits and the impact of this on survival.

Perhaps the most compelling finding in this study is a significant reduction in treatment adherence by patients in the Moderate-Severe study group. While it is known that substance abuse is common in the HNC population, and may therefore contribute to decreased treatment adherence, our results demonstrated that there was no difference in preoperative substance abuse between groups, yet treatment adherence was significantly worse in the Moderate-Severe group. A previous study by Lazure et al. [17] demonstrated that HNC patients with a diagnosis of major depressive disorder (MDD) have a 25 % greater mortality than non-depressed patients, independent of TNM staging. However, the cause for this significant reduction in survival was not clear. A multi-factorial explanation is probable, given the complexity of treatment modalities and postoperative rehabilitation in HNC. Failure of completion of adjuvant therapy is certain to contribute to this mortality rate, as it is known that timely completion of radiation therapy is an important predictor of successful disease control [18–20]. Our study demonstrated a significantly lower disease-specific (DSS) and overall survival (OS) in the Moderate-Severe group, however with only 12 months of follow-up. This suggests that any potential contribution to decreased survival rates imparted by depressive symptoms likely affects patients early, and potentially in the capacity of completion of adjuvant therapy. However, longer follow-up and further study is required to make this association.

The limitations of this study are its relatively small sample size and single-institution status. Future studies should aim to examine this condition in large cohorts in a multi-institutional manner. In addition, this was an exclusively surgical cohort of patients. We elected to include only surgical patients in our study due to the unique nature of their cosmetic concerns postoperatively and the potential differences in symptoms they may have compared to non-surgical patients. Future study should consider non-surgical patients to determine differences or similarities in optimal treatment regimens for both groups. As well, patients with "Mild" symptoms were included in analysis with "Normal" patients. This decision was made in psychiatric consult, as it was reasoned that the clinical manifestations of Moderate-Severe depression would be more likely to cause functional disability, and also be the cutoff for consideration of treatment. Lastly, this study involves relatively short follow-up of 12 months. This endpoint was chosen given the "acute" nature of the first 12 months after treatment, and the fact that often, 12 months postoperatively is often when patients consider a return to work. In addition, stated survival results are done so with cautionary connotation, as they apply in the context of 12-month follow-up. Continued study of the functional and survival status of the cohort is ongoing, and a screening and treatment algorithm has been integrated into the HNC clinical care pathway at the University of Alberta to ensure sustained progress.

## Conclusions

The prevalence of preoperative depressive symptoms is high in HNC patients. The effect of PDS on post-treatment functional status and rehabilitation, as well as treatment adherence, can act as significant contributing factors in postoperative course, and given these findings, early screening and intervention to avert the effects of moderate or severe depressive symptoms on postoperative rehabilitation should be considered.

**Abbreviations**
HNC: Head and neck cancer; PFPS: Postoperative functional performance status; PDS: Preoperative depressive symptoms;; QIDS: Quick Inventory of Depressive Symptoms; FACT-HN: Functional Assessment of Cancer Therapy for Head & Neck Cancer patients; RTOG: Radiation Therapy Oncology Group; CCI: Charlson Comorbidity Index; MDADI: MD Anderson Dysphagia Index; BDI-FS: Beck Depression Inventory Fast Screen; DSS: Disease-specific survival; OS: Overall survival.

**Competing interests**
The authors declare that they have no competing interests.

**Authors' contributions**
BB was involved in study design, data collection, distribution of questionnaires, data analysis, and manuscript preparation. JD was involved in data collection and distribution of questionnaires. MN was involved in distribution of questionnaires and enrolment. NM was involved in study design. JH and DAO were involved in study design and manuscript preparation. VB was involved in study design, manuscript preparation, and statistical analysis. HS was involved in study design, distribution of questionnaires, and manuscript preparation. All authors read and approved the final manuscript.

## Acknowledgments

The authors would like to acknowledge Dr. William Lydiatt of the University of Nebraska for his advice on the use of the data collected for this project. In addition, the authors would like to acknowledge the contributions of Dr. Hamdy El-Hakim of the University of Alberta for his advice pertaining to future directions for study.

## Author details

[1]Division of Otolaryngology-Head & Neck Surgery, University of Alberta Hospital, 1E4, Walter Mackenzie Centre, 8440-112 St, Edmonton, AB T6G 2B7, Canada. [2]Department of Psychiatry, University of Alberta Hospital, 1E1, Walter Mackenzie Centre, 8440-112 St, Edmonton, AB T6G 2B7, Canada.

## References

1. Sehlen S, Lenk M, Herschback P, Aydemir U, Dellian M, Schymura B, et al. Depressive symptoms after radiotherapy for head and neck cancer. Head Neck. 2003;25:1004–18.
2. Misono S, Weiss NS, Fann JR, Redman M, Yueh B. Incidence of suicide in persons with cancer. J Clin Oncol. 2008;26(29):4731–8.
3. Rush AJ, Trivedi MH, Ibrahim HM, Carmody TJ, Arnow B, Klein DN, et al. The 16-Item Quick Inventory of Depressive Symptomatology (QIDS), clinician rating (QIDS-C), and self-report (QIDSSR): a psychometric evaluation in patients with chronic major depression. Biol Psychiatry. 2003;54:573–83.
4. Trivedi MH, Rush AJ, Ibrahim HM, Carmody TJ, Biggs MM, Suppes T, et al. The inventory of depressive symptomatology, clinician rating (IDS-C) and self-report (IDS-SR), and the quick inventory of depressive symptomatology, clinician rating (QIDS-C) and self-report (QIDS-SR) in public sector patients with mood disorders: a psychometric evaluation. Psychol Med. 2004;34:73–82.
5. List MA, D'Antonio LL, Cella DF, Siston A, Mumby P, Haraf D, et al. The performance status scale for head and neck cancer patients and the Functional Assessment of Cancer Therapy-Head & Neck (FACT-H&N) scale: a study of utility and validity. Cancer. 1996;77:2294–301.
6. Movsas B, Scott C, Watkins-Bruner D. Pretreatment factors significantly influence quality of life in cancer patients: a Radiation Therapy Oncology (RTOG) analysis. Int J Radiat Oncol Biol Phys. 2006;65(3):830–5.
7. Coyne JC, Pajak TF, Harris J, Konski A, Movsas B, Ang K, et al. Emotional well-being does not predict survival in head and neck cancer patients: a Radiation Therapy Oncology Group study. Cancer. 2007;110(11):2569–75.
8. Yount S, List M, Du H, Yost K, Bode R, Brockstein B, et al. A randomized study comparing embedded versus enacted FACT – Head and Neck Symptom Index (FHNSI) scores. Qual Life Res. 2007;16(10):1615–26.
9. Arrieta O, Angulo L, Nunez-Valencia C, Dorantes-Gallereta Y, Macedo E, Martinez-Lopez D, et al. Association of depression and anxiety on quality of life, treatment adherence, and prognosis in patients with advanced non-small cell lung cancer. Ann Surg Oncol. 2013;20:1941–8.
10. Hu L, Ku F, Wang Y, Shen C, Hu Y, Yeh C, et al. Anxiety and depressive disorders among patients with esophageal cancer in Taiwan: a nationwide population-based study. Support Care Cancer 2015;23(3):733–40.
11. Lin B, Starmer H, Gourin C. The relationship between depressive symptoms, quality of life, and swallowing function in head and neck cancer patients 1 year after definitive therapy. Laryngoscope. 2012;122:1518–25.
12. Urba S, Gatz J, Shen W, Hossain A, Winfree K, Koustenis A, et al. Quality of life scores as prognostic factors of overall survival in advanced head and neck cacner: analysis of a phase III randomized trial of pemetrexed plus cisplatin versus cisplatin monotherapy. Oral Concol. 2012;48(8):723–9.
13. Shuman A, Terrell J, Light E, Wolf GT, Bradford CR, Chepeha D, et al. Predictors of pain among patients with head and neck cancer. Arch Otolaryngol Head Neck Surg. 2012;138(12):1147–54.
14. Moye J, June A, Martin LA, Gosian J, Herman L, Naik A. Pain is prevalent and persisting in cancer survivors: differential factors across age groups. J Geriatr Oncol. 2014;5(2):190–6.
15. Berg CJ, Thomas AN, Mertens AC, Schauer GL, Pinsker EA, Ahluwalia JS, et al. Correlates of continued smoking versus cessation among survivors of smoking-related cancers. Psychooncology. 2013;22(4):799–806.
16. Jerjes W, Upile T, Radhi H, Petrie A, Abiola J, Adams A, et al. The effect of tobacco and alcohol and their reduction/cessation on mortality in oral cancer patients: short communication. Head Neck Oncol. 2012;4(6):1–5.
17. Lazure KE, Lydiatt WM, Denman D, Burke W. Association between depression and survival or disease recurrence in patients with head and neck cancer enrolled in a depression prevention trial. Head Neck. 2009;31:888–92.
18. Peters LJ, Goepfert H, Ang KK, Byers RM, Maor MH, Guillamondegui O, et al. Evaluation of the dose for postoperative radiation therapy of head and neck cancer: first report of a prospective randomized trial. Int J Radiat Oncol Biol Phys. 1993;26(1):3–11.
19. Barton MB, Morgan G, Smee R, Tiver KW, Hamilton C, Gebski V. Does waiting time affect the outcome of larynx cancer treated by radiotherapy? Radiother Oncol. 1997;44(2):137–41.
20. Le Q, Fu KK, Kroll S. Influence of fraction size, total dose, and overall time on local control of T1-T2 glottic carcinoma. Int J Radiat Oncol Biol Phys. 1997;39(1):115–26.

# 4

# The Allen's test: revisiting the importance of bidirectional testing to determine candidacy and design of radial forearm free flap harvest in the era of trans radial endovascular access procedures

Andrew Foreman, John R. de Almeida, Ralph Gilbert and David P. Goldstein[*]

## Abstract

**Background:** The radial forearm free flap is a workhorse free flap. The radial artery, which supplies it, is increasingly being used for endovascular access. A complication of this is radial artery occlusion. Although often asymptomatic it can compromise future free tissue transfer.

**Case Presentation:** Two patients who underwent RFFF harvest for head and neck reconstruction are presented; both of who likely had distal radial artery occlusion.
The first patient had failure of flap perfusion, presumed secondary to radial artery occlusion from prior endovascular access at the distal radial artery. In the second case, we used the Allen's test in reverse to identify the same scenario and successfully redesigned the harvest.

**Conclusion:** The Allen's test is a simple bedside test that should be performed bidirectionally to exclude radial artery occlusion, which may compromise flap harvest. Radial artery occlusion will become increasingly common as the radial artery is used more frequently for endovascular access procedures.

**Keywords:** Allen's test, Radial artery, Reconstruction, Head and neck cancer, Endovascular

## Background

First described in 1929 by Edgar Allen, the Allen's test has become the most common method for assessing palmar arch patency [1]. Allen originally described his test for diagnosis of thromboangiitis obliterans of the ulnar artery however more recently it has been used to assess the adequacy of the ulnar collateral blood flow through the palmar arches prior to radial artery sacrifice during cardiac surgery and reconstructive surgery [2]. As a preoperative test it provides a degree of safety in preventing hand ischemia prior to undertaking these procedures. Its reported sensitivity and specificity are 54.5 and 91.7 %

respectively, which is acceptable given the simple and non-invasive nature of the test [3]. Given the dual arterial inflow to the hand, the Allen's test can be performed in both directions to assess either ulnar or radial artery patency individually. Whilst most commonly used to assess collateral flow through the ulnar artery, we believe this bedside assessment also has utility when performed in reverse to assess the flow through the radial artery (Fig. 1).

Cannulation of the radial artery for invasive monitoring and interventional procedures is becoming increasingly common. It places a significant number of patients at risk for asymptomatic radial artery occlusion, which may compromise subsequent radial forearm free flap (RFFF) harvest. We present a case of a compromised RFFF that was believed to be due to arterial injury from a prior radial arterial line and a second case where

* Correspondence: david.goldstein@uhn.ca
Department of Otolaryngology Head and Neck Surgery, University Health Network, Princess Margaret Cancer Centre, University of Toronto, Toronto, ON, Canada

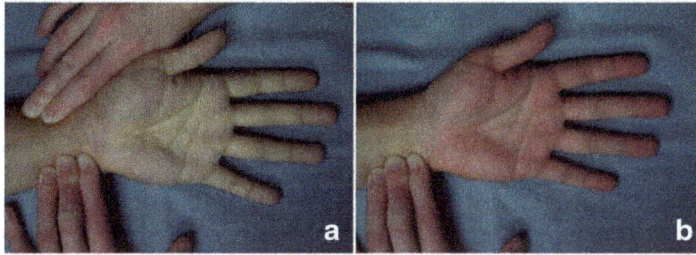

**Fig. 1** The 'reverse' Allen's test. **a**. The pallor associated with occlusion of both radial and ulnar artery inflow to the hand. **b**. Rapid return of redness to the hand following release of radial artery pressure confirming flow through the radial artery

bidirectional Allen's testing was able to pre-operatively identify a patient with radial artery occlusion that led to a change in RFFF design. These cases highlight the importance of performing the Allen's test in both directions prior to RFFF harvest to not only prevent hand ischemia but also to ensure adequacy of arterial inflow to the flap harvest site.

## Case Presentation

### Case Presentation: Illustrative case 1

A 66-year-old female presented to our head and neck clinic with a 2.5 cm left floor of mouth, biopsy-proven squamous cell carcinoma. The treatment recommendation was for primary surgery consisting of floor of mouth excision, bilateral selective neck dissections and radial forearm free flap (RFFF) reconstruction.

Her past history was significant for a colonic perforation approximately 2 years prior to her presentation to our clinic. At that time she required a laparotomy and colostomy followed by an extended intensive care unit stay. She was right-hand dominant and denied any trauma or surgery to the left forearm or hand. She was a 50-pack year smoker and a heavy alcohol drinker. Pre-operatively she was assessed for RFFF harvest with a standard Allen's test and pulse oximetry plythesmography, which were both normal. She had a palpable radial pulse and no visible evidence of trauma at the donor harvest site.

She was taken to the operating room and underwent resection of the primary site. A RFFF measuring 5 × 4 centimeters was designed overlying the radial artery with the distal aspect of the skin paddle placed approximately 3 cm proximal to the left flexor wrist crease. The flap was raised in standard fashion. During the flap elevation, significant fibrosis was encountered at the distal aspect of the pedicle as well as along the flexor retinaculum underlying the pedicle.

After the tourniquet was released, the skin paddle of the flap was not perfused. Assessment of the radial artery with pencil Doppler confirmed a pulse in the proximal artery but this was lost at the proximal end of the skin paddle. No pulse was obtainable within the borders of the flap. The distal artery clip was removed and there was no flow-through observed. A Fogarty catheter was then inserted from the distal end of the radial artery, however there was significant resistance towards the proximal end of the flap suggesting stenosis of the vessel. The catheter was passed proximal to the stenosis and on inflation and withdrawal of the catheter flow through the flap was able to be re-established however this was not sustained. A decision was made at this time to abort the RFFF. A left anterolateral thigh flap was raised without complication and used as reconstruction.

We hypothesized that during the prior surgery and ICU admission for management of her colonic perforation she had a left radial artery intra-arterial catheter placed for hemodynamic monitoring. This likely resulted in occlusion of the left radial artery, which was not appreciated on pre-operative assessment. Interestingly the location and length of radial artery occlusion in our case corresponds to the length of a standard intra-arterial catheter from its usual insertion site at the flexor wrist crease, as illustrated in Fig. 2.

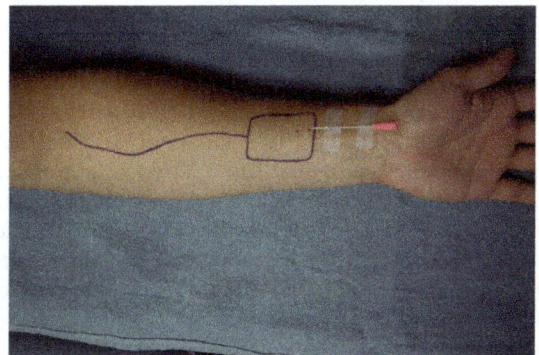

**Fig. 2** Redesigning a more proximal radial forearm free flap avoids the area of likely vessel trauma from an intra-arterial cannula. In this image, a standard intra-arterial cannula is positioned overlying the distal radial artery. The exact length of stenosis can be confirmed with Doppler ultrasonography

## Illustrative case 2

Following the first case we encountered a 69 year-old patient with an oral tongue cancer that required free-tissue reconstruction. He had a history of multiple medical comorbidities including diabetes, chronic renal failure and peripheral vascular disease, in addition to a history of prior surgeries. He had an arteriovenous fistula in his right arm and a left leg below-the-knee amputation. The Allen's test on the left hand was normal. We then assessed the patency of the radial artery by performing the Allen's test in reverse. Just as the radial artery occlusion is maintained with digital pressure in a standard Allen's test to assess the ulnar artery supply to the arches, palmar inflow through the radial artery is assessed in the 're-verse' Allen's test by maintaining ulnar artery compression. With normal radial artery patency the tester can expect rapid return of color to the hands and fingers upon release of the radial artery as illustrated in Fig. 1. In this case there was no evidence of hand reperfusion upon release of the radial artery. While maintaining ulnar compression the radial artery was assessed with the hand-held Doppler, which demonstrated that there was no Doppler signal of the radial artery at the flexor crease, however a Doppler signal was present more proximal on the artery, approximately 5 to 6 cm from the flexor crease. We therefore designed our flap in a more proximal location, an example of which is demonstrated in Fig. 2.

Flap harvest in this way was successful with a well-perfused flap transplanted to the hemi-glossectomy defect. The long pedicle length of the RFFF is advantageous in this situation, whereby shortening the pedicle length by moving the donor harvest site more proximal on the arm still permitted arterial and venous anastomoses to be performed in the neck without the need for vein grafts or deferring to an alternate donor site.

The RFFF has established itself as a workhorse reconstructive option for a multitude of head and neck defects providing thin, pliable tissue supplied by a long, large caliber vascular pedicle. Furthermore its attractiveness is enhanced by it being a reliable donor site with flap failure rates reported to be less than 3 % and an anatomical location that permits two-team harvest [4–6]. There are, however, potential morbidities associated with this flap harvest [7]. These may include a cosmetically displeasing donor site closure, skin graft loss with subsequent flexor tendon exposure along with alterations in range of movement, strength and sensation in the donor hand and forearm [8]. Despite their rarity, the most feared complications of RFFF harvest are the ischemic hand complications [9].

The vascular supply of the hand is derived from the superficial and deep palmar arches, which receive their arterial inflow from the radial and ulnar arteries. The ulnar artery is usually the dominant contributor to the superficial arch, anastomosing with the superficial branch of the radial artery over the thenar eminence [10]. Palmar digital arteries run distally from this arch to supply the fingers. A complete superficial arch is present in 84–90 % of patients, with considerable variation occurring. In contrast, the radial artery predominantly supplies the deep arch. It almost invariably forms a complete arch through anastomosis with the deep branch of the ulnar artery. The palmar metacarpal arteries arise from the deep arch and anastomose with the palmar digital arteries from the superficial arch. Hence the hand is supplied by an anastomosing network of arteries arising from both superficial and deep palmar arches, which in turn are supplied from a combination of the radial and ulnar arteries. These extensive anastomotic connections usually prevent the hand from ischemic damage in the face of injury to a single component of the network.

Following harvest of the radial artery during the RFFF harvest, the hand is solely perfused by the ulnar supply to the arches and the distal anastomotic connections ensure the hand and fingers remain perfused. However, inadequate flow through the ulnar artery may result in either acute or chronic hand ischemia [9]. The adequacy of flow through the palmar arches is routinely tested pre-operatively with the Allen's test to pre-emptively identify patients at risk of hand ischemia after radial artery sacrifice. Other tests such as Doppler ultrasonography and pulse oximetry with plythesmography have also been employed to improve accuracy of pre-operative clinical decision-making [11]. This dedicated assessment of the adequacy of the arch system reflects the seriousness of the morbidity should inadequate arch circulation be overlooked prior to RFFF harvest.

In contrast to the attention given to the potentially devastating donor site morbidity related to inadequate ulnar inflow, little has been published on the impact of radial artery occlusive disease in the setting of attempted RFFF harvest. The very nature of the arterial arcades within the hand may mask pre-existing radial artery damage as ulnar collateral circulation through the palmar arches can produce a palpable pulse on the radial side of the wrist crease in spite of radial artery occlusion more proximally. This may predispose to intra-operative flap failure. Performing the Allen's test in the reverse direction can ensure the adequacy of flow through the radial artery and prevent this potential complication.

Recently there has been increasing use of invasive monitoring during anesthesia and the intensive care setting as well as a dramatic expansion of therapeutic endovascular procedures. The radial artery has become an attractive option for arterial catheterization due to its superficial location and fewer access site complications. Whilst the complications of trans radial catheterization are reported to be lower than other sites, radial artery occlusion is the most frequently encountered [12]. The reported incidence of radial artery occlusion is 2 to 18 % [13], however it is recognized this may be an under-representation because this condition is usually asymptomatic and only detected with ultrasound or plethysmographic assessment of the radial artery or when the radial artery is re-accessed for another endovascular procedure.

As with ulnar artery disease, radial artery occlusion may be a silent disease given the arcade-like nature of the palmar vascular anatomy. Quite rightly, the vascular literature concludes that this condition is associated with essentially no major clinical sequelae, however it does limit the future utility of the radial artery as an arterial access site [14]. It is important to recognize that this also extends to its use in a free tissue transfer. It is interesting to note that the length of an intra-arterial catheter from the usual insertion site at the wrist corresponds to the area most commonly used to harvest a RFFF (Fig. 2).

As the use of the radial artery for diagnostic and therapeutic procedures continues to expand it is behest on the reconstructive surgeon to consider this potentially silent disease in planning head and neck reconstruction. To this end, we reiterate the importance of performing a detailed assessment of both ulnar and radial artery blood flow prior to RFFF harvest by performing the Allen's test in both directions, as already described. When the 'reverse' Allen's test demonstrates a complete lack of re-perfusion of the hand and digits then a lack of flow through the radial artery should be assumed. This is in contradistinction to the situation where there is reperfusion to the thumb and index finger, which is due to an incomplete arch with lack of communication with the ulnar system. In the latter situation a hand-held Doppler can be used to trace the flow in the radial artery in order to determine candidacy for a RFFF and when flow is present proximally it can aid in designing the flap more proximally over an area of skin that will be perfused by the radial artery. Alternatively, another donor site may be chosen, particularly if the injury to the radial artery extends proximally.

## Conclusion

In summary, the Allen's test is a time-honored, simple and non-invasive test to assess arterial flow through the palmar arches of the hand. It is important to remember that this is a bidirectional test and it should be performed in both directions prior to RFFF harvest. This can prevent both ischemic hand complications and

ensure that radial artery inflow to the distal forearm is sufficient to ensure a RFFF will perfuse after harvest. We highlight these technical details through two illustrative cases because we believe it is increasingly relevant in the current era where the radial artery is frequently being used as an access site for invasive monitoring and therapeutic endovascular procedures. This expansion of practice places an increasing number of patients at risk of radial artery occlusion a disease that is most often silent due to the extensive anastomotic connections of the palm. Furthermore patients may not recall they have had arterial cannulae placed during their prior hospital stays rendering history alone unreliable.

## Consent

Written informed consent was obtained from the patient for publication of this case report. A copy of the written consent is available for review by the Editor-in-Chief of this journal.

### Competing interests
The authors declare that they have no competing interests.

### Authors' contributions
All authors participated in the conception and design of the project. AF was involved with acquisition of the data. AF and DPG were involved with drafting the manuscript. All authors were involved in revising the manuscript critically for important intellectual content. All authors gave final approval of the version to be published. All authors agree to be accountable for all aspects of the work.

### Acknowledgements
Dr. Andrew Foreman was supported by the Margorie Hooper Scholarship from the Royal Australasian College of Surgeons.

### References
1. Cable DG, Mullany CJ, Schaff HV. The Allen test. Ann Thorac Surg. 1999;67:876–7.
2. Allen EV. Thromboangiitis obliterans: methods of diagnosis of chronic occlusive arterial lesions distal to the wrist with illustrative cases. Am J Med Sci. 1929;2:1–8.
3. Jarvis MA, Jarvis CL, Jones PR, Spyt TJ. Reliability of Allen's test in selection of patients for radial artery harvest. Ann Thorac Surg. 2000;70:1362–5.
4. Evans GR, Ainslie N, Robb GL, Reece GP, Miller MJ, Kroll SS, et al. The radial forearm free flap for head and neck reconstruction: a review. Am J Surg. 1994;168:446–50.
5. Avery CME. Review of the radial free flap: is it still evolving, or is it facing extinction? Part one: soft-tissue radial flap Br J Oral Maxillofac Surg. 2010;48:245–52.
6. Taylor SM, Hart R, Trites J, Bartlett C, Horwich P, Orlik JR, et al. Long-term functional donor site morbidity of the free radial forearm flap in head and neck cancer survivors. J Otolaryngol Head Neck Surg. 2014;43:1.
7. Brown MT, Couch ME, Huchton DM. Assessment of donor-site functional morbidity from radial forearm fasciocutaneous free flap harvest. Arch Otolaryngol Head Neck Surg. 1999;125:1371–4.
8. Sardesai MG, Fung K, Yoo JH, Bakker H. Donor-site morbidity following radial forearm free tissue transfer in head and neck surgery. J Otolaryngol Head Neck Surg. 2008;37:411–6.
9. Kanatas AN, Mitchell DA, Ong TK, Smith AB, Stead L, Ganesan K, et al. Duplex in the assessment of the free radial forearm flaps: Is it time to change practice? Br J Oral Maxillofac Surg. 2010;48:423–6.

10. Wood JW, Broussard KC, Burkey B. Preoperative testing for radial forearm free flaps to reduce donor site morbidity. JAMA Otolaryngol Head Neck Surg. 2013;139:183–6.

11. Khan AS, Henton JMD, Adams TST, Dwivedi RC, Harris PA. Evaluation of hand circulation before radial forearm free flap surgery. Laryngoscope. 2009;119:1679–81.

12. Garg K, Rockman CB, Maldonado TS, Mussa FF, Berland TL, Saltzberg SS, et al. Open surgical management of complications from indwelling radial artery catheters. J Vasc Surg. 2013;58:1325–30.

13. Chim H, Bakri K, Moran SL. Complications related to radial artery occlusion, radial artery harvest, and arterial lines. Hand Clin. 2015;31:93–100.

14. Honda T, Fujimoto K, Miyao Y, Koga H, Hirata Y. Access site-related complications after trans radial catheterization can be reduced with smaller sheath size and statins. Cardiovasc Interv Ther. 2012;27:174–80.

# 5

# 3-phase dual-energy CT scan as a feasible salvage imaging modality for the identification of non-localizing parathyroid adenomas

Michael Roskies[1], Xiaoyang Liu[2], Michael P. Hier[1], Richard J. Payne[1], Alex Mlynarek[1], Veronique Forest[1], Mark Levental[2] and Reza Forghani[2,3]*

## Abstract

**Objectives:** Accurate pre-operative imaging of parathyroid adenomas (PAs) is essential for successful minimally invasive surgery; however, rates of non-localizing PAs can be as high as 18 %. Multiphasic dual-energy CT (DECT) has the potential to increase accuracy of PA detection by enabling creation of paired material maps and spectral tissue characterization. This study prospectively evaluated the utility of 3-phase DECT for PA identification in patients with failed localizatio n via standard imaging.

**Methods:** Patients with primary hyperparathyroidism and non-localizing PAs underwent a 3 phase post-contrast DECT scan acquired at 25, 55, and 85 s. The scans were prospectively evaluated by two head and neck radiologists. Pre-operative localization was compared to intraoperative localization and final histopathology. A post-hoc DECT spectral density characterization was performed on pathologically-proven PAs.

**Results:** Out of 29 patients with primary hyperparathyroidism and non-localized PAs, DECT identified candidates in 26. Of the 23 patients who underwent parathyroidectomy, DECT provided precise anatomic localization in 20 patients (PPV = 87.0 %), one with multi-gland disease. The virtual unenhanced images were not found to be useful for diagnosis but successful diagnosis was made without an unenhanced phase regardless. Spectral analysis demonstrated a distinct spectral Hounsfield attenuation curve for PAs compared to lymph nodes on arterial phase images.

**Conclusion:** 3-phase DECT without an unenhanced phase is a feasible salvage imaging modality for previously non-localizing parathyroid adenomas. Optimal interpretation is achieved based on a combination of perfusion characteristics and other morphologic features. Advanced spectral DECT analysis has the potential for further increasing accuracy of PA identification in the future.

**Keywords:** Parathyroid adenoma, Head and neck surgery, Computed tomography, Dual-energy CT, 4D-CT, 4DCT, Minimally invasive parathyroidectomy

## Background

Accurate pre-operative localization of parathyroid adenomas (PAs) is essential for successful minimally invasive surgery. At many institutions, including ours, this is done based on two concordant studies. Typically, the most common approach for PA localization is by a combination of sestamibi and ultrasound [1, 2]. However, despite their popularity, these techniques have certain pitfalls. Limitations of sestamibi studies for parathyroid adenoma identification include absent radiotracer retention in some adenomas, diminishing sensitivity with decreasing adenomatous tissue, and potential confounding by concurrent thyroid disease or the occasional hot thyroid nodule [2]. Sestamibi also has low sensitivity for multiglandular disease. Ultrasound is operator dependent

* Correspondence: rforghani@jgh.mcgill.ca
[2]Department of Radiology, Jewish General Hospital & McGill University, Montreal, Quebec, Canada
[3]Segal Cancer Centre and Lady Davis Institute for Medical Research, Jewish General Hospital & McGillUniversity, Montreal, Quebec, Canada
Full list of author information is available at the end of the article

and, in addition, locations where ectopic PAs typically are located such as deep within the neck, the retropharyngeal space, and the mediastinum, tend to be areas that are blind-spots for ultrasound [2]. Reported sensitivities for the ability to lateralize (localize) PAs to the correct side of the neck are approximately 57 to 88 % for ultrasound and 65 to 86 % for sestamibi [3]. The addition of SPECT or SPECT/CT may further increase sensitivity for PAs to approximately 90 % or more according to some studies [2, 4], but that has not been the experience in our institution.

4-dimensional CT (4D-CT) is increasingly used for localization of PAs [3, 5–10]. 4D-CT enables characterization of perfusion characteristics of candidate PAs. The main principle behind 4D-CT is that PAs have different perfusion characteristics compared to lymph nodes and normal thyroid gland [3, 5]. In its original form, 4D-CT included a non-contrast acquisition followed by three post-contrast acquisitions that include an arterial phase (usually at 25 s) with two additional scans obtained after variable delays [2, 3, 5]. In general, PAs have more rapid and greater arterial phase enhancement and a more rapid rate of contrast wash-out compared to the normal thyroid gland [5]. Lymph nodes are typically hypoenhancing compared to PAs on arterial phase images, but demonstrate slow progressive enhancement on more delayed images, also a pattern different from typical PAs [5]. The combination of perfusion characteristics and high spatial resolution of CT technique accounts for the success of 4D-CT [5], with some studies reporting accuracy for lateralization of 94 % [5]. As a result, there is increasing interest and use of 4D-CT for PA identification and localization. However, one of the concerns about 4D-CT is radiation exposure because of multiple acquisitions. To this end, there are reports demonstrating that not all of the phases described in the original 4D-CT protocol may be necessary for accurate PA localization [11, 12]. Whereas one approach is to simply eliminate one or more phases from conventional multiphasic CT, another approach is to use more advanced techniques such as dual-energy CT for increasing the diagnostic yield and therefore potentially reducing the number of acquisition needed for a diagnostic exam.

Dual energy CT (DECT) is an advanced CT technique that evaluates tissues at different X-ray energies, enabling spectral evaluation and material tissue characterization beyond what is possible with conventional CT [13–16]. Normally, the attenuation of different tissues and materials varies when scanned at high and low tube voltages, depending on their specific elemental properties. With DECT, projection data are typically obtained simultaneously or near-simultaneously at 80 and 140 kVp (kilovolt peak) [14]. Using sophisticated computer algorithms, the data at different acquisition energies can then be normalized to specific combinations of two reference materials, such as iodine, water or calcium. Furthermore, the

spectral data can be used to generate image sets at different predicted energy levels (keV; kiloelectron volts), referred to as virtual monochromatic images (VMI). As such, DECT enables generation of virtual unenhanced images as well as other advanced tissue characterization not possible with conventional CT, all done by postprocessing and without the need for any additional scan acquisitions. There are emerging applications of DECT in all of the major subspecialties in radiology [16–22]. In the head and neck, there is increasing evidence that DECT can improve visualization of head and neck squamous cell carcinoma and increase accuracy for evaluation of thyroid cartilage invasion, among other applications [13, 22–28].

Currently, there are only isolated reports of DECT for localization of PAs [29] but no systematic evaluation of this technique. In this study, we prospectively evaluated the utility of multiphasic DECT for PA localization in a group of patients having discordant or unidentified PAs on a workup consisting at a minimum of ultrasound and sestamibi. A 3-phase DECT, without an unenhanced phase, was performed with the ability to create virtual unenhanced images as needed if needed for diagnostic evaluation. This was followed by a post-hoc spectral density evaluation of PAs and lymph nodes.

## Methods
### Patients
The study was approved by the institutional review board at the Jewish General Hospital. In the period from September 2013 to April 2014, after obtaining consent, we recruited all patients with primary hyperparathyroidism and non-concordant imaging studies (Table 1). At our institution, the standard studies used for PA localization are ultrasound and sestamibi SPECT/CT and all patients had undergone these studies. However, some patients had undergone additional investigations, including MRIs (15/29) and seven patients who had undergone a total of nine negative surgical explorations (Table 1). Non-concordance was defined as either unidentified (i.e. standard imaging fails to identify any PA) or discordant (i.e. standard imaging does not agree on the location). Demographic data was recorded and patients were divided into "unidentified" or "discordant" groups. Patients with a history of iodine allergy were excluded from the study.

### CT technique
All patients were scanned with the same 64-section dual-energy scanner (GE Discovery CT750HD; GE Healthcare, Milwaukee, WI). Scans were obtained at 25, 55, and 85 s after injection of 100 mL of iopamidol at 3.5 mL/s. The 25 and 55 s acquisitions were acquired in dual-energy rapid 80–140-kVp switching mode using the gemstone spectral imaging protocol [13]. These were acquired with a GSI preset 1, with a large scan field of view (up to 50 cm), 40-mm

**Table 1** Patient population and clinical presentation ($p > 0.05$ for all demographic data)

|  | Discordant | Unidentified |
|---|---|---|
| Subjects included | 18 | 11 |
| Average age | 63.61 | 54.36 |
| F:M ratio | 12:6 | 7:4 |
| Symptoms |  |  |
|    Incidental hypercalcemia | 14 | 8 |
|    Osteopenia/porosis | 2 | 2 |
|    Renal failure | 2 | 1 |
| Previous workup |  |  |
|    Ultrasound | 22 | 11 |
|    Sestamibi | 23 | 20 |
|    MRI | 10 | 5 |
|    Surgical exploration | 5 | 4 |

beam collimation, 0.6-second rotation time, and 0.984:1 helical pitch, resulting in a maximal tube current of approximately 640 mA. Images were reconstructed into 1.25 mm sections with 25-cm display field of view and $512 \times 512$ matrix. 70 keV VMIs, the VMI believed to simulate the standard 120 kVp single energy acquisition by extrapolation from abdominal CT studies, were reconstructed and transferred to PACS for interpretation. Source spectral images were transferred to a dedicated workstation (GE Advantage workstation 4.6; GE Healthcare, Milwaukee, WI) where virtual unenhanced image reconstruction or more advanced spectral analysis could be performed.

**Prospective PA identification**
The scans were prospectively reviewed by one of two attending head and neck radiologists with 5 (R.F.) and 15 (M.L.) years post-fellowship experience in head and neck radiology. Primary interpretation and prospective localization of PAs was performed using the multiphasic 70 keV VMIs. If needed, additional virtual unenhanced images were generated to help image interpretation at the discretion of the reporting radiologist. If virtual unenhanced images were used to assist interpretation, this was recorded. If patient was called back for additional imaging, such as to obtain true unenhanced images, this was also recorded. Potential candidate adenomas were described based on their size, shape, presence of an identifiable supplying artery (referred to as polar artery), and exact anatomic location with respect to the thyroid gland and associated cartilages. Depending on ability to localize a potential adenoma, the study was termed "DECT positive" or "DECT negative".

**Surgical confirmation**
The imaging findings were compared with localization during minimally invasive surgery and histopathologic confirmation. Sensitivity was calculated for pre-operative identification of correct side and quadrant. Successful surgical excision was considered based on histopathology and a decrease in the level of blood serum parathyroid hormone of greater than 50 % post-operatively.

**Post-hoc advanced DECT characterization**
Since little is known about the spectral characteristics of PAs, a post-hoc analysis of spectral curves of a subset of PAs [13] was performed and compared to lymph nodes in order to evaluate for potential differences in their spectral characteristics. Analysis was performed on the dedicated GE Advantage workstation (4.6; GE Healthcare, Milwaukee, WI). Quantitative image analysis was performed using region of interest (ROI) analysis. Scans were retrospectively reconstructed into different VMI energy levels ranging from 40 to 140 keV in 5 keV increments. PA and lymph node evaluation was performed by measuring mean CT attenuation (in Hounsfield units; HU) ± standard deviation (SD) within regions of interest (ROIs) across the entire range of VMI energy levels. All ROIs were placed by an attending head and neck radiologist (R.F.). ROIs were placed on the homogenous enhancing part of PAs or lymph nodes, excluding any heterogenous or cystic foci within the PA if present. Care was also taken not to overlap with adjacent tissues in order to avoid volume averaging with other tissues. Because of frequently small size of PAs and lymph nodes, small ROIs had to be used. However, to obtain a representative sample, 3 ROIs were obtained in each structure and the mean attenuation of the 3 ROIs calculated at each energy level for each structure. Each ROI was large enough to cover the enhancing area without overlap with heterogenous or cystic internal foci or adjacent tissue. For lymph nodes, normal lymph nodes were selected, avoiding areas obscured by artifact. When possible, nearby nodes (level VI or IV) were selected. If those were too small for analysis, then a level IB or IIA node was selected for analysis. The average area for each individual ROI used was 5.62 mm$^2$ (range 1.05–10.15 mm$^2$).

**Statistical analysis**
Positive predictive value was calculated for PA identification and final pathology in the unidentified and discordant studies. For quantitative ROI analysis, results were reported as mean ± SD. Spectral Hounsfield attenuation curves were generated from 40 to 140 keV, in 5 keV increments for comparison of PAs and LNs. For each structure (PA or lymph node), the average density was determined by calculating the average of the three ROIs

used per structure in that patient. Data from different patients were then pooled at each keV for comparison of PAs with lymph nodes. Comparison of means was performed using an unpaired two-tailed $t$-test. A $p$-value less than 0.05 was considered to be statistically significant. We used Graphpad Prism version 6.005 for statistical analysis (GraphPad Software, La Jolla California USA, www.graphpad.com, GraphPad Software, Inc., La Jolla, CA).

## Results

### Patient population and clinical presentation

In total, 29 patients were evaluated in this study, 11 in the unidentified and 18 in the discordant groups (Table 1). The average age of participants was 60.1 years old (range 39–76), consisting of 19 women and 10 men. The most common presenting complaint was asymptomatic incidental hypercalcemia with elevated parathyroid hormone, but presentations ranged from osteopenia to renal failure (Table 1). Total counts for imaging/procedures performed prior to DECT included: 33 ultrasounds, 43 sestamibi scans, 15 MRIs, and nine previous exploratory procedures (on seven patients).

### Prospective parathyroid adenoma identification and surgical outcome

Multiphasic dual-energy CTs localized potential PAs in 26 of 29 patients: 10/11 in the equivocal and 16/18 in the discordant group. One patient in the latter group had two candidate adenomas identified, corresponding to a 94.4 % "DECT positive" rate overall. Of the 26 DECT positive studies, 23 patients have undergone minimally invasive parathyroidectomy at this time and 20 operations were successful (PPV 87.0 %). Both adenomas in the patient with bilateral disease were histologically positive corresponding to 21 adenomas total and an 87.5 % PPV overall. Of the seven patients with previous negative surgical explorations, DECT found candidate adenomas in six. Operations were successful (positive localization and pathology) in four of the six patients. Of the three studies in which the DECT identified candidate could not be confirmed surgically, two were from the discordant and one from the unidentified group.

Among the 20 patients with pathologically proven PAs, DECT was concordant with the sestamibi SPECT/CT in seven cases but US in only one case. Basic characteristics of PAs are summarized in Table 2 and the location of the PAs in the discordant and unidentified groups is summarized in Table 3. Sizes ranged from 0.6 to 2.7 cm and means were similar in the two groups (1.43 cm discordant vs. 1.24 cm unidentified). Perfusion characteristics were a key component of PA identification, particularly on the 25 s arterial phase images (Fig. 1). However, not all PAs demonstrated typical robust arterial phase enhancement or rapid washout and

**Table 2** Basic characteristics of PAs on DECT

| Shape (%) | |
| --- | --- |
| Oval | 64.3 |
| Tear drop | 21.4 |
| Triangular | 7.1 |
| Tubular | 7.1 |
| Margins (%) | |
| Smooth | 78.6 |
| Lobulated | 21.4 |
| Other defining characteristics | |
| Low attenuation component (%) | 28.6 |
| Fat plane separating from thyroid (%) | 85.7 |
| Polar artery present (%) | 92.6 |
| Location (%) | |
| Perrier [37] | |
| Type A (4.8) | |
| Type B (9.5) | |
| Type C (23.8) | |
| Type D (28.6) | |
| Type E (4.8) | |
| Type F (19.0) | |
| Type G (9.5) | |

as such, other features were also important in identifying and localizing a PA (Table 2, Figs. 2 and 3). These included features that allowed confident separation of the PA from the thyroid gland, such as presence of fat plane between the PA and thyroid, perfusion pattern distinct from thyroid gland, and other morphologic characteristics enabling reliable distinction from lymph nodes (Table 2).

### Advanced DECT analysis

In the 29 patients evaluated here, the radiologists created virtual unenhanced images in only two of the cases

**Table 3** Location of PAs in the discordant and equivocal groups

| | Pathologically-proven ($N = 21$) | |
| --- | --- | --- |
| DECT characteristics | Discordant | Unidentified |
| Positive | 14 | 7 |
| Location (% of total (21); Perrier classification [37]) | A (4.8) | A (0) |
| | B (9.4) | B (0) |
| | C (18.9) | C (4.8) |
| | D (14.3) | D (14.3) |
| | E (0) | E (4.8) |
| | F (14.3) | F (4.8) |
| | G (4.8) | G (4.8) |

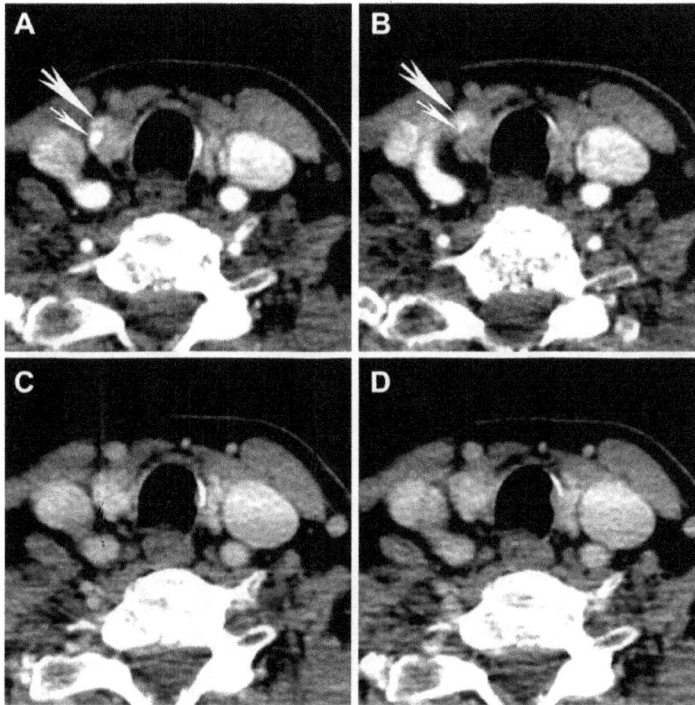

**Fig. 1** Typical perfusion characteristics in an intrathyroidal parathyroid adenoma. 70 keV VMIs at (**a**, **b**) 25 s and (**c**, **d**) 55 s are shown of a surgically and pathologically proven intrathyroidal parathyroid adenoma (*large arrow*). The feeding vessel supplying the adenoma is also seen (*small arrow*) and is helpful for diagnosis, sometimes referred to as the polar artery. There is the typical rapid and robust enhancement on arterial phase images (**a**, **b**). On the more delayed images, there is contrast washout from the adenoma but increased attenuation of the thyroid gland and the adenoma cannot be clearly distinguished from the thyroid gland (**c**, **d**)

and these were deemed not to be helpful. The limitation of virtual unenhanced images for PA localization is that in addition to the enhancing PA, the intrinsic iodine content of the thyroid gland is also suppressed (Fig. 4). As such, DECT virtual unenhanced images cannot be used as a complete substitute for the unenhanced CT for purposes of PA characterization. Early during recruitment, two out of 29 patients were called back in order to obtain actual unenhanced images. On retrospective evaluation, it was felt that these did not add significantly to the study and no patients were recalled for obtaining unenhanced CT during the work-up of the latter 20 patients in this study.

As part of this pilot study using DECT, a post-hoc quantitative spectral Hounsfield unit attenuation curve analysis was performed, comparing characteristics of PAs to lymph nodes (Fig. 5). On the 25 s arterial acquisition, there was a significant difference between the spectral attenuation curves of PAs compared to lymph nodes, with density separation in the low energy range ($P < 0.01$ - $P < 0.0001$; Fig. 5). Although there was a trend for density separation in the lower energy range on the 55 s acquisition, this was not statistically significant (Fig. 5).

## Discussion

Primary hyperparathyroidism (PHPT) is most commonly caused by a solitary benign parathyroid adenoma and the treatment is surgical excision [30]. In order to limit the extent of dissection in searching for the pathologic gland, preoperative localization studies are used [31]. These studies currently include sestamibi scanning, ultrasonography, computed tomography (CT), magnetic resonance imaging (MRI), positron emission tomography (PET) and angiography [2, 3, 32–34]. Pre-operative concordant images have a dramatic impact on success and associated morbidity of minimally invasive surgery [35].

There is increasing popularity of 4D-CT for localization of PAs although there are concerns about the radiation exposure associated with the classic 4 phase 4D-CT [3, 5–10]. While the effective dose of the typical 4D-CT protocol is greater than that of scintigraphy, studies have shown the lifetime incidence of cancer compared to baseline cancer risk for this population is negligible for either study [36]. Despite this and in order to minimize radiation exposure from the procedure to the extent possible, some groups are decreasing the number of acquisitions [11, 12]. DECT scans can be

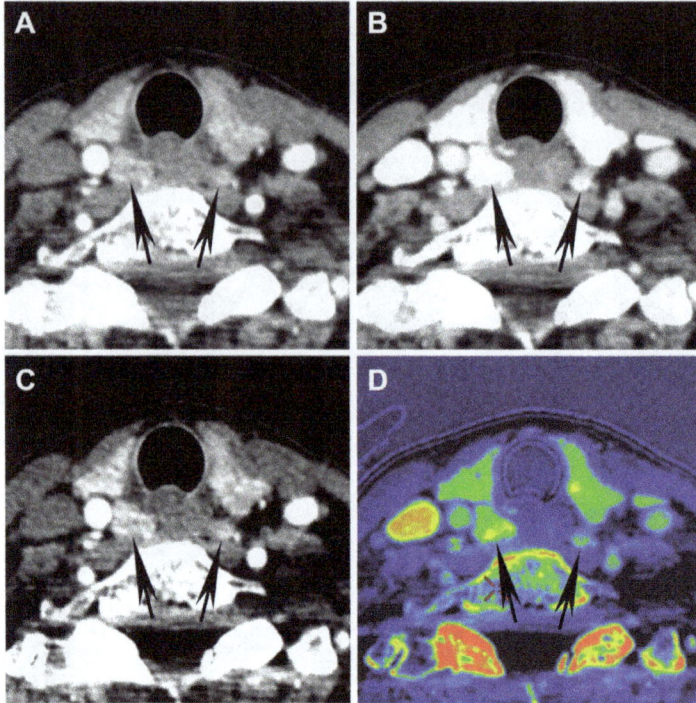

**Fig. 2** Atypical perfusion characteristics in bilateral parathyroid adenomas. (**a**) 25 s 70 keV VMI, (**b**) 55 s 70 keV VMI, (**c**) 25 s 50 keV VMI, and (**d**) 25 s iodine overlay map are shown demonstrating surgically and pathologically proven bilateral parathyroid adenomas (*arrows*). In this case, a typical robust arterial phase enhancement with rapid washout is not shown (adenoma attenuation on the 25 s images was less than 100 HU). However, the presence of a fat plane separating the adenomas from the thyroid gland, location, and different appearance from normal lymph nodes enabled a confident pre-operative diagnosis in this case. The 50 keV VMI (**c**) is shown as an example of how DECT low energy reconstructions can accentuate the density of enhancing/iodine containing structures (compare **c** to **a**). DECT also enables creation of iodine overlay maps (**d**), highlighting the iodine content of tissues and enabling a quantitative estimation of tissue iodine content

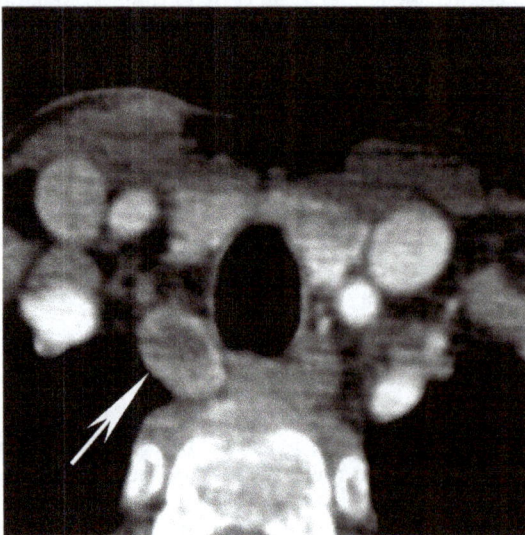

**Fig. 3** Parathyroid adenoma with cystic internal change. Example of surgically and pathologically proven parathyroid adenoma (*arrow*) extending to the right tracheo-esophageal groove

used to create virtual unenhanced images or iodine overlay maps that can estimate the iodine content of a structure based on a single acquisition [14, 15]. In addition, virtual monochromatic images can be created at different energy levels, and these can be evaluated quantitatively, potentially increasing the analytic capabilities of CT technique [13–15]. This could potentially improve accuracy and in turn enable a reduced number of acquisitions.

In this investigation, we used a 3 phase CT technique, with DECT acquisitions, to localize unidentified or discordant PAs prospectively. Consistent with other studies [3, 5–12], multiphasic CT was effective in localizing PAs in a significant percentage of cases, including cases of multi-gland disease and intrathyroidal PA. Although the radiologists had the ability to generate and use virtual unenhanced images, this was overall deemed not necessary and after the use for two cases in the early part of the study, without benefit, these were not created or used for the other cases. The problem of using virtual unenhanced images for PA identification is that both the iodinated contrast in the enhancing PA and the intrinsic iodine within the thyroid gland are suppressed (Fig. 4),

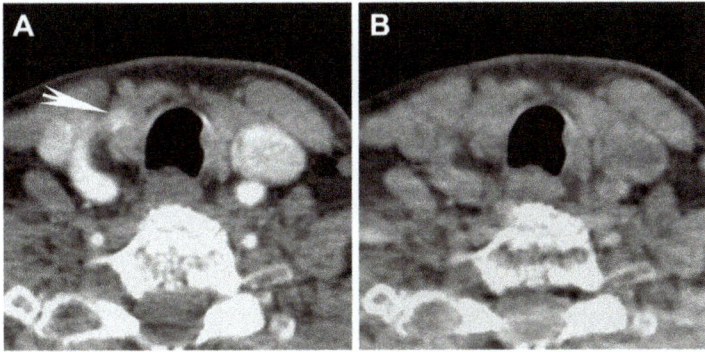

**Fig. 4** Virtual unenhanced DECT images. **a** 70 keV VMI and (**b**) virtual unenhanced image of the intrathyroidal parathyroid adenoma in Fig. 1 are shown. The parathyroid adenoma seen on the 70 keV VMI (*arrow*) cannot be seen on the virtual unenhanced image (**b**) because of suppression of iodinated contrast on that image. The iodinated contrast in the vessels as well as iodine within the thyroid gland are also suppressed

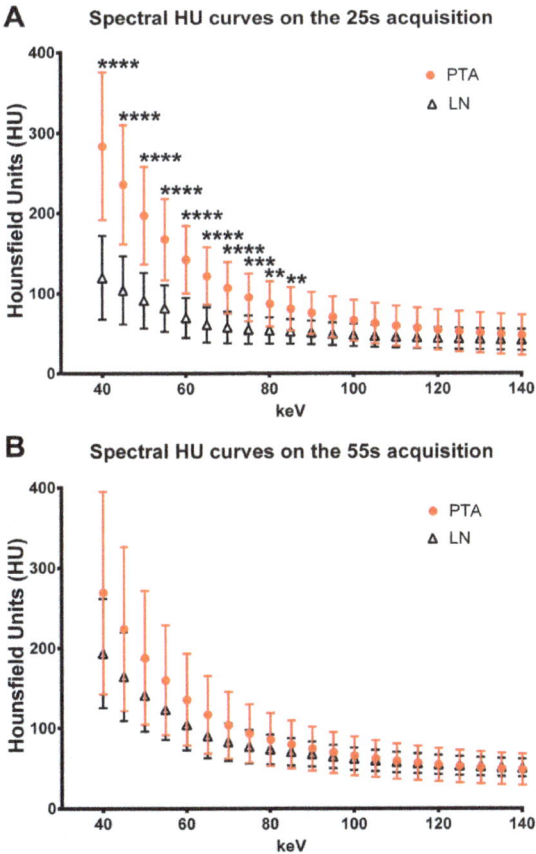

**Fig. 5** Spectral Hounsfield unit (HU) curve analysis of parathyroid adenomas compared to lymph nodes. Spectral HU analysis of 13 normal appearing lymph nodes (LN) and 14 surgical and pathologically proven adenomas (PA) from 13 patients are shown from the (**a**) 25 s and (**b**) 55 s DECT acquisitions. PA have different spectral HU characteristics compared to LN on the 25 s but not the 55 s acquisition with density separation on the left (lower energy) side of the curve. **$P < 0.01$, ***$P < 0.001$, ****$P < 0.0001$

defeating the purpose of the reconstructions for distinction of PA from thyroid tissue. On the other hand, we also demonstrate successful identification of PAs prospectively without the need for an unenhanced scan. During the early part of the study, two patients were called back for an unenhanced study. However, in retrospect these were deemed not necessary and were not performed in any of the patients later on. This is consistent with more recent reports demonstrating successful "4D-CT" with a reduced number of phases [11, 12].

Although our investigation did not reveal a role for the DECT virtual unenhanced images for PA localization, post-hoc spectral Hounsfield unit attenuation curve analysis demonstrated a difference in the characteristics of PAs compared to lymph nodes on arterial phase images (Fig. 5). Arterial phase images are one of the most important acquisitions in 4D-CT performed for PA localization and these preliminary observations suggest that DECT can further increase accuracy during this phase of the exam, which may in turn enable further reduction of the number of acquisitions without decreasing diagnostic accuracy in the future. Other potential applications of DECT could be improved PA visualization on low energy virtual monochromatic images and the use of estimated iodine content for PA identification (Fig. 2). These are topics of great interest for future research.

Although the perfusion characteristics are central in identifying PAs, other features such as location, presence of feeding or polar artery, and other characteristics that help distinguish PAs from normal lymph nodes such as cystic internal change were also important for accurate identification of PAs (Table 2). Furthermore, not all of the PAs demonstrated a typical robust arterial phase enhancement with rapid wash-out (Fig. 2). Therefore, rather than focusing on absolute thresholds, it may be more important to identify combinations of features that help distinguish PAs from potentially mimicking normal structures. Of course, it is possible that we observed a higher frequency of atypical appearing PAs because the study was used to evaluate unidentified or discordant PAs, resulting in a selection bias.

In this study, we were able to localize previously unidentified parathyroid adenomas in 26 of 29 patients. Twenty three of these patients have undergone surgical exploration at this time, and DECT correctly identified 21 PAs in 20 of those patients. We also demonstrate a high success-rate of minimally invasive parathyroidectomy on primary cases and even some secondary cases. Among the three false positives, two were in patients with prior surgery. Therefore, one must at least consider the possibility that these PAs may have not been found because of extensive scarring from the patient's prior surgery. One of the strengths of this study is that all PA identification was done prospectively. The limitation is that the numbers are relatively small. As many of these were outside referrals, another limitation could be that not all of the standard imaging was done at the institution were DECT was performed, potentially introducing a bias. However, among the 20 patients who successfully underwent surgery, 13 had sestamibi and 12 US at the same institution and therefore the proposed bias could not account for the success of DECT in these cases. In addition, a small number of patients could not be analyzed because they have not undergone surgery yet (either because of loss to follow-up or surgical waitlist time). Nonetheless, our results demonstrate the feasibility of a multiphasic study without an unenhanced phase and promising results for DECT spectral analysis for improving the diagnostic evaluation of PAs. The impact of more advanced DECT analysis will have to be tested in larger and ideally prospective use of these characteristics in future studies.

## Conclusion

In this prospective study, we demonstrate that a 3 phase CT technique, with DECT acquisitions and without an unenhanced phase, has high accuracy in identifying previously unidentified or discordant PAs. Furthermore, our post-hoc analysis demonstrates significant differences in the spectral characteristics of PAs compared to lymph nodes on arterial phase images. This suggests that advanced DECT analysis has the potential to further increase accuracy for PA identification, which could potentially enable a reduction in the number of CT acquisitions and associated radiation exposure. This is an interesting topic for future research.

## Abbreviations

PA: Parathyroid adenoma; CT: Computed tomography; 4D-CT: 4-dimensional CT; DECT: Dual-energy CT; PPV: Positive predictive value; VMI: Virtual monochromatic images; ROI: Region of interest; kVp: kilovolt peak; keV: kiloelectron volts.

## Competing interests

R.F. was speaker at a lunch and learn session titled "Dual-Energy CT Applications in Neuroradiology and Head and Neck Imaging" sponsored by GE Healthcare at the 27th Annual Meeting of the Eastern Neuroradiological Society in Sept 2015. The authors declare that they have no competing interests.

## Authors' contributions

MR carried out study conception and design, assisted on some parathyroidectomies, performed acquisition of data, analysis and interpretation and drafted the manuscript. XL participated in data acquisition, design, and spectral data analysis. ML participated in acquisition of data and was one of 2 radiologists reading all DECTs. MPH, RJP, VF and AM performed parathyroidectomies and revised the manuscript. RF supervised the entire project, carried out study conception and design, was one of 2 radiologists reading all DECTs, performed acquisition of data, analysis and interpretation and drafted the manuscript. All authors read and approved the final manuscript.

## References

1.  Munk RS, Payne RJ, Luria BJ, Hier MP, Black MJ. Preoperative localization in primary hyperparathyroidism. J Otolaryngol Head Neck Surg. 2008;37(3):347–54.
2.  Phillips CD, Shatzkes DR. Imaging of the parathyroid glands. Semin Ultrasound CT MR. 2012;33(2):123–9.
3.  Rodgers SE, Hunter GJ, Hamberg LM, Schellingerhout D, Doherty DB, Ayers GD, et al. Improved preoperative planning for directed parathyroidectomy with 4-dimensional computed tomography. Surgery. 2006;140(6):932–40. discussion 40–1.
4.  Patel CN, Salahudeen HM, Lansdown M, Scarsbrook AF. Clinical utility of ultrasound and 99mTc sestamibi SPECT/CT for preoperative localization of parathyroid adenoma in patients with primary hyperparathyroidism. Clin Radiol. 2010;65(4):278–87.
5.  Hunter GJ, Schellingerhout D, Vu TH, Perrier ND, Hamberg LM. Accuracy of four-dimensional CT for the localization of abnormal parathyroid glands in patients with primary hyperparathyroidism. Radiology. 2012;264(3):789–95.
6.  Hunter GJ, Ginat DT, Kelly HR, Halpern EF, Hamberg LM. Discriminating parathyroid adenoma from local mimics by using inherent tissue attenuation and vascular information obtained with four-dimensional CT: formulation of a multinomial logistic regression model. Radiology. 2014;270(1):168–75.
7.  Kelly HR, Hamberg LM, Hunter GJ. 4D-CT for preoperative localization of abnormal parathyroid glands in patients with hyperparathyroidism: accuracy and ability to stratify patients by unilateral versus bilateral disease in surgery-naive and re-exploration patients. AJNR Am J Neuroradiol. 2014;35(1):176–81.
8.  Hoang JK, Sung WK, Bahl M, Phillips CD. How to perform parathyroid 4D CT: tips and traps for technique and interpretation. Radiology. 2014;270(1):15–24.
9.  Mortenson MM, Evans DB, Lee JE, Hunter GJ, Shellingerhout D, Vu T, et al. Parathyroid exploration in the reoperative neck: improved preoperative localization with 4D-computed tomography. J Am Coll Surg. 2008;206(5):888–95. discussion 95–6.
10. Chazen JL, Gupta A, Dunning A, Phillips CD. Diagnostic accuracy of 4D-CT for parathyroid adenomas and hyperplasia. AJNR Am J Neuroradiol. 2012;33(3):429–33.
11. Welling RD, Olson Jr JA, Kranz PG, Eastwood JD, Hoang JK. Bilateral retropharyngeal parathyroid hyperplasia detected with 4D multidetector row CT. AJNR Am J Neuroradiol. 2011;32(5):E80–2.
12. Noureldine SI, Aygun N, Walden MJ, Hassoon A, Gujar SK, Tufano RP. Multiphase computed tomography for localization of parathyroid disease in patients with primary hyperparathyroidism: How many phases do we really need? Surgery. 2014;156(6):1300–6. discussion 13006–7.
13. Forghani R, Levental M, Gupta R, Lam S, Dadfar N, Curtin HD. Different Spectral Hounsfield Unit Curve and High-Energy Virtual Monochromatic Image Characteristics of Squamous Cell Carcinoma Compared with Nonossified Thyroid Cartilage. AJNR Am J Neuroradiol. 2015;36:1194–200.
14. Johnson T, Fink C, Schönberg SO, Reiser MF. Dual Energy CT in Clinical Practice. Berlin, Heidelberg: Springer; 2011.
15. Johnson TR. Dual-energy CT: general principles. AJR Am J Roentgenol. 2012;199(5 Suppl):S3–8.

16. Pomerantz SR, Kamalian S, Zhang D, Gupta R, Rapalino O, Sahani DV, et al. Virtual monochromatic reconstruction of dual-energy unenhanced head CT at 65–75 keV maximizes image quality compared with conventional polychromatic CT. Radiology. 2013;266(1):318–25.
17. De Cecco CN, Darnell A, Rengo M, Muscogiuri G, Bellini D, Ayuso C, et al. Dual-energy CT: oncologic applications. AJR Am J Roentgenol. 2012;199(5 Suppl):S98–S105.
18. Heye T, Nelson RC, Ho LM, Marin D, Boll DT. Dual-energy CT applications in the abdomen. AJR Am J Roentgenol. 2012;199(5 Suppl):S64–70.
19. Lu GM, Zhao Y, Zhang LJ, Schoepf UJ. Dual-energy CT of the lung. AJR Am J Roentgenol. 2012;199(5 Suppl):S40–53.
20. Postma AA, Hofman PA, Stadler AA, van Oostenbrugge RJ, Tijssen MP, Wildberger JE. Dual-energy CT of the brain and intracranial vessels. AJR Am J Roentgenol. 2012;199(5 Suppl):S26–33.
21. Vliegenthart R, Pelgrim GJ, Ebersberger U, Rowe GW, Oudkerk M, Schoepf UJ. Dual-energy CT of the heart. AJR Am J Roentgenol. 2012;199(5 Suppl):S54–63.
22. Forghani R. Advanced dual-energy CT for head and neck cancer imaging. Expert review of anticancer therapy. 2015;In press.
23. Albrecht MH, Scholtz JE, Kraft J, Bauer RW, Kaup M, Dewes P, et al. Assessment of an Advanced Monoenergetic Reconstruction Technique in Dual-Energy Computed Tomography of Head and Neck Cancer. Eur Radiol. 2015;25(8):2493–501.
24. Kuno H, Onaya H, Iwata R, Kobayashi T, Fujii S, Hayashi R, et al. Evaluation of cartilage invasion by laryngeal and hypopharyngeal squamous cell carcinoma with dual-energy CT. Radiology. 2012;265(2):488–96.
25. Lam S, Gupta R, Levental M, Yu E, Curtin HD, Forghani R. Optimal Virtual Monochromatic Images for Evaluation of Normal Tissues and Head and Neck Cancer Using Dual-Energy CT. AJNR Am J Neuroradiol. 2015;36:1518–24.
26. Liu X, Ouyang D, Li H, Zhang R, Lv Y, Yang A, et al. Papillary Thyroid Cancer: Dual-Energy Spectral CT Quantitative Parameters for Preoperative Diagnosis of Metastasis to the Cervical Lymph Nodes. Radiology. 2015;275(1):167–76.
27. Tawfik AM, Kerl JM, Bauer RW, Nour-Eldin NE, Naguib NN, Vogl TJ, et al. Dual-energy CT of head and neck cancer: average weighting of low- and high-voltage acquisitions to improve lesion delineation and image quality-initial clinical experience. Investig Radiol. 2012;47(5):306–11.
28. Tawfik AM, Razek AA, Kerl JM, Nour-Eldin NE, Bauer R, Vogl TJ. Comparison of dual-energy CT-derived iodine content and iodine overlay of normal, inflammatory and metastatic squamous cell carcinoma cervical lymph nodes. Eur Radiol. 2014;24(3):574–80.
29. Gimm O, Juhlin C, Morales O, Persson A. Dual-energy computed tomography localizes ectopic parathyroid adenoma. J Clin Endocrinol Metab. 2010;95(7):3092–3.
30. Eufrazino C, Veras A, Bandeira F. Epidemiology of Primary Hyperparathyroidism and its Non-classical Manifestations in the City of Recife, Brazil. Clin Med Insights Endocrinol Diabetes. 2013;6:69–74.
31. Akbaba G, Berker D, Isik S, Aydin Y, Ciliz D, Peksoy I, et al. A comparative study of pre-operative imaging methods in patients with primary hyperparathyroidism: ultrasonography, 99mTc sestamibi, single photon emission computed tomography, and magnetic resonance imaging. J Endocrinol Invest. 2012;35(4):359–64.
32. Lumachi F, Ermani M, Basso S, Zucchetta P, Borsato N, Favia G. Localization of parathyroid tumours in the minimally invasive era: which technique should be chosen? Population-based analysis of 253 patients undergoing parathyroidectomy and factors affecting parathyroid gland detection. Endocr Relat Cancer. 2001;8(1):63–9.
33. Schalin-Jantti C, Ryhanen E, Heiskanen I, Seppanen M, Arola J, Schildt J, et al. Planar scintigraphy with 123I/99mTc-sestamibi, 99mTc-sestamibi SPECT/CT, 11C-methionine PET/CT, or selective venous sampling before reoperation of primary hyperparathyroidism? J Nucl Med. 2013;54(5):739–47.
34. Herrmann K, Takei T, Kanegae K, Shiga T, Buck AK, Altomonte J, et al. Clinical value and limitations of [11C]-methionine PET for detection and localization of suspected parathyroid adenomas. Mol Imaging Biol. 2009;11(5):356–63.
35. Bergenfelz AO, Wallin G, Jansson S, Eriksson H, Martensson H, Christiansen P, et al. Results of surgery for sporadic primary hyperparathyroidism in patients with preoperatively negative sestamibi scintigraphy and ultrasound. Langenbecks Arch Surg. 2011;396(1):83–90.
36. Hoang JK, Reiman RE, Nguyen GB, Januzis N, Chin BB, Lowry C, et al. Lifetime Attributable Risk of Cancer From Radiation Exposure During Parathyroid Imaging: Comparison of 4D CT and Parathyroid Scintigraphy. AJR Am J Roentgenol. 2015;204(5):W579–85.
37. Perrier ND, Edeiken B, Nunez R, Gayed I, Jimenez C, Busaidy N, et al. A novel nomenclature to classify parathyroid adenomas. World J Surg. 2009;33(3):412–6.

# 6

# A retrospective study of head and neck re-irradiation for patients with recurrent or second primary head and neck cancer

Rolina Al-Wassia[1*], Siavosh Vakilian[2], Crystal Holly[3], Khalil Sultanem[4] and George Shenouda[2]

## Abstract

**Background:** We report our experience with patients who received re-irradiation to the head and neck area for locoregional recurrences (LRR) or second primaries (SP) in a previously irradiated field.

**Methods:** We reviewed 27 consecutive patients with a diagnosis of LRR or SP head and neck carcinoma treated with a second course of radiotherapy between April 2004 and July 2012. The main outcome measures were local control, overall survival, and complications. The results are expressed as actuarial values using the Kaplan–Meier estimates.

**Results:** The median follow-up time was 24.7 months (range: 11 days–79.3 months). There were 23 males and four females with a median age of 61 years (range: 40–87 years). The actuarial overall survival rates at 1, 2, and 5 years were 77, 59, and 57 %, respectively. The actuarial local control rate was 80, 52, and 52 % at 1, 2, and 5 years, respectively. Three patients developed systemic metastases. The rate of grade 3 toxicity was 26 %, and that of grade 4 toxicity was 3 %. There were two treatment-related deaths (grade 5 toxicity).

**Conclusions:** Continuous course re-irradiation in patients with LRR or SP head and neck cancer is feasible with acceptable toxicity. With current encouraging rates of local control and overall survival, this option should be discussed with patients who have few alternative therapeutic options.

**Keywords:** Re-irradiation, Head and neck, Squamous cell carcinoma

## Background

Surgical resection is typically considered the modality of choice in patients with locoregional recurrences (LRR) or second primary (SP) head and neck cancer who were previously treated with a full dose of radiation therapy [1]. Historically, patients who were deemed to have unresectable tumors, because of tumor location, extent, or medical comorbidities, were referred for palliative chemotherapy. However, the response rates achieved with chemotherapy for these patients ranged between 10 and 40 % [2]. In the last decade, re-irradiation (RI) has begun to gain conceptual acceptance, as experimental and clinical studies have demonstrated that high-dose RI can be administered with reasonable success and acceptable complication rates.

The management of LRR or SP head and neck cancer in patients who were previously treated with a full dose of irradiation remains a clinical challenge. The difficulty arises from the possibility of serious side effects following RI [3, 4]. Some of these toxicities, such as carotid rupture, fistula, or bleeding, can be life-threatening. In addition, other serious but non-life-threatening side effects can occur – for example, osteonecrosis, soft tissue fibrosis, carotid stenosis, severe xerostomia, and trismus.

In spite of these complications, accumulated data from different centers [5–7] showed increased local control and survival in patients treated with a tri-modality approach,

* Correspondence: ralwassia@kau.edu.sa
[1]Department of Radiation Oncology, King Abdulaziz University, Abdullah Suleiman Street, P.O Box 80200, 21589 Jeddah, Saudi Arabia
Full list of author information is available at the end of the article

including surgery followed by RI and chemotherapy (if indicated), over single modality or chemotherapy alone.

Reasonable survival has been reported with primary RI alone, with a median survival of 10 months and a 3-year overall survival of 22 % [8, 9]. More commonly, however, chemotherapy is given concurrently to overcome radioresistance and to improve outcomes. The leading multicenter Radiation Therapy Oncology Group (RTOG 9610) trial examining concurrent RI and chemotherapy showed OS at 1 and 2 years of 40 and 15 %, respectively. In the other RTOG study (RTOG 9911), the OS rates at 1 and 2 years were 50.2 and 25.9 %, respectively. Both trials used a hyperfractionated, twice-daily RI schedule, to a total dose of 60 Gy in 1.5 Gy fractions. The improvement in outcomes in the second trial could be a result of using different chemotherapy agents, such as platinum-based regimens, which are known to be more effective for squamous cell carcinoma than hydroxyuria and 5-fluorouracil. More recently, Kharofa *et al.* [10] published encouraging results of their experience with a continuous course of RI and concurrent carboplatin and paclitaxel for locally recurrent squamous cell carcinoma of the head and neck. The authors reported a median survival of 16 months, and an OS of 54 % at 1 year and 31 % at 2 years.

The purpose of this study is to describe our institutional outcomes in comparison to other published data on RI among a similar group of patients.

## Methods

We retrospectively reviewed the medical records of 30 consecutive patients who received RI for either LRR or for in-field SP cancers between 2004 and 2012. Permission for data abstraction was obtained from the institutional Ethics Review Board. Three patients received brachytherapy as their RI modality and were excluded. Thus, 27 patients were included in the analysis.

## Patients

Patients included in this retrospective study were aged between 40 and 87 years at the time of the second diagnosis, with a median age of 61 years. There were 23 males (85 %) and four females (15 %). Twenty-six patients received RI to the head and neck area with curative intent, whereas one patient with metastatic disease at second presentation was re-irradiated with a palliative intent. The RI volume was delivered to overlapping areas that had previously been irradiated at the time of the first cancer diagnosis. All patients had histological proof of LRR or SP squamous cell carcinoma.

The diagnostic evaluation included a physical examination, panendoscopy with biopsies, radiologic evaluation of the head and neck by computed tomography (CT) and/or magnetic resonance imaging (MRI), and screening for distant metastases using CT and/or positron emission tomography.

For previously irradiated patients presenting with LRR or SP tumors, surgical salvage has remained the standard of care in our institution. In cases of unresectable lesions, primary RI, with or without concurrent chemotherapy, was discussed with the multidisciplinary tumor board and, if deemed appropriate, the option was presented to the patient. Only patients with good performance status (Eastern Cooperative Oncology Group [ECOG] performance status of ≤2) were considered candidates for RI.

Postoperative RI was considered only if the pathological features of the surgical specimen indicated a high risk of subsequent recurrence [11, 12], such as positive margins, lymph node metastasis with extracapsular extension, and/or multiple lymph node metastases.

## Tumor

Primary head and neck tumor sites and the initial stage of disease are reported in Table 1. The recurrence was defined as local if the tumor recurred in the primary site in the previous radiation field, regional if it recurred in the previous radiation field but outside the primary site, and locoregional if the tumor recurred in both the primary

**Table 1** Patient and tumor characteristics at first presentation

|  | Number | Percent |
|---|---|---|
| Patient | 27 |  |
| Male | 23 | 85 |
| Female | 4 | 15 |
| Median age | 61 |  |
| Tumor site at first presentation |  |  |
| Larynx | 5 | 18 |
| Oropharynx | 7 | 26 |
| Nasopharynx | 7 | 26 |
| Maxillary sinus | 1 | 4 |
| Nasal cavity | 1 | 4 |
| Oral cavity | 2 | 7 |
| Unknown primary | 1 | 4 |
| Hypopharynx | 1 | 4 |
| Esophagus | 2 | 7 |
| Histology |  |  |
| Squamous cell carcinoma | 25 | 92 |
| Undifferentiated | 2 | 8 |
| Stage at first presentation |  |  |
| TxN0M0 | 1 | 4 |
| T1-4N0M0 | 8 | 30 |
| T1-4N1M0 | 7 | 26 |
| Tx-4N2M0 | 9 | 33 |
| Unknown | 2 | 7 |

site and in the regional nodes. After the first course of radiotherapy, 11 patients (41 %) had failed locally, four (15 %) had failed regionally, 10 (37 %) had failed locoregionally, and two had SP (7 %).

For tumor classification, the sixth edition of the Union Internationale Contre le Cancer (UICC) was used. Detailed information on staging is shown in Table 1. RI was not necessarily given at the time of the second diagnosis; in five patients, RI was given at the third diagnosis, as radiotherapy was not indicated in either the first or second courses of treatment. Of these five patients, four had recurrences and one patient had a SP.

Salvage surgery was performed in 12 patients (44 %) before RI and resulted in clear margins in four cases, close or positive margins in five cases, and gross residual disease in three cases. Concurrent chemotherapy or targeted therapy during RI was given in 21 patients (77 %) at the discretion of the treating physician, and it included various agents (cisplatin, carboplatin, 5-fluorouracil, or cetuximab). Six patients received RI alone.

## Treatment

In our present study, two different schedules for RI were used: one was similar to the RTOG bid schedule mentioned above, and the second consisted of a total dose of 60 Gy in 30 fractions once daily. Radiotherapy was given concurrently with chemotherapy, usually consisting of a platinum-based regimen, although targeted therapy such as cetuximab was also used; this was similar to other reports in the literature [13]. Radiotherapy was given with 4–6 MV photon linear accelerators using a head and neck thermoplastic immobilization mask. Treatment was given using either three-dimensional conformal radiotherapy, the intensity modulated radiotherapy (IMRT) technique, or Helical TomoTherapy, depending on the available resources at each of the two treatment sites. From 2004–2006, IMRT was mainly used (15 patients), whereas starting from 2007, 11 patients were treated with Helical TomoTherapy. The remaining patient received three-dimensional conformal radiotherapy.

The gross tumor volume (GTV) was defined as any macroscopically visible disease, detected by radiological investigations or by clinical exam, in both the primary tumor and the lymph nodes. A maximum margin of 1 cm was applied to the GTV to define the expansion to clinical target volume (CTV). The CTV to planning target volume margin was 5 mm in three-dimensional conformal radiotherapy and IMRT patients, and only 3 mm in TomoTherapy because of the image-guided radiotherapy function that allowed better day-to-day reproducibility of patient positioning. There was no attempt to treat any elective lymph node area or other areas at risk outside the CTV volume.

The most important organs at risk when RI was considered were the spinal cord, brainstem, salivary glands, optic apparatus, and mandible. For the spinal cord and brainstem, the dose was also calculated to a planning organ at risk volume (PRV), which was created by adding a 5 mm three-dimensional margin to the organ at risk. We limited the maximal spinal cord dose at retreatment to 20 Gy, with a maximum PRV dose of 22 Gy; a maximal dose to the brainstem of 20 Gy, with a maximum PRV dose of 22 Gy; a mandible dose of 40 Gy to <50 % of its volume; and 50 % of the parotids and salivary glands would receive no more than 25–30 Gy. Cumulative lifetime doses after RI were measured for all patients for whom complete information on the first treatment was available. Two patients received their first radiation treatment outside Canada, which precluded the calculation of cumulative doses to target volumes. Figure 1 illustrates how modern techniques such as IMRT allowed for excellent target coverage, while meeting strict constraints on the organs at risk, such as the brainstem and spinal cord.

In our series, RI was indicated in different clinical settings: as primary definitive treatment in 14 patients; as adjuvant treatment postoperatively in 12 patients; and as palliative treatment in one patient, as shown in Table 2.

### Statistics

All statistical analyses were performed using SPSS software version 10.0 (SPSS Inc, Chicago, IL, USA). Results were expressed as actuarial values using the Kaplan–Meier estimates. Actuarial and median survivals were calculated from the first day of the RI course.

## Results

From 2004–2012, 27 patients with LRR or SP head and neck cancer received RI at our institution. The median follow-up time was 24.7 months (range: 11 days–79.3 months).

The median maximal dose delivered to the spinal cord at retreatment was 15.5 Gy (range: 6–45 Gy), the median maximal dose delivered to the brainstem was 20 Gy (range: 1–63 Gy), and the median dose to the mandible was 63 Gy (range: 5–75 Gy). It is noteworthy to realize that these numbers represent median values of the maximal doses, which are often received by a very small volume of the irradiated organ. For both parotids, the mean dose was 28 Gy (range: 1–72 Gy).

### Disease control

The actuarial estimates of local control were 80, 52, and 52 % at 1, 2, and 5 years, as shown in Fig. 2. The median time to the first recurrence or the SP was 24.5 months (range: 4.6–283 months). The median time to the third diagnosis or second failure was 17 months (range: 3.5–192 months).

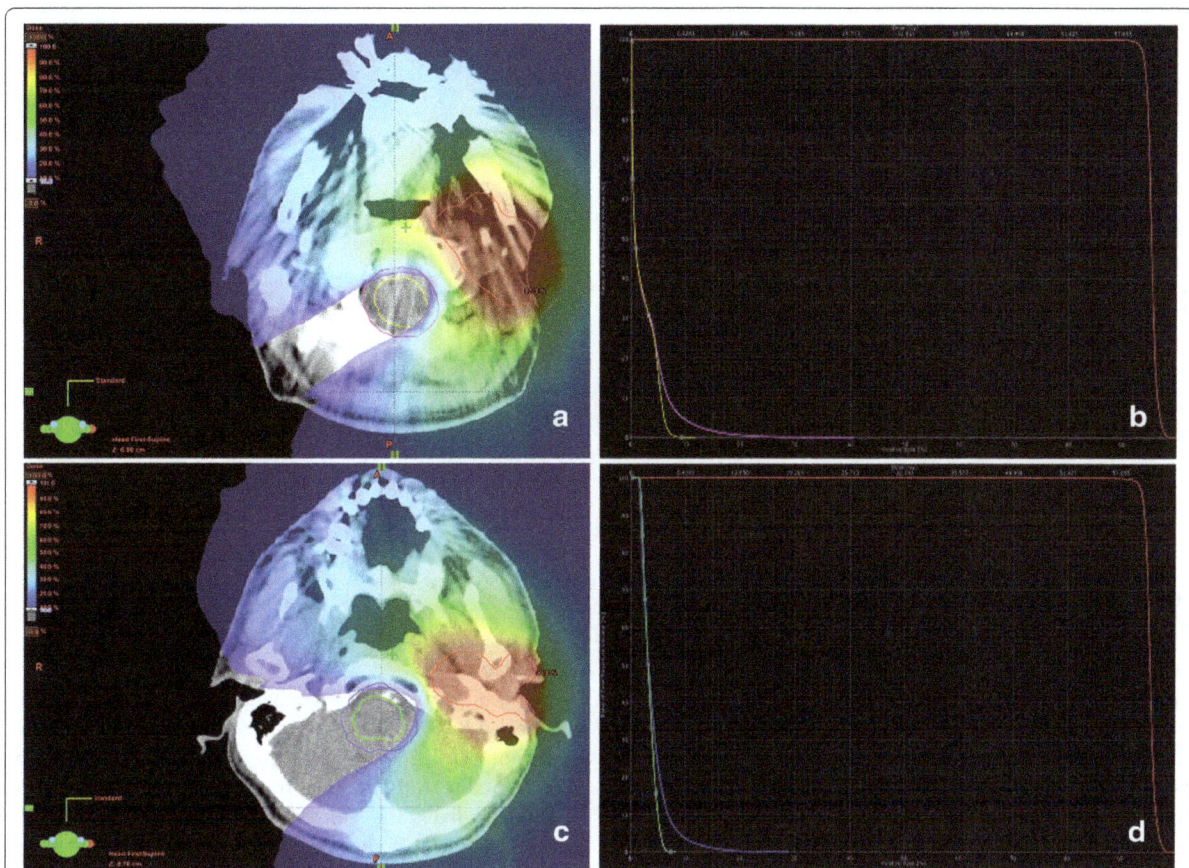

**Fig. 1 a** Color wash dose distribution and **b** dose volume histogram showing spinal cord and PRV sparing, **c** color wash dose distribution, and **d** dose volume histogram showing brainstem and PRV sparing. *PRV* planning organ at risk volume

**Table 2** Treatment characteristics at the time of RI

|  | Number | Percent |
|---|---|---|
| Surgery |  |  |
| Postoperative RI + systemic therapy | 9 | 33 |
| Postoperative RI alone | 3 | 11 |
| Definitive RI without surgery |  |  |
| RI + systemic therapy | 12 | 45 |
| RI alone | 2 | 7 |
| Palliative RI | 1 | 4 |
| Concurrent chemotherapy/targeted therapy |  |  |
| Cisplatin-based | 19 | 70 |
| Cetuximab | 2 | 7 |
| None | 6 | 22 |

*Abbreviation: RI re-irradiation*

Response to treatment after the second course of radiation was measured on either CT or MRI. The maximal radiation response was judged 6 months after the completion of radiation therapy. Nineteen patients (70 %) had a complete response, four patients (15 %) had a partial response, one patient (4 %) had no response, two patients (7 %) had progression of disease, and one patient had insufficient follow-up to evaluate response to treatment.

At a median follow-up of 24.7 months, 14 patients (52 %) had no evidence of failure, four patients (15 %) had local failure, three (11 %) had regional failure, two (7 %) had locoregional failure, two (7 %) had SP, and two (7 %) had persistent disease. Five patients received their second course of radiation at the third diagnosis. Two of these patients were diagnosed with a SP, while the other three had local failures. Four out of these five patients had received high-dose radiotherapy. All four remained locally controlled. The remaining patient with esophageal cancer had received a palliative dose and had immediate local progression; the patient died shortly after.

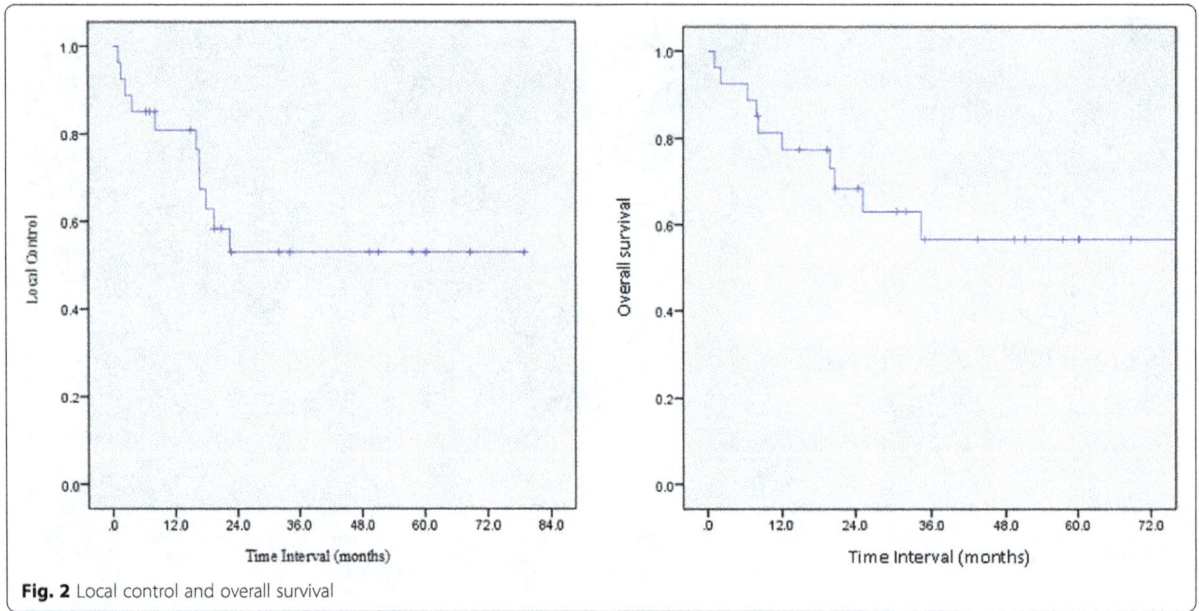

**Fig. 2** Local control and overall survival

## Overall survival and distant metastasis

The actuarial OS rates at 1, 2, and 5 years were 77, 59, and 57 %, respectively (Fig. 2), calculated from the first day of the RI course. At a median follow-up of 24.7 months, 17 patients (64 %) were alive. Only three patients (11 %) developed systemic metastases; one patient developed metastasis and died during the treatment course.

## Toxicity

The National Cancer Institute Common Toxicity Criteria for Adverse Events version 3.0 (CTCAE) was used for toxicity grading. Overall late grade 1–3 toxicity was reported in 25 (93 %) of the treated patients. Details of toxicity are presented in Tables 3 and 4. Two grade 5 toxicities occurred: one as a result of carotid rupture leading to death, and one death secondary to mucosal bleeding (in a patient with locally recurrent disease). No brainstem or spinal cord injuries or brain necrosis were observed.

**Table 3** Late toxicities

| Toxicity | Grade 1 | Grade 2 | Grade 3 | Grade 4 | Grade 5 |
|---|---|---|---|---|---|
| Dry mouth | 21 % | 52 % | 7 % | | |
| Dysphagia | 29 % | 36 % | 11 % | | |
| Trismus | 28 % | 31 % | 7 % | | |
| Muscle fibrosis | 25 % | 25 % | 11 % | | |
| Vascular | | | | | 7 % |
| Loss of taste | 43 % | 11 % | | | |
| Hearing loss | 7 % | 21 % | 3 % | | |
| Radio-osteonecrosis | | 7 % | 7 % | 3 % | |

## Discussion

In our group of patients receiving high-dose RI for head and neck LRR or SP tumors, we found excellent actuarial local control of 52 % and OS of 57 % at 5 years. These compare favorably with findings from the reported literature. The report from the University of Texas MD Anderson Cancer Center [14] showed a median time to progression of 7 months and progression-free rates at 1, 2, and 5 years of 44, 34, and 29 %, respectively. The median OS was 16 months, and the OS at 1, 3, and 5 years was 54, 31, and 20 %, respectively. Sher *et al.* [15] reported the results of 35 patients with recurrent head and neck cancer treated with continuous course RI, while using platinum-based chemotherapy and an IMRT technique. The actuarial 2-year survival was 48 %, with a 2-year locoregional control rate of 67 % and a median OS of 1.9 years. Lee *et al.* [16] reported the Memorial Sloan–Kettering Cancer Center's experience of 105 patients with recurrent head and neck cancer who underwent RI with chemotherapy in 75 % of patients. An IMRT technique was used in 70 % of patients. The 2-year locoregional progression-free and OS rates were 42 and 37 %, respectively.

A few reasons could account for our good results. Unlike some other studies [5, 7], all but one of our patients received some form of IMRT, either on a linear accelerator or on a Helical TomoTherapy unit. This has allowed for the delivery of RI in a more conformal fashion, minimizing acute toxicities and thus reducing treatment interruptions. The fact that our long-term toxicity data compare favorably with those of the reported literature (only three grade 4 or 5 toxicities, despite the relatively common grade 3 toxicities) again reinforces the positive effect of IMRT

**Table 4** Grade 4 and 5 severe adverse events

| Primary site | Primary stage | Initial treatment | Primary response | Second diagnosis | Interval between first and second diagnosis (months) | Life time accumulated dose | Toxicity description | Interval between second radiation and toxicity (months) |
|---|---|---|---|---|---|---|---|---|
| Oropharynx cancer | T4N2b | Concurrent Platinum-based chemotherapy + radiation 70/35 Gy | Complete | Local recurrence | 17.7 | 134 Gy | Carotid rupture Causing death | 6 months |
| Maxillary cancer | T3N2 | Radiation 74/32 Gy | Complete | Second primary, oropharynx cancer | 51.8 | 144 Gy | 1 – osteonecrosis, fractured mandible, disabling; 2 – skin fistula with bone exposed to air | 24 months |
| Oropharynx cancer | T2N1 | Surgical resection followed by adjuvant radiation of 60 Gy | Complete | Locoregional recurrence | 29 | 120 Gy | Mucositis, 5 × 6 cm ulceration causing bleeding, leading to death | 5 months |

techniques employed in our group of patients, allowing for the delivery of radical doses of RI to tumor-bearing volumes, with significant sparing of the critical normal previously irradiated organs. Also, 78 % of patients in the current report received some form of concomitant systemic therapy, most of them with cisplatin. Our results can also be attributed, at least partially, to careful patient selection. In the current series, one-third of the patients had node-negative disease at first presentation, and almost one-half had recurrences that were only local, without lymph node involvement, and all patients had an ECOG of ≤2.

The current series is limited by the relatively small sample size of 27 patients. Also, given the different practices at our two affiliated institutions, our patients did not all receive the same dose/fractionation schedule. Fifteen patients were treated to 60 Gy in 2 Gy fractions once daily; however, a significant minority (six patients) received twice-daily fractionation. In addition, 12 % of patients did not receive concurrent systemic treatment. On the other hand, irradiation techniques were homogeneous, with all but one patient receiving IMRT.

In the current series, the planning target volume based on the GTV was re-irradiated with no attempts to treat any elective nodal sites. This approach was similar to that of previous series that reported on their experiences from different centers [17–20], and which showed that the majority of failures after RI were local at the site of the recurrent GTVs (rGTV). In the Michigan series [21], where RI included the rGTV with no elective neck nodal irradiation, the authors studied 66 patients at a median follow-up of 42 months and found that all LRRs occurred within the rGTVs except for two (4 %). Sher et al. [15] reported that 73 % of LRRs occurred within the RI volumes in patients treated with an IMRT technique to the rGTV alone. In the series by Popovtzer et al., [21], 71 % of patients had presented with evidence of local failure after RI, while neck-only failures occurred in two patients (5 %). These results confirm that recurrent local disease continues to be a significant challenge in patients with RI for LRR or SP tumors in the head and neck region.

Most of the reported series currently tend to use a continuous RI course using once-daily fractionation schedules [22–24]. A recent report from the Beth Israel Medical Center was published on the use of Intra-Operative-Radiotherapy (IORT) in patients with loco-regional recurrent head and neck cancer. Seventy-six patients were identified who underwent treatment to a total of 87 sites after gross-total resection. The 2-year estimate loco-regional control was 62 % with a median survival of 19 months and a 2-year survival rate of 42 %. The authors concluded that IORT was well tolerated and was associated with an encouraging local-regional disease control and an improved overall survival [25].

## Conclusions

In conclusion, our results reinforce the emerging view in the scientific community that RI with concomitant chemotherapy for LRR or SPs, in a region that previously received high-dose irradiation, is feasible, and it produces good local control with chances of long-term survival; it also features acceptable, albeit not negligible, long-term toxicity. More importantly, clinical judgment and careful patient selection, as well as the judicious use of modern IMRT/image-guided radiotherapy techniques are critical components for the safe delivery of RI. The care of these patients requiring RI to the head and neck region is complex and should be carried out by centers where necessary multidisciplinary expertise and support are available.

### Abbreviations
CT: Computed tomography; CTV: Clinical target volume; ECOG: Eastern Cooperative Oncology Group; GTV: Gross tumor volume; LRR: Locoregional recurrences; MRI: Magnetic resonance imaging; OS: Overall survival; PRV: Planning organ at risk volume; rGTV: recurrent gross tumor volume; RI: Re-irradiation; SP: Second primary.

### Competing interests
The authors declare that they have no conflicts of interest or financial contributions to disclose.

### Authors' contributions
RAW and GS contributed to the study design and conception; RAW and SV were responsible for data acquisition; RAW and CH were involved in data analysis and interpretation; RAW and SV were involved in drafting the manuscript; GS provided a critical revision of the manuscript. All authors read and approved the final manuscript.

### Acknowledgements
I would like to take this opportunity to express my gratitude to the authors who have been instrumental in the successful completion of this project. I would like to show my greatest appreciation to Dr George Shenouda – I cannot say "thank you" enough for his tremendous support and help. Also, my deepest thanks to all the nurses and therapists working in the Radiation Oncology Department at the McGill Health Center who contributed to the management of our patients.
English-language editing of this manuscript was provided by Journal Prep.

### Author details
$^1$Department of Radiation Oncology, King Abdulaziz University, Abdullah Suleiman Street, P.O Box 80200, 21589 Jeddah, Saudi Arabia. $^2$Department of Radiation Oncology, McGill University Health Centre, McGill University, Montreal, Québec, Canada. $^3$Department of Clinical Epidemiology, McGill University, Montreal, Québec, Canada. $^4$Radiation Oncology, Segal Cancer Centre, Sir Mortimer B. Davis Jewish General Hospital, McGill University, Montreal, Québec, Canada.

### References
1.  Bachar GY, Goh C, Goldstein DP, O'Sullivan B, Irish JC. Long-term outcome analysis after surgical salvage for recurrent tonsil carcinoma following radical radiotherapy. Eur Arch Otorhinolaryngol. 2010;267:295–301.
2.  Caponigro F, Massa E, Manzione L, Rosati G, Biglietto M, De Lucia L, et al. Docetaxel and cisplatin in locally advanced or metastatic squamous-cell carcinoma of the head and neck: a phase II study of the Southern Italy Cooperative Oncology Group (SICOG). Ann Oncol. 2001;12:199–202.
3.  Kasperts N, Slotman B, Leemans CR, Langendijk JA. A review on re-irradiation for recurrent and second primary head and neck cancer. Oral Oncol. 2005;41:225–43.

4. McDonald MW, Moore MG, Johnstone PA. Risk of carotid blowout after reirradiation of the head and neck: a systematic review. Int J Radiat Oncol Biol Phys. 2012;82:1083–9.

5. Biagioli MC, Harvey M, Roman E, Raez LE, Wolfson AH, Mutyala S, et al. Intensity-modulated radiotherapy with concurrent chemotherapy for previously irradiated, recurrent head and neck cancer. Int J Radiat Oncol Biol Phys. 2007;69:1067–73.

6. Janot F, de Raucourt D, Benhamou E, Ferron C, Dolivet G, Bensadoun RJ, et al. Randomized trial of postoperative reirradiation combined with chemotherapy after salvage surgery compared with salvage surgery alone in head and neck carcinoma. J Clin Oncol. 2008;26:5518–23.

7. Salama JK, Vokes EE, Chmura SJ, Milano MT, Kao J, Stenson KM, et al. Long-term outcome of concurrent chemotherapy and reirradiation for recurrent and second primary head-and-neck squamous cell carcinoma. Int J Radiat Oncol Biol Phys. 2006;64:382–91.

8. Goldstein DP, Karnell LH, Yao M, Chamberlin GP, Nguyen TX, Funk GF. Outcomes following reirradiation of patients with head and neck cancer. Head Neck. 2008;30:765–70.

9. Langendijk JA, Kasperts N, Leemans CR, Doornaert P, Slotman BJ. A phase II study of primary reirradiation in squamous cell carcinoma of head and neck. Radiother Oncol. 2006;78:306–12.

10. Kharofa J, Choong N, Wang D, Firat S, Schultz C, Sadasiwan C, et al. Continuous-course reirradiation with concurrent carboplatin and paclitaxel for locally recurrent, nonmetastatic squamous cell carcinoma of the head-and-neck. Int J Radiat Oncol Biol Phys. 2012;83:690–5.

11. Berger B, Belka C, Weinmann M, Bamberg M, Budach W, Hehr T. Reirradiation with alternating docetaxel-based chemotherapy for recurrent head and neck squamous cell carcinoma: update of a single-center prospective phase II protocol. Strahlenther Onkol. 2010;186:255–61.

12. Bernier J, Cooper JS, Pajak TF, van Glabbeke M, Bourhis J, Forastiere A, et al. Defining risk levels in locally advanced head and neck cancers: a comparative analysis of concurrent postoperative radiation plus chemotherapy trials of the EORTC (#22931) and RTOG (# 9501). Head Neck. 2005;27:843–50.

13. Balermpas P, Keller C, Hambek M, Wagenblast J, Seitz O, Rödel C, et al. Reirradiation with cetuximab in locoregional recurrent and inoperable squamous cell carcinoma of the head and neck: feasibility and first efficacy results. Int J Radiat Oncol Biol Phys. 2012;83:e377–83.

14. Sulman EP, Schwartz DL, Le TT, Ang KK, Morrison WH, Rosenthal DI, et al. IMRT reirradiation of head and neck cancer-disease control and morbidity outcomes. Int J Radiat Oncol Biol Phys. 2009;73:399–409.

15. Sher DJ, Haddad RI, Norris Jr CM, Posner MR, Wirth LJ, Goguen LA, et al. Efficacy and toxicity of reirradiation using intensity-modulated radiotherapy for recurrent or second primary head and neck cancer. Cancer. 2010;116:4761–8.

16. Lee N, Chan K, Bekelman JE, Zhung J, Mechalakos J, Narayana A, et al. Salvage re-irradiation for recurrent head and neck cancer. Int J Radiat Oncol Biol Phys. 2007;68:731–40.

17. Benchalal M, Bachaud JM, François P, Alzieu C, Giraud P, David JM, et al. Hyperfractionation in the reirradiation of head and neck cancers. Result of a pilot study. Radiother Oncol. 1995;36:203–10.

18. Chen AM, Farwell DG, Luu Q, Cheng S, Donald PJ, Purdy JA. Prospective trial of high-dose reirradiation using daily image guidance with intensity-modulated radiotherapy for recurrent and second primary head-and-neck cancer. Int J Radiat Oncol Biol Phys. 2011;80:669–76.

19. Comet B, Kramar A, Faivre-Pierret M, Dewas S, Coche-Dequeant B, Degardin M, et al. Salvage stereotactic reirradiation with or without cetuximab for locally recurrent head-and-neck cancer: a feasibility study. Int J Radiat Oncol Biol Phys. 2012;84:203–9.

20. Hoebers F, Heemsbergen W, Moor S, Lopez M, Klop M, Tesselaar M, et al. Reirradiation for head-and-neck cancer: delicate balance between effectiveness and toxicity. Int J Radiat Oncol Biol Phys. 2011;81:e111–8.

21. Popovtzer A, Gluck I, Chepeha DB, Teknos TN, Moyer JS, Prince ME, et al. The pattern of failure after reirradiation of recurrent squamous cell head and neck cancer: implications for defining the targets. Int J Radiat Oncol Biol Phys. 2009;74:1342–7.

22. Creak AL, Harrington K, Nutting C. Treatment of recurrent head and neck cancer: re-irradiation or chemotherapy? Clin Oncol (R Coll Radiol). 2005;17:138–47.

23. Mendenhall WM, Mendenhall CM, Malyapa RS, Palta JR, Mendenhall NP. Re-irradiation of head and neck carcinoma. Am J Clin Oncol. 2008;31:393–8.

24. Wong SJ, Machtay M, Li Y. Locally recurrent, previously irradiated head and neck cancer: concurrent re-irradiation and chemotherapy, or chemotherapy alone? J Clin Oncol. 2006;24:2653–8.

25. Scala LM, Hu K, Urken ML, Jacobson AS, Persky MS, Tran TN, et al. Intraoperative high-dose-rate radiotherapy in the management of locoregionally recurrent head and neck cancer. Head Neck. 2013;35(4):485–92.

# 7

# Incidence of cutaneous malignant melanoma by socioeconomic status in Canada: 1992–2006

Stephanie E. Johnson-Obaseki[1*], Varant Labajian[1], Martin J. Corsten[2] and James T. McDonald[3]

## Abstract

**Background:** There are no nationwide studies documenting changes in cutaneous malignant melanoma incidence or association of incidence with socioeconomic status (SES) in Canada. We sought to determine whether melanoma incidence increased from 1992 to 2006 and if there was an association between SES and melanoma incidence. Additionally, we studied whether there was a correlation between province of residence and melanoma incidence.

**Methods:** Cases from the Canadian Cancer Registry were reviewed. Demographic and socioeconomic information were extracted from the Canadian Census of Population data. Cases were linked to income quintiles by postal code. A negative binomial regression was performed to identify relationships among these variables.

**Results:** Overall incidence of melanoma in Canada increased by 67 % from 1992 to 2006 ($p < 0.0001$). The increase in incidence was greater for melanoma in situ compared with invasive melanoma (136 % versus 52 % [$p < 0.0001$]). Incidence was positively correlated with higher income quintiles; the incidence rates among patients in the lowest income quintiles were 67 % of that for the highest income quintiles ($p < 0.0001$).

**Discussion:** A wide variety of explanations have been postulated for an increased incidence in melanoma among persons of higher SES, including access to and awareness of screening, more access to vacations in sunny climates, and increased leisure time. Variations in incidence of melanoma by urban vs. rural location and province may indicate differences in access to dermatologists across Canada.

**Conclusions:** Melanoma incidence is increasing in Canada and is higher among people in high SES groups. This rise is likely due to a combination of factors including a true rise in incidence due to increases in sun exposure, and also an increased detection rate, particularly in those who are more aware of the disease and have access to resources for detection.

**Keywords:** Melanoma, Socioeconomic status, Income, Incidence, Urban residence, Rural residence

## Background

Worldwide incidence of cutaneous malignant melanoma (hereafter referred to as 'melanoma') has continued to rise over the past several decades, with about 160,000 new cases diagnosed each year in the United States alone [1–3]. Most of the increased incidence has occurred in countries with predominately fair-skinned people. The countries with the highest incidence include Australia [4], New Zealand [5], Western European countries [6] and North American countries [7, 8]. Though melanoma is less common than other skin cancers, it causes 75 % of deaths from skin cancer [2].

Ongoing depletion of the ozone layer and increased solar ultraviolet radiation reaching the earth's surface is causing a continued rise in skin cancer incidence. The World Health Organization estimates that there is an increase of 4500 skin cancer cases for each 10 % decrease in ozone levels [1]. The risk of melanoma is associated with increases in sun holidays [9, 10] and use of indoor tanning beds [11, 12]. Earlier detection of thinner melanomas accounts for a substantial proportion of the increase in melanoma incidence [13–15]. This can likely

* Correspondence: sjohnsonobaseki@gmail.com
[1]Department of Otolaryngology-Head and Neck Surgery, University of Ottawa, S3 – 501 Smyth Road, Ottawa, ON K1H 8L6, Canada
Full list of author information is available at the end of the article

be explained by improved education and screening strategies [16]. As melanoma results from cumulative exposure to the sun, people have more time to accumulate sun damage and subsequent cancers with increased longevity [17, 18].

Socioeconomic status (SES) is known to be associated with both melanoma incidence and survival [10, 19–21]. High SES is associated with increased incidence of melanoma, thinner tumors, increased survival and decreased mortality [19–21]. Singh et al. examined the incidence of cutaneous melanoma in the United States by merging population-based central cancer registries with county-level SES estimates from the U.S. Census Bureau [21]. They found that counties with lower poverty, higher education, higher income and lower unemployment had higher age-adjusted melanoma incidence rates for early stage disease [21]. Similarly, Perez-Gomez et al. examined the association of SES and melanoma in Sweden using the Swedish Cancer Environment Registry and the Background Population Registry, which contain information on occupation, residence and date of death [20]. They used these data to determine association between SES (using occupation as a proxy) and melanoma and found a marked increase in the risk of melanoma in white-collar workers, particularly for men [20]. Other studies have yielded similar results. Theories explaining the increased incidence of melanoma among higher SES individuals include intense intermittent ultraviolet exposure (sun holidays) [20] and increased knowledge of and access to screening [16]. The reason for decreased mortality in this group may be related to an earlier stage at diagnosis [16].

Haider et al. used a population-based, cross-sectional study of administrative health care databases in a single Canadian province (Ontario) to determine if there was an association between melanoma prevalence and income level (used as a proxy for SES) [22]. They found an increased prevalence of 225 % in the highest compared with the lowest income groups. The Western Canada Melanoma study was performed by Gallagher et al. to determine the association between SES and risk of melanoma in four Canadian provinces (British Columbia, Alberta, Saskatchewan and Manitoba) [23]. Their study consisted of a detailed, multivariate analysis of 261 male cases as well as age- and sex-matched controls, using usual occupation as their proxy for SES. In their univariate analysis they found a strong positive association between SES and risk of melanoma. However, using multivariate analysis, they found that this association was substantially explained by host constitutional factors and sunlight exposure.

There has been conflicting evidence in the literature regarding how urban or rural residence affects the incidence of melanoma. Aase et al. used Norwegian Cancer Registry data from 1955 to 1989 and found urban residence to be associated with high melanoma incidence [24]. Conversely, Wesseling et al. analyzed the Costa Rica Cancer Registry data from 1981 to 1993 and found an increase in melanoma incidence in rural areas [25]. Perez-Gomez et al. also included an analysis of melanoma incidence by urban versus rural place of residence [20]. They found that there was an increased risk in men living in larger towns. The pattern for women living in urban areas showed an increase only in melanomas of the leg. Increase in intermittent sun exposure (a known significant risk factor for melanoma) and, perhaps, improved access to health care for screening and detection may cause increased incidence [20].

To our knowledge, there has not been a Canadian study using nationwide Cancer Registry data to examine the relationship between melanoma cancer incidence, SES and geographic location in Canada. The purpose of this study was to determine whether there was an increased incidence of melanoma in Canada from 1992 to 2006 and if there was an association between SES and incidence. Additionally, we studied whether there was an association between urban versus rural residence and incidence of melanoma and if there was a correlation between province of residence and incidence of cutaneous melanoma.

## Methods

Data for this study were extracted from the Canadian Cancer Registry data file and the Canadian Census of Population from Statistics Canada. The registry data file contains patient demographic and tumor-specific information on each tumor included in provincial and territorial cancer registries from 1992 to 2006 inclusively, while the census files provide neighborhood-level (dissemination area, DA) data on age/sex composition, average household income and location of residence. The reason that newer data is not included is due to the fact that 2006 is the last year that the long form census was used. Data sources, the methods employed to generate income quintiles and demographic characteristics, and the methods used to construct the dataset for estimation have been described in detail elsewhere [26, 27]. Since census data are available only every 5 years, cases diagnosed in 1992–1995 were associated with data from the 1991 census year (CY); cases diagnosed in the 1996–2000 period, the 1996 CY; cases diagnosed in the 2001–2005 period, the 2001 CY; and cases diagnosed in the 2006–2007 period, the 2006 CY. The number of DAs for which census information was available was 32,825 in 1991, 38,016 in 1996, 46,909 in 2001 and 52,443 in 2006. Income quintile (InQ) for each DA was defined relative to other DAs in the associated census division, which Statistics Canada defines as a group of neighboring municipalities joined together for the purposes of regional planning and managing of common services. Dissemination areas within each census division were sorted by average household income then assigned to one of five InQs. All analysis was within the University of New Brunswick Research Data Centre (NB-RDC) and all output was vetted for release using enhanced vetting methods required by Statistics Canada. Ethics approval is not required for research projects using data stored in the NB-RDC.

For each CY, the unit of observation for the analysis of incidence was the DA, and the key variable of interest was the number of cases of melanoma (International Classification of Diseases codes: O2/3 C44.0-C44.9), including both malignant melanoma and melanoma in situ, diagnosed in adults over the age of 18 in each DA over a relevant period of time corresponding to the CY. Unfortunately, data on in situ melanoma cases are not available for Ontario in the data provided by Statistics Canada, which necessitates estimation of the main model for a number of alternative sample specifications. These include: 1) all cases of melanoma, invasive melanoma and in situ melanoma for all provinces and territories except Ontario and 2) invasive melanoma for all provinces and territories including Ontario.

The exposure variable was the adult population in the DA during the CY multiplied by the number of years in the corresponding time interval for that census (2, 4 or 5 years). Negative binomial regression models were estimated where neighborhood SES, as measured by the InQ of the DA, was captured by a 0/1 binary variable for each InQ, with the highest InQ specified as the baseline. Indicator variables for each CY from 1996 to 2006 with 1991 as the reference year were included to reflect changes over time. The regressions also included indicator variables for province of residence of the individual at the time of diagnosis as well as whether the DA of residence was a larger urban center (census metropolitan area with a total population of at least 100,000 of which 50,000 or more must live in an urban core), smaller urban center (census agglomeration with a total population of between 10,000 and 100,000) and rural, if the DA was not located in either a census metropolitan area or census agglomeration.

To control for differences in the ethnic/racial composition across DA populations and over time, the total adult population in each DA that identify as 1) black, 2) south Asian, 3) east Asian and 4) other visible minority group were extracted from each census file. Each of these measures was included as controls in the analysis.

## Results
### Incidence by census year
Using multivariate regression, the incidence of invasive melanoma increased with time over the study period of CY 1991 to CY 2006 after controlling for age, sex and race

(Table 1). For invasive melanoma (excluding Ontario) the incidence rate ratio (IRR) increased from 1.0 in the reference CY (1991) to 1.52 in the 2006 CY (IRR 1.52, $p < 0.000$, 95 % confidence interval [CI] 1.46–1.59). Most of the increase in incidence occurred between the 2001 and 2006 CYs (IRR 2001 1.05, $p < 0.00$), 95 % CI 1.01–1.09). The results were not materially different when Ontario was included in the analysis. For melanoma in situ, a similar but more pronounced pattern of increasing IRRs with later CYs was identified, with the 2006 CY showing an incidence rate 136 % greater than the 1991 CY (IRR 2.36, $p < 0.000$, 95 % CI 2.17–2.57). Table 2 displays the multivariate analysis regression results broken down by controls for the age/sex composition of the DA as well as controls for the various race proportions in the DA.

### Incidence by socioeconomic status
Table 1 shows that, for invasive melanoma, individuals in the lowest InQ had an incidence rate that was 82 % of the incidence rate of individuals in the highest InQ (IRR 0.82, $p < 0.000$, 95 % CI 0.78–0.85) after controlling for age, sex and race distribution and other factors. A similar, but stronger, association existed for melanoma in situ; again, a progressively lower incidence rate ratio was identified for progressively lower InQs, with the lowest InQ having an incidence rate that was 68 % of that for the highest InQ (IRR 0.68, $p < 0.000$, 95 % CI 0.62–0.73). The analysis was repeated with the Ontario data and showed no significant difference from the results excluding Ontario. In the first column of results from Table 1, determinants of the diagnosis of both invasive and in situ melanoma for all provinces and territories except Ontario (as in situ data was not available for Ontario) were estimated. Progressively lower InQs were associated with a progressively lower diagnosis of melanoma and the IRR of each InQ relative to the highest was significantly <1.

### Incidence by province of residence
There were wide disparities in the incidence rate of melanoma across the various provinces of Canada, as seen in Table 1. British Columbia was used as the reference province. Ontario was omitted to facilitate comparisons between in situ and invasive melanoma (only results for invasive melanoma in Ontario were available). Again, age, sex and race were controlled for multivariate regression analysis. For invasive melanoma, several provinces had IRRs that were significantly less than for British Columbia, with the most significant difference occurring in the province of Quebec, with an incidence rate only 44 % of that for the reference province (IRR 0.44, $p < 0.000$, 95 % CI 0.42–0.45). Other provinces with significantly lower IRRs included Newfoundland (IRR 0.66, $p < 0.000$, 95 % CI 0.61–0.71), Manitoba (IRR 0.74, $p < 0.000$, 95 % CI 0.70–0.78), Saskatchewan (IRR 0.75,

**Table 1** Incidence rate ratios of the diagnosis of melanoma[a] (excludes Ontario)[b]

| | All melanoma (n = 105,681) | | | In situ | | | Invasive | | |
|---|---|---|---|---|---|---|---|---|---|
| | IRR | P value | 95 % CI | IRR | P value | 95 % CI | IRR | P value | 95 % CI |
| Place of residence | | | | | | | | | |
| City (census metropolitan area) | 1 | | | 1 | | | 1 | | |
| Town (census agglomeration) | 0.80 | 0.00 | (0.77–0.82) | 0.69 | 0.00 | (0.65–0.74) | 0.82 | 0.00 | (0.79–0.85) |
| Rural | 0.80 | 0.00 | (0.78–0.82) | 0.71 | 0.00 | (0.67–0.75) | 0.82 | 0.00 | (0.79–0.85) |
| Income quintile | | | | | | | | | |
| Highest | 1 | | | 1 | | | 1 | | |
| 2nd highest | 0.89 | 0.00 | (0.86–0.91) | 0.86 | 0.00 | (0.81–0.92) | 0.89 | 0.00 | (0.86–0.92) |
| Middle | 0.85 | 0.00 | (0.83–0.88) | 0.79 | 0.00 | (0.74–0.85) | 0.86 | 0.00 | (0.83–0.90) |
| 2nd lowest | 0.83 | 0.00 | (0.81–0.86) | 0.76 | 0.00 | (0.71–0.82) | 0.85 | 0.00 | (0.82–0.88) |
| Lowest | 0.79 | 0.00 | (0.76–0.81) | 0.68 | 0.00 | (0.62–0.73) | 0.82 | 0.00 | (0.78–0.85) |
| Census year | | | | | | | | | |
| 2006 | 1.67 | 0.00 | (1.62–1.73) | 2.36 | 0.00 | (2.17–2.57) | 1.52 | 0.00 | (1.46–1.59) |
| 2001 | 1.10 | 0.00 | (1.07–1.13) | 1.38 | 0.00 | (1.28–1.49) | 1.05 | 0.02 | (1.01–1.09) |
| 1996 | 1.01 | 0.61 | (0.98–1.04) | 1.09 | 0.02 | (1.01–1.18) | 1.00 | 0.89 | (0.96–1.03) |
| 1991 | 1 | | | 1 | | | 1 | | |
| Province | | | | | | | | | |
| Newfoundland and Labrador | 0.67 | 0.00 | (0.63–0.72) | 0.73 | 0.00 | (0.63–0.84) | 0.66 | 0.00 | (0.61–0.71) |
| Prince Edward Island | 1.16 | 0.00 | (1.06–1.26) | 1.59 | 0.00 | (1.31–1.92) | 1.07 | 0.26 | (0.95–1.20) |
| Nova Scotia | 1.12 | 0.00 | (1.08–1.17) | 1.65 | 0.00 | (1.52–1.79) | 1.00 | 0.94 | (0.95–1.05) |
| New Brunswick | 0.99 | 0.69 | (0.95–1.04) | 1.20 | 0.00 | (1.08–1.32) | 0.94 | 0.04 | (0.89–1.00) |
| Quebec | 0.39 | 0.00 | (0.37–0.40) | 0.17 | 0.00 | (0.15–0.18) | 0.44 | 0.00 | (0.42–0.45) |
| Ontario | b | | | b | | | b | | |
| Manitoba | 0.78 | 0.00 | (0.75–0.81) | 0.90 | 0.03 | (0.83–0.99) | 0.74 | 0.00 | (0.70–0.78) |
| Saskatchewan | 0.74 | 0.00 | (0.71–0.78) | 0.69 | 0.00 | (0.61–0.77) | 0.75 | 0.00 | (0.71–0.80) |
| Alberta | 0.95 | 0.00 | (0.92–0.98) | 1.36 | 0.00 | (1.27–1.45) | 0.85 | 0.00 | (0.82–0.89) |
| British Columbia | 1 | | | 1 | | | 1 | | |
| Territories | 0.45 | 0.00 | (0.37–0.57) | 0.55 | 0.02 | (0.34–0.90) | 0.43 | 0.00 | (0.33–0.56) |

CI confidence interval, IRR incidence rate ratio

[a]Negative binomial regressions on the incidence of diagnosed cases of melanoma by dissemination area (DA) and census year. Regressions include detailed controls for the age/sex composition of the DA as well as controls for the proportions of adults in the DA who are 1) black, 2) South Asian, 3) other Asian and 4) other visible minority groups

[b]Cases of in situ melanoma are not available for Ontario in the Canadian Cancer Registry dataset in the Statistics Canada Research Data Centre so Ontario DAs are excluded from these regressions

p < 0.000, 95 % CI 0.70–0.80), Alberta (IRR 0.85, p < 0.000, 95 % CI 0.82–0.89) and the Territories (IRR 0.43, p < 0.000, 95 % CI 0.33–0.56). For melanoma in situ, different provincial patterns exist; several provinces had IRRs significantly greater than British Columbia, including Prince Edward Island, New Brunswick, Nova Scotia and Alberta, while Quebec, Saskatchewan and the Territories had IRRs markedly less than reference (e.g., Quebec [IRR 0.17, p < 0.000, 95 % CI 0.15–0.18]).

### Incidence by urban/rural residence

Table 1 demonstrates the results of our analysis of melanoma incidence by residence population density. For invasive melanoma (again, excluding Ontario, but controlling for age, sex and race), individuals living in rural areas had incidence rates significantly less than individuals in cities (IRR 0.82, p < 0.000, 95 % CI 0.79–0.85). Similar results were seen for individuals living in towns (IRR 0.82, p < 0.000, 95 % CI 0.79–0.85). Again, similar, but more dramatic, differences were seen for in situ melanoma; for rural residence, the incidence rate was 71 % of that for cities (IRR 0.71, p < 0.000, 95 % CI 0.67–0.75) and for towns, the incidence rate was 69 % of that for cities (IRR 0.69, p < 0.000, 95 % CI 0.65–0.74). Reintroducing Ontario into the analysis did not significantly change these results.

**Table 2** Incidence rate ratios of the diagnosis of melanoma[a] (excludes Ontario)[b]–other controls

| | All melanoma (n–105,681) | | | In situ | | | Invasive | | |
|---|---|---|---|---|---|---|---|---|---|
| | IRR | P value | 95 % CI | IRR | P value | 95 % CI | IRR | P value | 95 % CI |
| Proportion of Population by age/sex | | | | | | | | | |
| Male 20–29 | 1 | | | 1 | | | 1 | | |
| Male 30–39 | 0.99 | 0.01 | (0.99–1.00) | 0.98 | 0.01 | (0.97–0.99) | 1.00 | 0.25 | (0.99–1.00) |
| Male 40–49 | 0.99 | 0.00 | (0.98–0.99) | 0.98 | 0.01 | (0.97–1.00) | 0.99 | 0.01 | (0.98–1.00) |
| Male 50–59 | 0.99 | 0.01 | (0.99–1.00) | 0.99 | 0.48 | (0.98–1.01) | 0.99 | 0.02 | (0.98–1.00) |
| Male 60–69 | 1.00 | 0.42 | (0.99–1.01) | 1.00 | 0.99 | (0.98–1.02) | 0.99 | 0.34 | (0.98–1.01) |
| Male 70–79 | 1.01 | 0.00 | (1.01–1.02) | 1.01 | 0.32 | (0.99–1.03) | 1.01 | 0.00 | (1.01–1.02) |
| Male 80+ | 1.02 | 0.00 | (1.02–1.03) | 1.04 | 0.00 | (1.02–1.06) | 1.02 | 0.00 | (1.01–1.03) |
| Female 20–29 | 0.99 | 0.07 | (0.99–1.00) | 0.99 | 0.04 | (0.97–1.00) | 1.00 | 0.23 | (0.99–1.00) |
| Female 30–39 | 1.00 | 0.56 | (0.99–1.00) | 1.00 | 0.91 | (0.99–1.01) | 1.00 | 0.39 | (0.99–1.00) |
| Female 40–49 | 1.01 | 0.00 | (1.01–1.02) | 1.02 | 0.01 | (1.00–1.03) | 1.01 | 0.00 | (1.01–1.02) |
| Female 50–59 | 1.02 | 0.00 | (1.01–1.03) | 1.03 | 0.00 | (1.01–1.04) | 1.02 | 0.00 | (1.01–1.02) |
| Female 60–69 | 1.02 | 0.00 | (1.01–1.03) | 1.02 | 0.09 | (1.00–1.04) | 1.02 | 0.00 | (1.01–1.03) |
| Female 70–79 | 1.01 | 0.00 | (1.01–1.02) | 1.02 | 0.01 | (1.00–1.03) | 1.01 | 0.00 | (1.01–1.02) |
| Female 80+ | 1.01 | 0.00 | (1.00–1.01) | 1.00 | 0.70 | (0.99–1.01) | 1.01 | 0.00 | (1.01–1.01) |
| Proportion of Population by race | | | | | | | | | |
| White | 1 | | | 1 | | | 1 | | |
| Black | 0.91 | 0.00 | (0.88–0.95) | 0.81 | 0.00 | (0.73–0.89) | 0.93 | 0.00 | (0.90–0.97) |
| East/Southeast Asian | 0.91 | 0.00 | (0.90–0.92) | 0.88 | 0.00 | (0.86–0.91) | 0.92 | 0.00 | (0.90–0.93) |
| South Asian | 0.88 | 0.00 | (0.87–0.90) | 0.90 | 0.00 | (0.86–0.94) | 0.88 | 0.00 | (0.86–0.90) |
| Other groups | 0.98 | 0.09 | (0.95–1.00) | 0.99 | 0.69 | (0.92–1.05) | 0.98 | 0.16 | (0.95–1.01) |

CI confidence interval, IRR incidence rate ratio
[a]Negative binomial regressions on the incidence of diagnosed cases of melanoma by dissemination area (DA) and census year. Table presents regression results for control variables not reported in Table 1
[b]Cases of in situ melanoma are not available for Ontario in the Canadian Cancer Registry dataset in the Statistics Canada Research Data Centre so Ontario DAs are excluded from these regressions

## Discussion

Our study confirmed that within Canada, like in other developed countries, the incidence of melanoma has risen dramatically in the 15 years spanned by these data [1–7]. Interestingly, our data showed that the rate of increase in melanoma incidence has accelerated between the 2001 and 2006 CYs. Multiple factors have been attributed to this overall rise in melanoma incidence, including depletion of the ozone layer (and its attendant protection from solar ultraviolet-B radiation) [1]. In addition, societal attitudes toward tanning have changed over the past several decades, with an increased association between tanned skin and physical attractiveness. The availability of tanning beds, and the exposure to them among young people, has also been associated with an increase in the incidence of melanoma [11, 12]. An increase in leisure time in developed societies is thought to have led to more vacations spent in southern climes as well as an increase in outdoor tanning [22]. The increased aging of our population also is likely a factor in higher melanoma rates [17, 18].

Other authors have pointed to changing criteria for the diagnosis of melanoma, which have increased the number of melanomas being diagnosed. Weyers et al. refers to this increase in melanoma incidence as a "pseudoepidemic," and argues that melanomas are being detected now that would otherwise have regressed naturally [28]. An increased awareness about melanoma screening has led to cases being diagnosed at earlier stages; this was illustrated in our data by the fact that the increase in incidence for melanoma in situ was substantially larger than that of melanoma as a whole.

The second finding in our study was a strong association between higher SES and increased melanoma incidence. This association between high SES and higher incidence of melanoma is likely also multifactorial, as many of the explanations for the increased incidence of melanoma may impact individuals of different socioeconomic status differently [10, 19–21, 24]. Factors like access to tanning beds, vacation travel to warmer climates and the availability of leisure time, which may be spent sunbathing, are plausibly more prevalent in individuals from more advantaged socioeconomic circumstances. It is even plausible that attitudes about physical attractiveness and sun tanning are different between different socioeconomic strata. Many studies have also shown that awareness of, and access to, screening for cancer is disproportionately higher in individuals with higher SES [29]. Individuals of higher SES may be more likely to see a dermatologist and to investigate abnormal pigmented lesions. It should be noted that the effects of race on SES and melanoma incidence may represent an important confounder; we did attempt to eliminate the possibility of such confounding by including race in our logistic regression analysis.

The third finding in our study was a higher incidence of melanoma, even when controlling for SES and other factors, in urban residents of Canada. Our own previous study with thyroid cancer, another malignancy frequently detected during screening exams, found that urban residence (rather than in towns or rural areas) correlates with increased detection of cancer in Canada [26]. This may be due to access to a physician in general or more specifically to a dermatologist. Di Quinzio et al found that family physician visits correlated with earlier stage melanoma [30]. Certainly, dermatologists are typically concentrated in urban centers in Canada, and patients may be more likely to be referred to a specialist such as a dermatologist regarding suspicious pigmented lesions if they live in an urban area. Whether individuals who live in cities spend more time in the sun than town or rural residents is unclear at present.

Finally, our study found substantial discrepancies in melanoma incidence across different Canadian provinces. This is similar to what was previously found by Gaudette and Gao [31]. Further studies are needed to help elucidate the reasons for this large discrepancy, but access to screening for melanoma and access to specialists such as dermatologists may also differ from province to province, in the same way that they differ for urban and rural residences.

Our study had several important limitations. Not all data for the incidence of melanoma was available in some provinces, and in situ data was not available for Ontario. Second, while we did control for race using the techniques described, race was not included in the Canadian Cancer Registry data. Thirdly, we similarly do not possess data within the Canadian Cancer Registry on such important characteristics as tanning bed use, time spent in sun or awareness of/access to screening tests for melanoma on the individual level. Finally, our data is only up until 2006, as the long form census was not used in 2011.

## Conclusions

The incidence of melanoma rose significantly in our study from 1992 to 2006; this rise was most striking in melanoma in situ. Individuals with higher SES and patients in urban centers had significantly higher incidence rates of melanoma than individuals with lower SES or who resided in towns or rural areas. Finally, there were differences, in some cases quite dramatic, between the various provinces of Canada with respect to melanoma incidence.

**Abbreviations**
CY: census year; DA: dissemination area; InQ: income quintile; NB-RDC: New Brunswick Research Data Centre; SES: socioeconomic status.

**Competing interests**
The authors declare that they have no competing interests.

**Authors' contributions**
SEJ-O conception and design, drafting the article and final approval. VL analysis and interpretation of data, drafting the article and final approval. MJC conception and design, drafting the article and final approval. JTM analysis and interpretation of data, revising the article critically for important intellectual content and final approval. All authors read and approved the final manuscript.

**Author details**
¹Department of Otolaryngology-Head and Neck Surgery, University of Ottawa, S3 – 501 Smyth Road, Ottawa, ON K1H 8L6, Canada. ²Department of Otolaryngology – Head and Neck Surgery, Aurora Health Care, Aurora St. Luke's Medical Center, 2801 W. Kinnickinnic River Parkway, Suite 630, Milwaukee, WI 53215, USA. ³Department of Economics, University of New Brunswick, PO Box 4400, Fredericton, NB E3B6C4, Canada.

**References**
1. World Health Organization. Skin cancers. Available at: http://www.who.int/uv/faq/skincancer/en/index1.html. [Accessed Nov. 14, 2014].
2. Surveillance, Epidemiology, and End Results Program. SEER Cancer Statistics Review, 1975–2009 (Vintage 2009 Populations). Available at: http://seer.cancer.gov/csr/1975_2009_pops09/. [Accessed Nov. 14, 2014].
3. American Cancer Society. Cancer Facts & Figure 2013. Available at: http://www.cancer.org/acs/groups/content/@epidemiologysurveilance/documents/document/acspc-036845.pdf. Accessed Nov. 14, 2014].
4. Coory M, Baade P, Aitken J, Smithers M, McLeod GR, Ring I. Trends for in situ and invasive melanoma in Queensland, Australia, 1982–2002. Cancer Causes Control. 2006;17(1):21–7.
5. Bulliard JL, Cox B. Cutaneous malignant melanoma in New Zealand: trends by anatomical site, 1969-1993. Int J Epidemiol. 2000;29(3):416–23.
6. de Vries E, Bray FI, Coebergh JW, Parkin DM. Changing epidemiology of malignant cutaneous melanoma in Europe 1953–1997: rising trends in incidence and mortality but recent stabilizations in western Europe and decreases in Scandinavia. Int J Cancer. 2003;107(1):119–26.
7. Garbe C, Leiter U. Melanoma epidemiology and trends. Clin Dermatol. 2009;27(1):3–9.
8. Erdmann F, Lortet-Tieulent J, Schüz J, Zeeb H, Greinert R, Breitbart EW, et al. International trends in the incidence of malignant melanoma 1953–2008– are recent generations at higher or lower risk? Int J Cancer. 2013;132(2):385–400.
9. Veierød MB, Weiderpass E, Thörn M, Hansson J, Lund E, Armstrong B, et al. A prospective study of pigmentation, sun exposure, and risk of cutaneous malignant melanoma in women. J Natl Cancer Inst. 2003;95(20):1530–8.
10. Bentham G, Aase A. Incidence of malignant melanoma of the skin in Norway, 1955–1989: associations with solar ultraviolet radiation, income and holidays abroad. Int J Epidemiol. 1996;25(6):1132–8.
11. Boniol M, Autier P, Boyle P, Gandini S. Cutaneous melanoma attributable to sunbed use: systematic review and meta-analysis. BMJ. 2012;345:e4757.
12. International Agency for Research on Cancer Working Group on artificial ultraviolet (UV) light and skin cancer. The association of use of sunbeds with cutaneous malignant melanoma and other skin cancers: a systematic

review. Int J Cancer. 2007;120(5):1116–22. Erratum in: Int J Cancer 2007;120(11):2526.

13. Lipsker DM, Hedelin G, Heid E, Grosshans EM, Cribier BJ. Striking increase of thin melanomas contrasts with stable incidence of thick melanomas. Arch Dermatol. 1999;135(12):1451–6.

14. Downing A, Newton-Bishop JA, Forman D. Recent trends in cutaneous malignant melanoma in the Yorkshire region of England; incidence, mortality and survival in relation to stage of disease, 1993–2003. Br J Cancer. 2006;95(1):91–5.

15. MacKie RM, Bray CA, Hole DJ, Morris A, Nicolson M, Evans A, et al. Incidence of and survival from malignant melanoma in Scotland: an epidemiological study. Lancet. 2002;360(9333):587–91.

16. Bataille V, de Vries E. Melanoma–Part 1: epidemiology, risk factors, and prevention. BMJ. 2008;337:a2249.

17. Macdonald JB, Dueck AC, Gray RJ, Wasif N, Swanson DL, Sekulic A, et al. Malignant melanoma in the elderly: different regional disease and poorer prognosis. J Cancer Educ. 2011;2:538–43.

18. Anderson WF, Pfeiffer RM, Tucker MA, Rosenberg PS. Divergent cancer pathways for early-onset and late-onset cutaneous malignant melanoma. Cancer. 2009;115(18):4176–85.

19. Idorn LW, Wulf HC. Socioeconomic status and cutaneous malignant melanoma in Northern Europe. Br J Dermatol. 2014;170(4):787–93.

20. Pérez-Gómez B, Aragonés N, Gustavsson P, Lope V, López-Abente G, Pollán M. Socio-economic class, rurality and risk of cutaneous melanoma by site and gender in Sweden. BMC Public Health. 2008;8:33.

21. Singh SD, Ajani UA, Johnson CJ, Roland KB, Eide M, Jemal A, et al. Association of cutaneous melanoma incidence with area-based socioeconomic indicators-United States, 2004–2006. J Am Acad Dermatol. 2011;65(5 Suppl 1):S58–68.

22. Haider A, Mamdani M, Shear NH. Socioeconomic status and the prevalence of melanoma in Ontario, Canada. J Cutan Med Surg. 2007;11(1):1–3.

23. Gallagher RP, Elwood JM, Threlfall WJ, Spinelli JJ, Fincham S, Hill GB. Socioeconomic status, sunlight exposure, and risk of malignant melanoma: the Western Canada Melanoma Study. J Natl Cancer Inst. 1987;79(4):647–52.

24. Aase A, Bentham G. Gender, geography and socio-economic status in the diffusion of malignant melanoma risk. Soc Sci Med. 1996;42(12):1621–37.

25. Wesseling C, Antich D, Hogstedt C, Rodríguez AC, Ahlbom A. Geographical differences of cancer incidence in Costa Rica in relation to environmental and occupational pesticide exposure. Int J Epidemiol. 1999;28(3):365–74.

26. Guay B, Johnson-Obaseki S, McDonald JT, Connell C, Corsten M. Incidence of differentiated thyroid cancer by socioeconomic status and urban residence: Canada 1991–2006. Thyroid. 2014;24(3):552–5.

27. Hwang E, Johnson-Obaseki S, McDonald JT, Connell C, Corsten M. Incidence of head and neck cancer and socioeconomic status in Canada from 1992 to 2007. Oral Oncol. 2013;49(11):1072–6.

28. Weyers W. The 'epidemic' of melanoma between under- and overdiagnosis. J Cutan Pathol. 2012;39(1):9–16.

29. Johnson S, McDonald JT, Corsten M. Oral cancer screening and socioeconomic status. J Otolaryngol Head Neck Surg. 2012;41(2):102–7.

30. Di Quinzio ML, Dewar RA, Burge FI, Veugelers PJ. Family physician visits and early recognition of melanoma. Can J Public Health. 2005;96:136.

31. Gaudette LA, Gao RN. Changing trends in melanoma incidence and mortality. Health Rep. 1998;10:29.

# 8

# Outcome analysis of 215 patients with parotid gland tumors

Boban M. Erovic[1], Manish D. Shah[1], Guillem Bruch[1], Meredith Johnston[2], John Kim[2], Brian O'Sullivan[2], Bayardo Perez-Ordonez[3], Ilan Weinreb[3], Eshetu G. Atenafu[4], John R. de Almeida[1], Patrick J. Gullane[1], Dale Brown[1], Ralph W. Gilbert[1], Jonathan C. Irish[1] and David P. Goldstein[1,5*]

## Abstract

**Background:** To identify prognostic factors in patients with parotid gland carcinomas who were treated at the Princess Margaret Hospital.

**Methods:** Clinical outcome of two hundred fifteen patients with malignancies of the parotid gland was evaluated over a 16-year period.

**Results:** Two-hundred-fifteen patients with adenoid cystic carcinoma ($n = 20$), adenocarcinoma ($n = 19$), acinic cell carcinoma ($n = 62$), basal cell adenocarcinoma ($n = 7$), carcinoma-ex-pleomorphic adenoma ($n = 18$), mucoepidermoid carcinoma ($n = 70$) and salivary duct carcinoma ($n = 19$) have been included. The 5- and 10-year overall and disease-free survivals were 80.62 %/69.48 % and 74.37 %/62.42 %, respectively. Multivariable analysis showed that age greater than 60 years, advanced pN classification, histopathological grade and the presence of lymphovascular invasion significantly worsened overall and disease-free survival. Univariable analysis revealed periparotid lymph node involvement was associated with decreased overall ($p < 0.0001$) and disease-free survival ($p < 0.0001$).

**Conclusions:** In addition to age, pN classification, histopathological grade, perineural invasion, and lymphovascular involvement, periparotid lymph node metastasis appears to be an important prognosticator in parotid gland malignancy.

**Keywords:** Prognostic factors, Salivary gland tumors, Periparotid lymph node metastases

## Introduction

Malignant salivary glands tumors are rare, representing only 2 % of all head and neck malignancies [1]. Salivary gland carcinomas represent a heterogeneous group of malignancies with diverse biological behaviors [2, 3], rendering standardization of management extremely difficult. In the first large published case series of 2807 patients with salivary gland malignancies over a 35 year period, Spiro [3] reported that the site of origin, histologic subtype, grading, and clinical stage were significant prognostic factors for overall survival. Wahlberg *et al.* [4] analyzed a Swedish cohort of 2465 patients treated between 1960 and 1998 for malignant parotid tumors and found that histopathological subtype, age and sex were also significant clinical predictors for survival [4]. Other studies have demonstrated the importance of regional lymph node involvement, positive surgical margins, perineural invasion, and facial nerve palsy as significant clinical predictors of outcome [4–7]. Recent studies have investigated molecular prognosticators associated with less favorable outcomes in those with salivary gland malignancy [8–11]. Interpretation of the literature is often difficult as patients in a given case series have typically been treated over extended periods of time, and using non-uniform treatment modalities [12].

The primary objective of this study was to analyze the outcome and patterns of failure in 215 patients with malignant parotid gland tumors managed at the Princess Margaret Cancer Centre (Toronto, Canada). The secondary objective was to evaluate whether previously

* Correspondence: david.goldstein@uhn.ca
[1]Department of Otolaryngology-Head and Neck Surgery, Wharton Head and Neck Program, University Health Network, Princess Margaret Cancer Centre, Toronto, ON, Canada
[5]Princess Margaret Hospital, Wharton Head and Neck Centre, 610 University Avenue, 3rd Floor, Toronto, ON M5G 2 M9, Canada
Full list of author information is available at the end of the article

reported clinical and pathologic factors were significant predictors of survival.

## Material and patients

A retrospective review of 215 consecutive patients with primary parotid gland cancers treated at the Princess Margaret Cancer Center between 1989 and 2005 was performed. Patients were identified through the Princess Margaret Cancer Registry and cross-referenced with a head and neck surgical registry. Approval was obtained from the Institutional Research Ethics Board prior to data collection. Patients with a newly diagnosed malignancy arising within the parotid were included in the study if they received some or all of their treatment at the Princess Margaret. A subset of patients included were those that had their initial surgery at an outside institution that were referred in shortly after their initial procedure for either further resection followed by radiation or for post-operative radiation alone. Patients with submandibular, sublingual and minor salivary gland cancers, lymphomas or malignancies metastatic to the salivary glands were excluded. Patients were also excluded if they were treated with palliative intent.

The management approach at the Princess Margaret for patients with parotid gland malignancy has been surgical resection with adjuvant radiotherapy used in those patients with positive margins, high-grade histology, perineural invasion/spread or nodal metastases, or where uncertainty existed about completeness of resection, usually arising from very close juxtaposition of the tumor to the facial nerve. Generally, in cases where the tumor was abutting but not invading the facial nerve and nerve function was normal pre-operatively, the facial nerve was preserved with the addition of post-operative radiotherapy. Therapeutic neck dissections were performed when there was clinical or radiographic evidence of nodal metastases. In patients without any evidence of nodal metastases, prophylactic neck dissection was performed in those patients with high-grade malignancies. For all patients undergoing surgery, the surrounding lymph nodes were examined, including the upper neck in parotid tumors. Enlarged nodes were sampled and if frozen section examination confirmed metastases, an appropriate neck dissection was performed. Patients that had an initial surgery at an outside center were offered revision surgery prior to post-operative radiotherapy if they had residual disease on MRI, otherwise they were managed with post-operative radiotherapy alone.

Diagnosis of all tumors was performed by head and neck pathologists and classified according to the World Health Organization (WHO) classification of salivary gland malignancies [2]. Demographic, clinical, and pathological data was obtained from hospital records. The pathological parameters included histologic subtype,

perineural invasion (PNI), lymphovascular invasion (LVI), margin status, extra capsular extension and metastases to the peri-parotid lymph nodes. Peri-parotid and intra-parotid lymph nodes were defined as those nodes attached to or within the parotid gland, respectively. The grade of the tumour when reported by the pathologist was recorded. Disease was staged at the time of initial presentation using the American Joint Committee on Cancer (AJCC) classification staging system.

## Statistical analysis

Descriptive statistics were used for describing patient demographics and pathological characteristics. Categorical variables were expressed as counts and proportions, whereas continuous variables were expressed as means with standard deviations (SD). Outcome measures included control rates, overall survival (OS) and disease-free survival (DFS), which were estimated using the Kaplan-Meier product method. Time to event outcomes were calculated from the date of diagnosis to the event of interest. Differences between survival curves were analyzed using the log-rank test.

Potential prognostic variables achieving significance level of 0.20 or less on univariable analysis were subsequently entered into a multivariable Cox-proportional hazards model and stepwise model-building was used to determine the simplest model that best described the association in the data. Histologic subtype was not incorporated into the multivariable analysis for either OS or DFS as this would lead to excessive stratification of the data given the number of patients in the study. Grade was included in the multivariable analysis; however, since the majority of patients were either low or high grade, the intermediate grade patients were grouped with the high-grade patients. All $p$-values were 2-sided. Results were considered significant if $p < 0.05$. Statistical analyses were performed using SAS (Version 9.3, SAS Institute, Inc., Cary, NC).

## Results

A total of 215 patients with parotid gland cancers managed with primary surgery were included in the study. The mean (median) age of the patients was 55 (56) years (range 15–91) and 112 patients (52 %) were female. Out of the 215 patients only 12 (5.6 %) patients presented with a facial paralysis.

Facial nerve preserving surgery was performed in 179 patients with 28 patients undergoing a total parotidectomy with nerve sacrifice and an additional 8 had a total parotidectomy, nerve sacrifice and temporal bone resection. Adjuvant post-operative radiotherapy was given to 168 (78 %) patients. The mean and median radiation dose was 58 and 60 Gy, respectively (range from 35 to 70Gy). Neck dissections were performed in 105 (48.8 %)

patients. Selective and modified radical neck dissection was performed in 81 (37.7 %) and 19 (8.8 %) patients, respectively. An additional 90 patients that did not have planned neck dissection had pathologic assessment of the intraparotid or periparotid lymph nodes.

Tumor characteristics, including T and N classification, are summarized in Table 1. Mucoepidermoid carcinoma (MEC) was the most common histologic variant of parotid gland cancer, accounting for 32.5 % percent of cases, followed in frequency by acinic cell (28.8 %) and adenoid cystic carcinoma (ACC) (9.3 %). Histopathological grade for each histologic subtype of parotid cancer, if specified is presented in Table 2.

Positive surgical margins (i.e. tumor extending to the inked margin of specimen) were identified in 38.9 % ($n = 77/198$) of patients who underwent parotidectomy. Margin status was not available for 17 patients. Positive margins were reported in 12 patients with ACC, 10 patients with salivary duct carcinoma, and 6 patients with carcinoma ex-pleomorphic adenoma. Positive margins were noted in 34.8 % of patients (31/89) with grade 1 tumors, 32.3 % of patients (10/31) with grade II tumors, and 45.1 % of patients (32/71) with grade III tumors. Of the patients with positive margins, 36 (46.8 %) had their initial surgery performed at an outside center and were referred for further management. Eight of these patients underwent a repeat surgical resection as part of their management.

Perineural invasion (PNI) was reported in 53 (26.9 %) patients. Salivary duct carcinoma had the highest frequency (72.2 %, $n = 13/18$), followed by ACC (45 %, 9/20), adenocarcinoma (52.6 %, 10/19), carcinoma ex-pleomorphic adenoma (21.4 %, 3/14), MEC (16.4 %, 10/61), and acinic cell carcinoma (8.3 %, 5/58). The incidence of perineural invasion increased with histopathological grade. PNI was reported in 4.4 % (4/90) of grade I tumors, 26.7 % (8/30) of grade II tumors, and 55.7 % (39/70) of grade III tumors ($p$-value < 0.0001). Lymphovascular invasion (LVI) was reported in 40 (20.6 %) patients. It occurred most commonly in salivary duct carcinomas (61.1 %, $n = 11/18$), followed by adenocarcinoma (52.6 %, 10/19), carcinoma ex-pleomorphic adenoma (42.9 %, 6/14), acinic cell carcinoma (14.0 %, 8/57), ACC (10.5 %, 2/19), and MEC (5 %, 3/60). LVI was uncommon in grade I and grade II tumors (7.9 % and 6.7 %, respectively); however, it was frequently found in grade III tumors 31/40 (45.6 %) ($p$-value <0.0001).

Overall, 52 patients had nodal metastases. Thirty-five (67.3 %) of these patients had positive periparotid lymph nodes noted on final pathology, 29 (82.9 %) of which had extranodal extension. Periparotid nodal metastases were most commonly noted with salivary duct carcinomas (61 %; 11/18). This was followed in frequency by adenocarcinoma (22.7 %; 5/22), MEC (17.9 %; 12/67), acinic cell carcinoma (8.2 %; 5/61), carcinoma ex-pleomorphic adenoma (6.7 %; 1/15), and ACC (3.9 %; 1/26) ($p$-value < 0.0001). The incidence of periparotid nodal metastases increased with histological grade; 7.5 % of grade I tumors demonstrated periparotid nodal metastases, 11.8 % of grade II tumors, and 30 % of grade III tumors ($p$-value = 0.0003). Among the 35 patients with positive periparotid nodes 17 (56.7 %) were staged clinically as N0 (clinical nodal staging was not available for 5 patients). Moreover, of the 35 patients, with a positive periparotid node 38.8 % also had lateral neck nodal metastases, in contrast to 2.7 % of patients with negative periparotid nodes.

## Outcome

The mean and median follow-up durations for the entire cohort were 85.2 and 80.7 months, respectively. The mean and median follow-up durations of living patients were 101 and 102 months, respectively. At the time of last follow-up, 148 (68.8 %) patients were alive without disease, 7 (3.3 %) were alive with disease, and 4 (1.9 %) were lost to follow up (patients alive at last visit but with less than 2 months of follow-up). During the observation period, 36 patients (16.7 %) died of disease and 6 (2.8 %) died of other causes. The mean time to death was 39.9 months (range 1.77-129.64 months).

## Recurrence

During the study period 48 patients (22.3 %) developed a recurrence. Twelve developed local recurrence, 7 developed regional recurrence and 29 developed distant metastases. Eleven of these patients had two sites of recurrence, with the most frequent combination ($n = 9$, 4.2 %) being local and distant failure. The recurrence rate for node positive and node negative patients was 63.5 % and 23.0 %, respectively ($p < 0.0001$). The odds ratio of developing recurrent disease in the node positive compared to the node negative group was 5.80 (95 % CI 2.88-11.70). Furthermore, the incidence of distant metastases was significantly higher in the node positive group (30.8 %) than for the node negative group (6.35 %; $p$-value <0.0001). The odds ratio of detecting distant metastatic disease in the node positive group was 6.55 (95 % CI 2.59-18.56) compared to the node negative group. Patients with lymphovascular invasion had a significantly higher chance of having distant metastases (72.2 %) compared to those without lymphovascular invasion (39.1 %, $p = 0.023$).

## Survival

For the entire cohort, the mean and median follow-up time was 85 and 81 months (range 1–256 months), respectively. The 5- and 10-year OS was 80.6 % and

**Table 1** Demographic and clinicopathological data of 215 patients with major salivary gland carcinoma

| Variable | | Number of patients (%) Total = 215 |
|---|---|---|
| Morphology | Acinic carcinoma | 62 (28.84 %) |
| | Adenocarcinoma | 19 (8.84 %) |
| | Adenoid cystic carcinoma | 20 (9.30 %) |
| | Basal cell adenocarcinoma | 7 (3.26 %) |
| | Carcinoma-ex pleomorphic | 18 (8.37 %) |
| | Mucoepidermoid carcinoma | 70 (32.56 %) |
| | Salivary duct carcinoma | 19 (8.84 %) |
| Pathological Tumor classification | T1 | 68 (34.17 %) |
| | T2 | 61 (30.65 %) |
| | T3 | 48 (24.12 %) |
| | T4a | 20 (10.05 %) |
| | T4b | 2 (1.01 %) |
| | na | 16 (7.44 %) |
| Pathological Lymph node status | N0 | 126 (70.79 %) |
| | N+ | 52 (29.21 %) |
| | na | 37 (17.2 %) |
| Pathological Staging | I | 64 (33.51 %) |
| | II | 46 (24.08 %) |
| | III | 40 (20.94 %) |
| | IVa | 41 (21.47 %) |
| | na | 24 (11.16 %) |
| Pathological Grading | I | 94 (45.41 %) |
| | II | 34 (16.43 %) |
| | III | 79 (38.16 %) |
| | na | 8 (3.72 %) |
| Margin status | negative | 121 (61.11 %) |
| | positive | 77 (38.89 %) |
| | na | 17 (7.90 %) |
| Perineural invasion | negative | 144 (73.10 %) |
| | positive | 53 (26.90 %) |
| | na | 18 (8.37 %) |
| Lymphovascular invasion | negative | 154 (79.38 %) |
| | positive | 40 (20.62 %) |
| | na | 21 (9.76 %) |
| Extracapsular extension | negative | 169 (88.48 %) |
| | positive | 22 (11.52 %) |
| | na | 24 (11.16 %) |

**Table 1** Demographic and clinicopathological data of 215 patients with major salivary gland carcinoma *(Continued)*

| Periparotid lymph node involvement | negative | 167 (82.67 %) |
|---|---|---|
| | positive | 35 (17.33 %) |
| | na | 13 (6.04 %) |

na = not available

69.5 %, respectively. The 5- and 10-year DFS was 74.4 % and 62.4 %, respectively.

Histological subtype was a clear predictor of OS (Fig. 1) on univariable analysis. Other predictors of OS are summarized in Table 3. Significant predictors of OS on multivariable analysis are summarized in Table 4. Lymphovascular invasion, histopathologic grade, nodal status, age >60 and adjuvant radiation therapy was shown to be a significant predictor for overall survival. Patients who received radiotherapy postoperatively had a significant prolonged overall survival compared to patients who had no adjuvant radiotherapy ($p = 0.007$).

Predictors of disease-free survival (DFS) on univariable analysis are summarized in Table 3. Margin status was not a significant predictor of outcomes on UVA for either OS or DFS. Predictors of DFS on multivariable analysis were lymphovascular invasion, pathologic N classification, perineural invasion and age > 60 years (Table 5). Fig. 2 presents the Kaplan Meier DFS curves for the histologic subtype ($p < 0.0001$).

## Discussion

The heterogeneous nature of parotid gland malignancies, along with their diverse biological behavior and relative rarity can make their management very challenging. Knowledge of clinical and histopathologic prognostic factors is critical to making appropriate decisions regarding therapeutic options [4, 12, 13]. We sought to perform a review of outcomes of parotid cancer outcomes managed at a single tertiary care oncology center in the modern era and assess for predictors of outcome.

Our study cohort was comparable in demographic and clinicopathologic data to other recently published reports

**Table 2** Histopathological grading for each histologic subtype of parotid cancer

| Histology | Grade I (%) | Grade II (%) | Grade III (%) |
|---|---|---|---|
| Acinic Cell Carcinoma | 53 (87) | 2 (3) | 6 (10) |
| Adenocarcinoma NOS | 1 (5) | 3 (16) | 15 (79) |
| Adenoid Cystic Carcinoma | 6 (35) | 4 (24) | 7 (41) |
| Basal Cell Adenocarcinoma | 4 (80) | 0 | 1 (20) |
| Carcinoma-ex Pleomorphic Adenoma | 4 (22) | 1 (6) | 13 (72) |
| Mucoepidermoid carcinoma | 26 (38) | 24 (35) | 18 (26) |
| Salivary duct Carcinoma | 0 | 0 | 19 (100) |

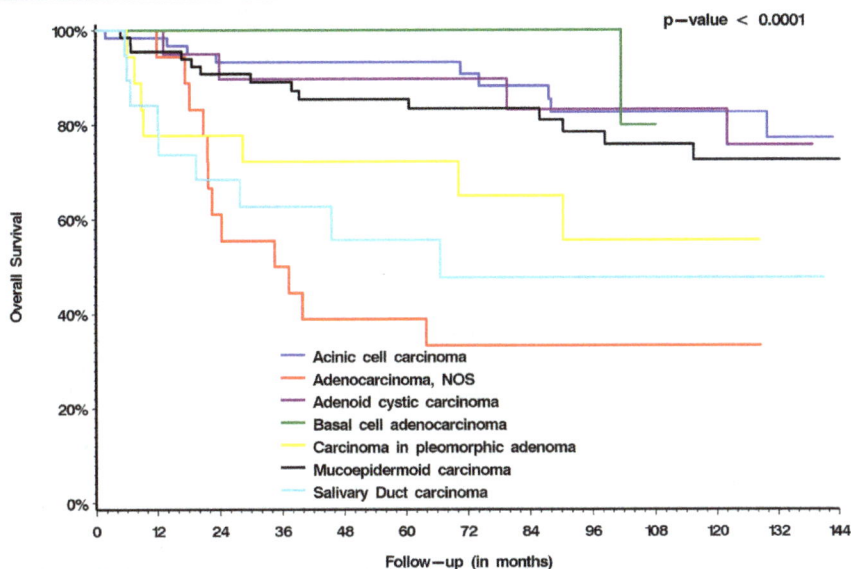

**Fig. 1** Kaplan-Meier curves for overall survival of 215 patients with parotid gland malignancies stratified by morphology

[7, 14]. Mucoepidermoid carcinoma and acinic cell carcinoma were the two most common variants. Patients with acinic cell, adenoid cystic and mucoepidermoid carcinoma had a better overall and recurrence-free survival compared to patients diagnosed with salivary duct carcinoma, carcinoma-ex-pleomorphic adenoma and adenocarcinoma. As has been demonstrated by the data in this study and others, patients can be stratified to high or low risk for survival according to their histology, as well as to their grade.

**Table 3** Univariable analysis of overall-, and disease-free survival and clinicopathological parameters of patients with parotid gland carcinomas

| Variable | Univariable testing | |
|---|---|---|
| | Overall survival = | Disease-free survival |
| | p-value | |
| pT classification (T1/2 vs. T3/4) | <0.0001 | <0.0001 |
| pN status (N+ vs. N0) | <0.0001 | <0.0001 |
| Histopathological grade | <0.0001 | <0.0001 |
| Perineural invasion | <0.0001 | <0.0001 |
| Lymphovascular invasion | <0.0001 | <0.0001 |
| Extracapsular extension | <0.0001 | <0.0001 |
| Age <60y | <0.0001 | 0.0011 |
| Histological subtype | <0.0001 | 0.0003 |
| Periparotid node involvement | <0.0001 | <0.0001 |
| Positive Margins | 0.37 | 0.08 |

pT and pN = pathological T and N classification

In concert with prior studies, we have also observed that patients with positive neck nodes, perineural, and lymphovascular invasion have lower overall and disease free-survival [7, 15, 16]. Similar to previous reports, patients younger than 60 years have a better disease-free survival than older patients. The explanation for this finding is unclear, although immunologic or other age-associated factors may play a role [17, 18].

Controversy exists as to the most appropriate management of the neck in patients with primary malignancies of the parotid. One of the complicating factors is the frequent lack of a preoperative histological subtype diagnosis. While most head and neck oncologists agree that elective neck dissection is warranted in those undergoing parotidectomy for high-risk or high-grade disease, stratification is often unknown at the time of primary surgery. Furthermore, in the setting of known malignancy, clinical nodal evaluation appears to significantly underestimate the true incidence of cervical nodal metastases [19]. Indeed, our study agreed with others that there is a significantly higher incidence of pathologic positivity in the neck then can be expected by exam or imaging. A recent meta-analysis has demonstrated that 23 % of patients with cN0 neck had positive disease [19]. However, there does appear to be an association between periparotid nodes and cervical lymphadenopathy. Klussman et al. [20] similarly noted of 36 patients with intraparotid nodes, 12 had positive cervical nodes (33 %). This raises the possibility that evidence of periparotid lymph node metastases may be a marker for more lateral neck nodal disease. In the current study

**Table 4** Multivariable analysis of overall survival and clinicopathological parameters of patients with parotid gland carcinomas

| Variable | | Multivariable analysis for overall survival | | |
|---|---|---|---|---|
| | p-value | Hazard ratio | 95 % Confidence Interval | |
| Lymphovascular invasion | 0.0020 | 3.217 | 1.532 | 6.755 |
| Histopathological grade | 0.0293 | 3.774 | 1.312 | 10.858 |
| pN status | 0.0430 | 1.060 | 1.002 | 1.122 |
| Age >60 | 0.0352 | 1.990 | 1.049 | 3.775 |
| Radiation yes/no | 0.0056 | 0.272 | 0.106 | 0.696 |

pN = pathological N classification

lateral neck nodes were more common in those that had positive periparotid nodes than those that did not. In addition, almost half of the patients with a positive periparotid node were staged clinically as being N0. Thus, a decision for a lateral neck dissection may need to made at the time of surgery based on identifying a periparotid node and evaluating for metastases on frozen section analysis.

Multiple studies, including this one, have shown significantly worse outcomes with pathologically positive neck disease [3, 4, 7, 14]. In this cohort of patients, neck node positivity was a strong predictive factor for recurrent disease, in particularly for distant metastatic recurrence. In particular, 31 % of patients with nodal metastases have developed simultaneously distant metastases, primarily to the lungs. Looking at the nodal disease of all patients that have been included in this study we observed that subsequently the rate of patients who died of disease was significantly higher in the neck node positive group compared to patients with negative nodes in the neck. Furthermore, the disparity in outcomes may be underestimated due to a relatively high incidence of patients with occult cervical metastatic disease not undergoing elective neck dissection.

Lymphovascular invasion was also found to be a strong predictor of distant metastases and survival. On multivariable analysis with nodal metastases and grade included in the model LVI was still found to be a significant predictor of survival. One of the limitations was that the lymphatic and vascular invasion was not

separated in pathology reports to determine whether one or both are associated with distant metastases and reduced survival [21, 22]. The high rate of distant metastases in patients with high-grade tumors, nodal metastases and LVI, points to the need for evaluating systemic therapies to be used alongside current treatment paradigms in patients with these high risk features.

As with most series facial nerve paralysis at presentation in our series was uncommon. While only 12 patients presented with facial paralysis 36 ultimately required facial nerve resection. Thus, patients with pre-operatively functioning nerves do need to be made aware of the possibility of nerve resection when there is evidence of nerve invasion or encasement intra-operatively.

Positive margins were reported in our series in almost 40 % of patients. This included patients that were managed elsewhere and referred in for further management, as well as cases where tumor was found to be extending to the margin of the specimen, in regions where the tumor is intimately related to the facial nerve. On analysis positive margin status was not a significant predictor of RFS. Almost all these patients would have received postoperative adjuvant therapy, thus highlighting the excellent control rates that can be achieved with adjuvant radiotherapy in the setting of microscopic positive margins. Lin and coworkers [26] compared the clinical outcome among 101 patients with salivary gland carcinomas after adjuvant radiotherapy. Although patients with positive margins had a shortened disease-free survival their clinical outcome was equal to those patients with negative margins [23].

**Table 5** Multivariable analysis of recurrence-free survival and clinicopathological parameters of patients with parotid carcinomas

| Variable | | Multivariable analysis for recurrence-free survival | | |
|---|---|---|---|---|
| | p-value | Hazard ratio | 95 % Confidence Interval | |
| Lymphovascular invasion | 0.0482 | 1.953 | 1.005 | 3.794 |
| pN status | 0.0076 | 1.069 | 1.018 | 1.122 |
| Perineural invasion | 0.0040 | 2.526 | 1.345 | 4.745 |
| Age >60 | 0.0447 | 1.749 | 1.013 | 3.018 |
| Radiation yes/no | 0.6233 | 0.822 | 0.375 | 1.798 |
| Histopathological grade | NS | | | |

pN = pathological N classification
NS = not significant

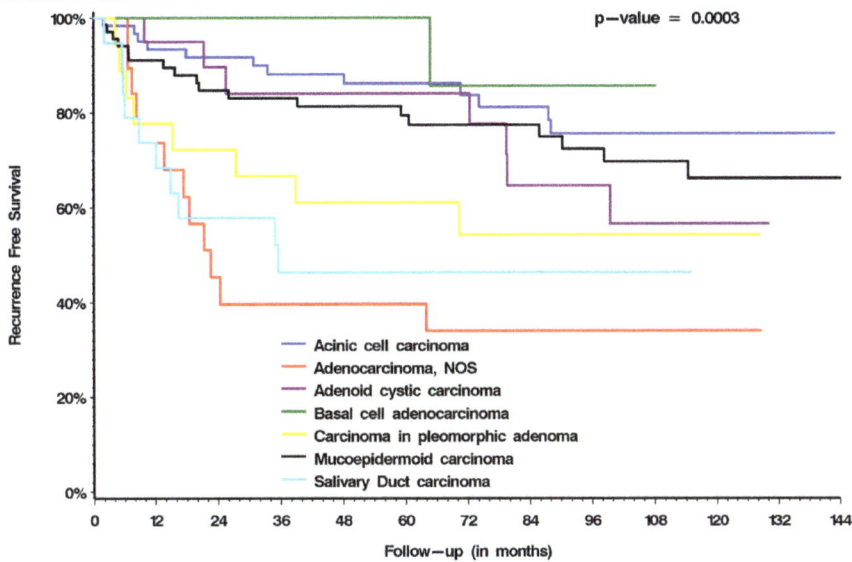

**Fig. 2** Kaplan-Meier curves for recurrence-free survival of 215 patients with parotid gland malignancies stratified by morphology

While the inclusion of the diverse group of pathologies can be regarded as a limitation to the study we feel that the study provides an overview of the differences in the patterns of behaviour. In terms of outcomes, even within groups there is variability in biology based on tumor grade and thus tumor grade may provide more prognostic information than the type of parotid cancer.

## Conclusions

Our single institution experience has demonstrated that advanced age, lymph node status, perineural and lymphovascular invasion were the strongest predictors of oncologic outcome. Moreover we have shown that periparotid lymph node involvement has a major impact on disease-free and overall survival in patients with parotid carcinomas. The presence of periparotid lymph node involvement should alert the surgeon to the probability of advanced disease and the need for more aggressive treatment and follow up. Nevertheless, multi-institutional prospective studies are needed to further address this question. Currently, there is a phase II RTOG (1008) trial comparing adjuvant radiation versus chemoradiation in accruing patients with intermediate to high grade salivary gland carcinomas who have undergone curative intent surgical resection and are found to have the following risk factors for recurrence: T3-4, or N1-3 disease, or T1-2 N0 patients with positive or close (≤1 mm) microscopic margins of resection.

**Competing interests**
The authors declare that they have no competing interests.

**Authors' contributions**
DPG JCI and GB participated in the conception and design of the project. BE MS and GB were involved with acquisition of the data. BE DPG and EA were involved in the analysis and interpretation of the data. BE MS GB JI and DPG were involved with drafting the manuscript. All authors were involved in revising the manuscript critically for important intellectual content. All authors gave final approval of the version to be published. All authors agree to be accountable for all aspects of the work.

**Author details**
[1]Department of Otolaryngology-Head and Neck Surgery, Wharton Head and Neck Program, University Health Network, Princess Margaret Cancer Centre, Toronto, ON, Canada. [2]Department of Radiation Oncology, Princess Margaret Cancer Centre, University of Toronto, Toronto, ON, Canada. [3]Department of Pathology, University Health Network, Princess Margaret Cancer Centre, Toronto, ON, Canada. [4]Department of Biostatistics, University Health Network, Princess Margaret Cancer Centre, Toronto, ON, Canada. [5]Princess Margaret Hospital, Wharton Head and Neck Centre, 610 University Avenue, 3rd Floor, Toronto, ON M5G 2 M9, Canada.

**References**
1.  Siegel R, Naishadham D, Jemal A. Cancer statistics. CA Cancer J Clin. 2012;62:10–29.
2.  Seifert G, Sobin LH. Histological typing of salivary gland tumours. World Health Organization International Histological Classification of Tumours. 2nd ed. New York: Springer; 1991.
3.  Spiro RH. Salivary neoplasms: overview of a 35-year experience with 2,807 patients. Head Neck. 1986;8:177–84.
4.  Wahlberg P, Anderson H, Biörklund A, Möller T, Perfekt R. Carcinoma of the parotid and submandibular glands–a study of survival in 2465 patients. Oral Oncol. 2002;38:706–13.
5.  Carrillo JF, Vázquez R, Ramírez-Ortega MC, Cano A, Ochoa-Carrillo FJ, Oñate-Ocaña LF. Multivariate prediction of the probability of recurrence in patients with carcinoma of the parotid gland. Cancer. 2007;109:2043–51.
6.  Cederblad L, Johansson S, Enblad G, Engström M, Blomquist E. Cancer of the parotid gland; long-term follow-up. A single centre experience on recurrence and survival. Acta Oncol. 2009;48:549–55.

7.  Vander Poorten VL, Hart A, van der Laan BF, Baatenburg de Jong RJ, Manni JJ, Marres HA, et al. Prognostic index for patients with parotid carcinoma: external validation using the nationwide 1985–1994 Dutch Head and Neck Oncology Cooperative Group database. Cancer. 2003;97(6):1453–63.

8.  Camelo-Piragua SI, Habib C, Kanumuri P, Lago CE, Mason HS, Otis CN. Mucoepidermoid carcinoma of the breast shares cytogenetic abnormality with mucoepidermoid carcinoma of the salivary gland: a case report with molecular analysis and review of the literature. Hum Pathol. 2009;40:887–92.

9.  Miyabe S, Okabe M, Nagatsuka H, Hasegawa Y, Inagaki A, Ijichi K, et al. Prognostic significance of p27Kip1, Ki-67, and CRTC1-MAML2 fusion transcript in mucoepidermoid carcinoma: a molecular and clinicopathologic study of 101 cases. Oral Maxillofac Surg. 2009;67:1432–41.

10. Rao PH, Roberts D, Zhao YJ, Bell D, Harris CP, Weber RS, et al. Deletion of 1p32-p36 is the most frequent genetic change and poor prognostic marker in adenoid cystic carcinoma of the salivary glands. Clin Cancer Res. 2008;14:5181–7.

11. Hamakawa H, Nakashiro K, Sumida T, Shintani S, Myers JN, Takes RP, et al. Basic evidence of molecular targeted therapy for oral cancer and salivary gland cancer. Head Neck. 2008;30:800–9.

12. Loh KS, Barker E, Bruch G, O'Sullivan B, Brown DH, Goldstein DP, et al. Prognostic factors in malignancy of the minor salivary glands. Head Neck. 2009;1:58–63.

13. Koul R, Dubey A, Butler J, Cooke AL, Abdoh A, Nason R. Prognostic factors depicting disease-specific survival in parotid-gland tumors. Int J Radiat Oncol Biol Phys. 2007;68:714–8.

14. Takahama Jr A, Sanabria A, Benevides GM, de Almeida OP, Kowalski LP. Comparison of two prognostic scores for patients with parotid carcinoma. Head Neck. 2009;31:1188–95.

15. Vander Poorten VL, Balm AJ, Hilgers FJ, Tan IB, Keus RB, Hart AA. Stage as major long term outcome predictor in minor salivary gland carcinoma. Cancer. 2000;89:1195–204.

16. Roh JL, Choi SH, Lee SW, Cho KJ, Nam SY, Kim SY. Carcinomas arising in the submandibular gland: high propensity for systemic failure. J Surg Oncol. 2008;97:533–7.

17. Saito H, Osaki T, Murakami D, Sakamoto T, Kanaji S, Tatebe S, et al. Effect of age on prognosis in patients with gastric cancer. ANZ J Surg. 2006;76:458–61.

18. Rosenberg J, Chia YL, Plevritis S. The effect of age, race, tumor size, tumor grade, and disease stage on invasive ductal breast cancer survival in the U.S. SEER database. Breast Cancer Res Treat. 2005;89:47–54.

19. Valstar MH, van den Brekel MW, Smeele LE. Interpretation of treatment outcome in the clinically node-negative neck in primary parotid carcinoma: a systematic review of the literature. Head Neck. 2010;32:1402–11.

20. Klussmann JP, Ponert T, Mueller RP, Dienes HP, Guntinas-Lichius O. Patterns of lymph node spread and its influence on outcome in resectable parotid cancer. Eur J Surg Oncol. 2008;34:932–7.

21. Ali S, Palmer FL, Yu C, DiLorenzo M, Shah JP, Kattan MW, et al. A predictive nomogram for recurrence of carcinoma of the major salivary glands. JAMA Otolaryngol Head Neck Surg. 2013;139:698–705.

22. Ali S, Bryant R, Palmer FL, DiLorenzo M, Shah JP, Patel SG, Ganly I. Distant Metastases in Patients with Carcinoma of the Major Salivary Glands. Ann Surg Oncol. 2015;22(12):4014–19.

23. Lin YC, Chen KC, Lin CH, Kuo KT, Ko JY, Hong RL. Clinicopathological features of salivary and non-salivary adenoid cystic carcinomas. Int J Oral Maxillofac Surg. 2012;41:354–60s.

# 9

# Adjuvant Radioactive iodine 131 ablation in papillary microcarcinoma of thyroid

Khalid Hussain AL-Qahtani[1], Mushabbab Al Asiri[2], Mutahir A. Tunio[2*], Naji J. Aljohani[3], Yasser Bayoumi[4], Hanadi Fatani[5] and Abdulrehman AlHadab[6]

## Abstract

**Background:** Papillary Microcarcinoma (PMC) of thyroid is a rare type of differentiated thyroid cancer (DTC), which according to the World Health Organization measures 1.0 cm or less. The gold standard of treatment of PMC is still controversy. Our aim was to contribute in resolving the debate on the therapeutic choices of the surgical and adjuvant I-131 (RAI) treatment in PMC.

**Methods:** From 2000 to 2012, 326 patients were found to have PMC and were retrospectively reviewed for clinicopathological characteristics, treatment outcomes and prognostic factors.

**Results:** Mean age of cohort was 42.6 years (range: 18–76) and the mean tumor size was 0.61 cm ± 0.24; lymph node involvement was seen in 12.9 % of cases. Median follow up period was 8.05 years (1.62–11.4). Total 23 all site recurrences (7.13 %) were observed; more observed in patients without I-131 ablation (*p <0.0001*). Ten year DFS rates were 89.6 %. Cox regression Model analysis revealed size, histopathologic variants, multifocality, extrathyroidal extension, lymphovascular space invasion, nodal status, and adjuvant RAI ablation the important prognostic factors affecting DFS.

**Discussion:** Despite excellent DFS rates, a small proportion of patients with PMC develop recurrences after treatment. Adjuvant RAI therapy improves DFS in PMC patients with aggressive histopathologic variants, multifocality, ETE, LVSI, tumor size (> 0.5 cm) and lymph node involvement. Failure of RAI ablation to decrease risk in N1a/b supports prophylactic central neck dissection during thyroidectomy, however more trials are warranted.

**Conclusion:** Adjuvant I-131 ablation following thyroidectomy in PMC patients, particularly with poor prognostic factors improves DFS rates.

**Keywords:** Papillary microcarcinoma, Optimal treatment, Adjuvant radioiodine ablation, Disease free survival, Saudi Population

## Background

In Saudi Arabia, the incidence of differentiated thyroid cancers (DTC) especially papillary thyroid cancers (PTC) is increasing exponentially over the past years accounting for more than 10 % of all cancers among females [1, 2]. Higher rates for identification of PTC in recent years are attributed to the use of high resolution neck ultrasonography (USG) and USG-guided fine needle aspiration biopsy (FNAB) [3].

With the use of these high resolution transducers, papillary microcarcinoma (PMC), i.e. tumor size 1 cm or less can easily be detected [4, 5]. Patients with PMC have generally an excellent outlook with use of surgery, radioactive iodine-131 (RAI) ablation, suppression of thyroid-stimulating hormone (TSH) secretion with levothyroxine, with long term disease-free survival (DFS) of 84–97 % [6]. However, still there is much debate regarding the most appropriate treatment of PMC ranging from observation alone to over-treatment with surgery followed by adjuvant RAI ablation [7–10].

* Correspondence: drmutahirtonio@hotmail.com
[2]Radiation Oncology, Comprehensive Cancer Center, King Fahad Medical City, Riyadh 59046, Saudi Arabia
Full list of author information is available at the end of the article

In the present study, we aimed to evaluate the different prognostic factors for DFS in PMC patients in our population, and also to determine the DFS in patients with PMC treated with or without adjuvant RAI ablation following thyroidectomy.

## Methods

After formal approval from the institutional ethical committee, medical records of 1192 patients with confirmed papillary thyroid cancers (PTC) who were treated or followed up in two major referral hospitals of Riyadh, Saudi Arabia, during the period of July 2000 and December 2012 were reviewed using computer based departmental database system. Patients with PMC were retrieved in following manner;

### Definition

PMC was defined according WHO classification system for thyroid tumors as "PTC is measuring ≤ 1 cm in greatest dimension" [5].

### Demographic, clinicopathological and radiological variables

Demographic and clinical data including age at the diagnosis, gender, and symptomatology were reviewed. A detailed second review of all histopathological specimens was performed by experienced histopathologist. Different histopathological parameters, including the location of tumor, tumor size, histopathologic variants, multifocality, extrathyroidal extension (ETE), lymphovascular space invasion (LVSI), surgical margin status, and cervical lymph node status and background thyroid tissue were also recorded. Data from different imaging modalities, including neck ultrasonography, whole body I-131 scintigraphy (WBS), computed tomography (CT) scan of neck and chest, flourodeoxyglucose positron emission tomography (FDG-PET) was collected. Periodic postoperative thyroid function tests (TFTs), thyroid antibodies and stimulated thyroglobulin (TG) levels (off thyroxin or thyrotropin-Alfa injection) were also reviewed. Different treatment modalities, including hemi-thyroidectomy (removal of lobe and isthmus), total thyroidectomy (removal of entire gland), neck dissection, adjuvant RAI ablation, different doses used in millicurie (mCi) and the details of neck irradiation details (if given) were also reviewed.

The primary endpoint was the disease free survival (DFS). Secondary points were; the frequency of PMC and histologic variants, local recurrence free survival (LRFS), distant metastasis free survival (DMFS) and overall survival (OS) according to (a) treatment with or without adjuvant I-131 ablation and (b) according to primary tumor size (≤0.5 cm vs. > 0.5 cm).

Local recurrence was defined as, clinically or radiologically detectable recurrences in the thyroid bed or in cervical

lymph nodes on imaging (ultrasonography, WBS and CT-PET) after evaluating for elevated thyroglobulin (TG) levels. Distant metastasis was defined as, clinically or radiologically detectable disease outside the neck on imaging (WBS, CT imaging and CT-PET) after evaluating for elevated thyroglobulin (TG) levels. The DFS was defined as, the duration between the surgery date and the date of documented disease reappearance/relapse, death from cancer and/or last follow-up (censored). The OS was defined as, the duration between the surgery date and the date of patient death or last follow-up (censored).

### Statistical analysis

Chi-square test, Student's $t$ test, or Fisher exact tests were used to determine the differences in various clinical variables. Multivariate logistic regression was done using Cox proportional hazards modeling. Probabilities of LRFS, DMFS, DFS and OS were shown with the Kaplan-Meier method and the comparisons for various survival curves were performed using log rank. All statistical analyses were performed using the computer program SPSS version 16.0.

## Results

### Demographic and clinicopathological features of cohort

Among the 1192 PTC patients in our departmental database, 377 (31.6 %) patients were found to have PMC. Fifty one (13.3 %) patients with insufficient data regarding size, treatment and follow-up period were excluded. The remaining study cohort ($n = 326$) consisted of 271 (83.1 %) women and 55 (16.9 %) men; the median age at diagnosis was 42.6 years ±11.6. The majority of patients had total thyroidectomy ($n = 299$, 91.7 %); only 27 (8.3 %) patients underwent lobectomy. The mean tumor size was 0.61 cm ± 0.24, with 12.9 % ($n = 42$) involvement of cervical lymph nodes (level VI in 34 patients). The predominant histopathologic variants were, classic (265 patients), follicular (41 patients), and tall cell (11 patients). Other clinicopathological features are described in Table 1.

### Clinicopathological features and DFS Comparison in PMC patients treated with and without I-131 ablation

Among 326 patients, 182 (55.8 %) patients were given adjuvant RAI ablation as shown in Table 1. Major indications for adjuvant RAI ablation were multifocality (67.1 %), extra-thyroidal extension (ETE) in 31.3 % of cases, aggressive histopathologic variants (tall cell, sclerosing), lymph node metastasis (23.1 %) and distant metastasis at time of presentation (1.65 %). Primary tumor size was not a primary indication in our series; however the observed mean tumor size was bigger in patients treated with adjuvant RAI ablation (0.72 cm vs. 0.44 cm). RAI ablation doses were as; 30 m-curie (mCi)

**Table 1** Patients characteristics

| Variable | Whole cohort N (%) | RAI ablation N (%) | Without RAI ablation N (%) | P value* |
|---|---|---|---|---|
| Total patients | 326/1192 (27.4 %) | 182/326 (55.8) | 144/326 (44.2) | 0.06 |
| Age (years) | 42.6 (18–76) SD ±11.6 | 43.2 (18–76) SD ± 12.4 | 41.8 (19–71) SD ± 10.2 | |
| ≤45 years | 201 (61.7) | 110 (60.4) | 94 (65.3) | 0.81 |
| ≥45 years | 125 (38.3) | 72 (39.6) | 50 (34.7) | |
| Gender | | | | |
| Female | 271 (83.1) | 146 (80.2) | 125 (86.8) | 0.06 |
| Male | 55 (16.9) | 36 (19.8) | 19 (13.2) | |
| Female to male ratio | 4.9 | 4.0 | 6.5 | |
| Type of surgery | | | | |
| Total thyroidectomy | 299 (91.7) | 182 (100) | 117 (81.3) | 0.04 |
| Hemi-thyroidectomy | 27 (8.3) | - | 27 (18.7) | |
| Lymph node surgery | | | | |
| Central neck dissection | 88 (27.0) | 54 (29.7) | 34 (23.6) | |
| Lateral neck dissection | 18 (5.5) | 9 (4.9) | 9 (6.3) | 0.9 |
| Sampling | 55 (16.9) | 25 (13.7) | 30 (20.8) | |
| None | 165 (50.6) | 94 (51.7) | 71 (49.3) | |
| Mean size (cm) | 0.61 (0.1–1.0) ± 0.24 | 0.72 (0.2–1.0) ± 0.21 | 0.44 (0.1–0.9) ± 0.2 | |
| ≤0.5 cm | 161 (49.4) | 50 (27.5) | 111 (77.1) | <0.0001 |
| ≥0.5 cm | 165 (50.6) | 132 (72.5) | 33 (22.9) | |
| Histopathologic variants | | | | |
| Classic | 265 (81.3) | 143 (78.6) | 122 (84.7) | |
| Follicular | 41 (12.6) | 21 (11.5) | 20 (13.9) | |
| Hurthle cell | 8 (2.5) | 6 (3.3) | 2 (1.4) | |
| Tall cell | 11 (3.4) | 11 (6.0) | - | 0.001 |
| Sclerosing | 1 (0.3) | 1 (0.5) | - | |
| Multifocal | | | | |
| Yes | 125 (38.3) | 122 (67.1) | 3 (2.1) | <0.0001 |
| No | 201 (61.7) | 60 (32.9) | 141 (97.9) | |
| ETE | | | | |
| Yes | 62 (19.0) | 57 (31.3) | 5 (3.5) | <0.0001 |
| No | 264 (81.0) | 125 (68.7) | 139 (96.5) | |
| LVSI | | | | |
| Yes | 55 (16.9) | 49 (26.9) | 6 (4.2) | <0.0001 |
| No | 271 (83.1) | 133 (73.1) | 138 (95.8) | |
| Surgical margins | | | | |
| Positive | 35 (10.7) | 30 (16.5) | 5 (3.5) | <0.0001 |
| Negative | 291 (89.3) | 152 (83.5) | 139 (96.5) | |
| Lymph node metastasis | | | | |
| Yes | 42 (12.9) | 42 (23.1) | - | <0.0001 |
| N1a | 34 (73.8) | 34 (73.8) | | |
| N1b | 8 (19.2) | 8 (19.2) | | |
| No | 284 (87.1) | 140 (76.9) | 144 (100) | |

**Table 1** Patients characteristics *(Continued)*

| | | | | |
|---|---|---|---|---|
| Background thyroid tissue | | | | |
| Normal | 98 (30.1) | 47 (25.8) | 51 (35.4) | |
| Multi-nodular goiter | 106 (32.5) | 60 (32.9) | 46 (31.9) | |
| Lymphocytic thyroiditis/Hashimotos' thyroiditis | 122 (37.5) | 75 (41.3) | 47 (32.6) | *0.052* |
| Distant Metastasis at presentation | 3 (0.9) | 3 (1.65) | - | *<0.0001* |
| AJCC staging | | | | |
| I | 217 (66.5) | 73 (40.1) | 139 (96.5) | |
| II | - | - | - | |
| III | 96 (29.5) | 96 (52.6) | 5 (3.5) | *<0.0001* |
| IVA | 10 (3.1) | 10 (5.6) | - | |
| IVB | - | - | - | |
| IVC | 3 (0.9) | 3 (1.7) | - | |
| Mean postoperative TG (ng/ml) | 1.39 (0.1–42890) | 2.44 (0.1–42890) | 0.39 (0.1–8.9) | *0.62* |
| RAI dose | | | | |
| 30 mCi | | 50 (27.5) | - | *<0.0001* |
| 100 mCi | | 85 (46.7) | - | |
| 150-200 mCi | | 47 (25.8) | - | |
| RT to Neck | 2 (0.61) | 2 (1.1) | - | *<0.0001* |
| Recurrences | | | | |
| Locoregional | 13 (3.9) | 4 (2.2) | 9 (6.2) | *<0.001* |
| Distant | 10 (3.1) | 4 (2.2) | 6 (4.2) | |

*P value pertaining to the variation in clinicopathological characteristics between two groups

*RAI* radioactive iodine 131, *N* number, *SD* standard deviation, *ETE* extra-thyroidal extension, *LVSI* lymphovascular space invasion, *AJCC* American joint committee on cancer, *TG* thyroglobulin, *mCi* millicurie, *RT* radiation therapy

for tumors with multifocality and focal ETE (27.5 %); 100 mCi for tumors with multifocality, ETE, LVSI, positive surgical margins, poor histopathologic variants, and elevated postoperative stimulated TG levels (>2 ng/ml) (46.7 %); 150 mCi for positive lymph nodes (24.7 %), and 200 mCi for distant metastasis at the time of diagnosis (1.65 %). RAI ablation was tolerated well without any grade 3 or 4 side effects. Additional neck irradiation was given in two patients with adherent tumors; trachea (one patient; 0.5 %) and skeletal muscle (one patient; 0.5 %).

A median follow-up period was 8.05 years (range: 1.62–11.4). For whole cohort, the 5 and 10 years LRFS were 98.4 % and 96.8 % respectively; DMFS rates were 92.4 % at 5 years and 90 % at 10 years. Five and 10 years OS rates were 99.3 % and 98.6 % (two deaths) and the 5 and 10 years DFS rates were 94.7 % and 89.6 %.

Total 23 recurrences (7.13 %) were observed; 8/182 in patients with RAI ablation and 15/144 in patients without RAI ablation. The pattern of recurrences was as: three patients had disease in thyroid bed only, 10 had cervical nodes, and 10 failed at distant sites (9 patients

in lungs and one patient in bones). Combined locoregional and distant recurrences were seen in 3 patients. The elevated TG levels were always seen with local recurrences and distant metastasis. The isolated locoregional recurrences were salvaged by surgery (lateral neck dissection; 7 patients, completion thyroidectomy; 2 patients and excision in one patient), followed by RAI ablation (12 patients) and distant failures were salvaged by RAI ablation (9 patients) and palliative irradiation for bony lesion (one patient). Time to initial local recurrence was 0.8 years and time to initial distant metastasis was 1.5 year. The 5 and 10 year DFS rates were 95.7 % vs. 90.9 % and 92.2 % vs. 84 % in patients with and without RAI ablation respectively (*p = 0.04*) Fig. 1a. The 5 and 10 year DFS rates according to different prognostic factors are summarized in Table 2. The overall 5 and 10 year DFS rates were significantly dropped in the presence of poor histopathologic variants (*p < 0.001*) and ETE. In addition to these factors, multifocality (*p < 0.001*) LVSI (*p = 0.001*) and elevated postoperative thyroglobulin levels > 2 ng/ml (*p = 0.04*) resulted in inferior 5 and 10 year DFS in patients treated without RAI ablation.

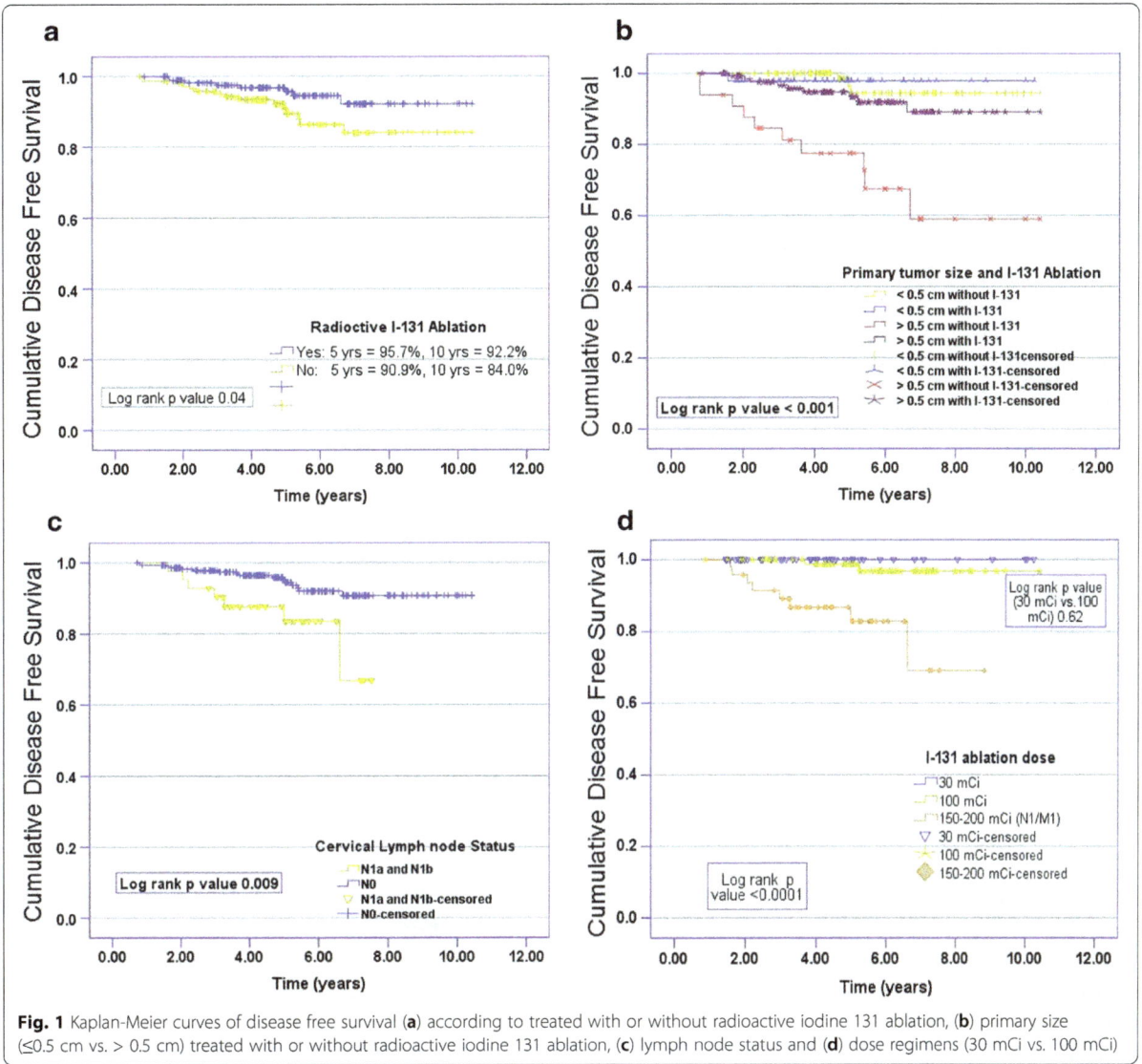

**Fig. 1** Kaplan-Meier curves of disease free survival (**a**) according to treated with or without radioactive iodine 131 ablation, (**b**) primary size (≤0.5 cm vs. > 0.5 cm) treated with or without radioactive iodine 131 ablation, (**c**) lymph node status and (**d**) dose regimens (30 mCi vs. 100 mCi)

## Clinicopathological features and DFS comparison among PMC of size ≤ 0.5 cm and > 0.5 cm

With regard to the difference in DFS (locoregional and distant failure), a comparative analysis was performed according to primary tumor size (≤0.5 cm vs. > 0.5 cm) as described in the Table 3. About 161 (49.4 %) patients had tumors of size ≤ 0.5 cm and 165 (50.6 %) patients had tumors of size above 0.5 cm in greatest dimension. Significant demographic and clinicopathological differences were observed between two groups. Patients with tumor size ≤ 0.5 cm were younger (mean age 36.7 years), with higher female to male ratio (6.3), and with more aggressive histopathologic variants (tall cell, sclerosing). The cervical lymph node metastases were seen in 9.3 % of patients with tumor size ≤ 0.5 cm as compared to

patients with tumor size > 0.5 cm (16.4 %) with $p < 0.001$. Patients with tumor size ≤ 0.5 cm had high rates of hemithyroidectomy (18.7 %), less adjuvant RAI ablation (31.1 %) with low recurrence rates. There was also no significant difference in 5 and 10 year DFS rates in in patients with tumor size ≤ 0.5 cm treated with or without adjuvant RAI ablation ($p = 0.71$) Fig. 1b. Further it was seen that adjuvant RAI ablation did better in N0 as compared to N1 neck status Fig. 1c. Also in patients treated with adjuvant RAI ablation, no significant difference was observed between two dose regimens (30 mCi vs. 100 mCi) with $p = 0.62$ (Fig. 1d).

### Prognostic factors

Cox regression Model using univariate and multivariate analysis for DFS to predict important prognostic factors

**Table 2** Disease free survival according to different prognostic factors

| Variable | RAI ablation | | | | Without RAI ablation | | | |
|---|---|---|---|---|---|---|---|---|
| | 5 years-DFS | p | 10 years-DFS | p | 5 years-DFS | p | 10 years-DFS | p |
| Age | | | | | | | | |
| ≤45 years | 97.8 % | | 93.5 % | | 87.6 % | | 83.6 % | |
| ≥45 years | 92.5 % | NS | 85.3 % | NS | 88.5 % | NS | 84.5 % | NS |
| Gender | | | | | | | | |
| Female | 95.4 % | | 91.2 % | | 93.8 % | | 82.2 % | |
| Male | 96.8 % | NS | 89.4 % | NS | 90.4 % | NS | 82.0 % | NS |
| Histopathologic variants | | | | | | | | |
| Classic | 96.1 % | | 93.5 % | | 95.5 % | | 92.3 % | |
| Follicular | 94.7 % | | 90.9 % | | 78.9 % | | 59.6 % | |
| Hurthle cell | 96.1 % | | 92.7 % | | 90.0 % | 0.001 | 78.9 % | <0.001 |
| Tall cell | 68.2 % | | - | | | | - | |
| Sclerosing | 55.0 % | 0.002 | - | <0.001 | | | - | |
| Multifocal | | | | | | | | |
| Yes | 95.2 % | | 90.9 % | | 66.7 % | | 33.3 % | |
| No | 96.6 % | NS | 93.4 % | NS | 90.0 % | <0.001 | 88.3 % | <0.0001 |
| Surgical margins | | | | | | | | |
| Positive | 96.6 % | | 91.5 % | | 86.3 % | | 84.0 % | |
| Negative | 96.8 % | NS | 95.3 % | NS | 93.2 % | NS | 87.9 % | NS |
| ETE | | | | | | | | |
| Yes | 89.5 % | | 85.5 % | | 40.0 % | | 0.0 % | |
| No | 98.2 % | 0.03 | 95.1 % | 0.02 | 91.7 % | <0.0001 | 80.1 % | <0.0001 |
| LVSI | | | | | | | | |
| Yes | 89.5 % | | 85.5 % | | 80.0 % | | 60.0 % | |
| No | 92.5 % | NS | 89.4 % | NS | 93.2 % | 0.02 | 84.4 % | 0.001 |
| Mean postoperative TG | | | | | | | | |
| ≤2 ng/ml | 96.6 % | | 93.4 % | | 93.2 % | | 91.7 % | |
| >2 ng/ml | 89.5 % | NS | 85.5 % | NS | 87.9 % | NS | 80.1 % | 0.04 |
| Surgery | | | | | | | | |
| Total thyroidectomy | 96.0 % | | 94.4 % | | 93.2 % | | 87.5 % | |
| Hemi-thyroidectomy | 91.5 % | 0.03 | 86.0 % | 0.03 | 85.1 % | 0.04 | 80.2 % | 0.02 |

*RAI* radioactive iodine 131, *yr* year, *DFS* disease free survival, *SD* standard deviation, *ETE* extra-thyroidal extension, *LVSI* lymphovascular space invasion, *TG* thyroglobulin

Table 4. Important prognostic factors were, histopathologic variants ($p < 0.0001$), multifocality ($p < 0.0001$), ETE ($p < 0.0001$), LVSI ($p =0.03$), nodal status ($p < 0.0001$), and adjuvant RAI ablation ($p < 0.0001$).

## Discussion

Despite excellent DFS rates in patients with PMC, about 3–16 % of patients develop local and distant failures [11]. In present study, we were able to determine overall five and ten year DFS rates of 94.7 % and 89.6 % respectively after aggressive treatment by total thyroidectomy followed by RAI ablation in the majority of cases. These results were found in consistent with similar reported data [12–15]. Several clinicopathological and treatments related prognostic factors were observed. An important prognostic factor, the age > 45 years was not found a prognosticator to predict DFS in our study, suggesting that other risk factors, such as aggressive histopathologic variants, multifocality, ETE, and LVSI are more important clinicopathological predictors than age in PMC [16]. Similarly, in contrast to other reported data, gender was also not found an important predictor of DFS [17]. Improved DFS was observed in patients who underwent total thyroidectomy. Possible explanation for this could be (a) high percentage of multifocality, and (b) more aggressive histopathological variants (tall cell and diffuse

**Table 3** Comparative analysis of clinicopathological characteristics based on the size of primary tumors

| Variable | Tumor size ≤ 0.5 cm N (%) | Tumor size > 0.5 cm N (%) | P value |
|---|---|---|---|
| Total patients | 161/326 (49.4) | 165/326 (50.6) | - |
| Age (years) | 36.7 (8–71) | 47.8 (8–76) | |
| ≤45 years | 107 (66.5) | 94 (56.9) | 0.034 |
| ≥45 years | 54 (33.5) | 71 (43.1) | |
| Gender | | | |
| Female | 139 (86.4) | 132 (80.0) | 0.08 |
| Male | 22 (13.6) | 33 (20.0) | |
| Mean size (cm) | 0.38 (0.1–0.5) | 0.68 (0.6–1.0) | <0.001 |
| Histopathologic variants | | | |
| Classic | 126 (78.2) | 139 (84.3) | |
| Follicular | 26 (16.2) | 14 (8.5) | |
| Hurthle cell | 4 (2.5) | 4 (2.4) | 0.023 |
| Tall cell | 4 (2.5) | 7 (4.3) | |
| Sclerosing | 1 (0.6) | - | |
| Multifocal | | | |
| Yes | 36 (22.4) | 89 (53.9) | |
| No | 125 (77.6) | 76 (46.1) | <0.001 |
| ETE | | | |
| Yes | 16 (9.9) | 46 (27.9) | <0.001 |
| No | 145 (90.1) | 119 (72.1) | |
| LVSI | | | |
| Yes | 14 (8.7) | 41 (24.9) | <0.001 |
| No | 147 (91.3) | 124 (75.1) | |
| Surgical margins | | | |
| Positive | 5 (3.1) | 30 (18.2) | |
| Negative | 156 (96.9) | 135 (81.8) | <0.001 |
| Background thyroid tissue | | | |
| Normal | 60 (37.3) | 38 (23.0) | |
| Multi-nodular goiter | 48 (29.8) | 58 (35.2) | |
| Lymphocytic thyroiditis/Hashimotos' thyroiditis | 53 (32.9) | 69 (41.8) | 0.05 |
| Lymph node metastasis | | | |
| Yes | 15 (9.3) | 27 (16.4) | |
| No | 146 (90.7) | 138 (83.6) | <0.001 |
| RAI ablation | | | |
| Yes | 50 (31.1) | 132 (67.3) | <0.001 |
| No | 111 (68.9) | 22 (13.3) | |
| Recurrences | | | |
| Locoregional | 4 (2.5) | 9 (5.5) | |
| *Thyroid bed* | *1/4* | *2/9* | |
| *Lymph nodes* | *3/4* | *7/9* | <0.001 |
| Distant | 2 (1.3) | 8 (4.9) | |
| *Lungs* | *2* | *7/8* | |
| *Bone* | *-* | *1/8* | |

*I-131* radioactive iodine 131, *N* number, *ETE* extra-thyroidal extension, *LVSI* lymphovascular space invasion, *RAI* radioactive iodine

**Table 4** Cox regression model of various prognostic factors for disease specific survival

| Variable | All patients | | | |
|---|---|---|---|---|
| | Univariate analysis | | Multivariate analysis | |
| | RR (95 % CI) | p | RR (95 % CI) | p |
| Age | | | | |
| ≤45 years | 1.05 (0.7–1.3) | | 1.07 (0.8–1.3) | |
| ≥45 years | 1.10 (0.8–1.4) | 0.6 | 1.10 (0.9–1.3) | 0.06 |
| Gender | | | | |
| Female | 1.07 (0.9–1.4) | | 1.05 (0.7–1.3) | |
| Male | 1.05 (0.7–1.3) | 0.6 | 1.40 (1.2–1.6) | 0.05 |
| Histopathologic variants | | | | |
| Classic | 1.05 (0.7–1.2) | | 1.20 (0.8–1.6) | |
| Follicular | 1.00 (0.6–1.8) | | 1.18 (0.7–1.5) | |
| Hurthle cell | 1.30 (1.1–1.7) | | 2.00 (1.6–2.4) | |
| Tall cell | 2.70 (1.6–4.5) | | 2.82 (2.4–4.6) | |
| Sclerosing | 1.80 (1.6–2.9) | <0.0001 | 2.00 (1.6–3.0) | <0.0001 |
| Multifocal | | | | |
| Yes | 3.1 (2.8–4.2) | | 2.94 (2.2–3.4) | |
| No | 1.0 (0.8–1.2) | <0.0001 | 1.07 (0.9–1.3) | <0.0001 |
| Surgical margins | | | | |
| Positive | 1.10 (0.9–1.4) | | 1.20 (0.8–1.6) | |
| Negative | 1.07 (0.9–1.4) | 0.7 | 1.17 (0.6–1.2) | 0.68 |
| ETE | | | | |
| Yes | 4.2 (3.5–5.1) | | 3.31 (1.7–4.2) | |
| No | 1.05 (0.7–1.1) | <0.0001 | 1.17 (0.9–1.4) | <0.0001 |
| LVSI | | | | |
| Yes | 2.0 (1.7–2.9) | | 1.81 (1.6–2.8) | |
| No | 1.0 (0.8–1.2) | 0.02 | 1.04 (0.9–1.5) | 0.03 |
| Lymph nodes | | | | |
| Positive | 4.45 (3.7–6.8) | | 3.74 (3.4–5.9) | |
| Negative | 1.17 (0.9–1.4) | <0.0001 | 1.01 (0.8–1.3) | <0.0001 |
| Mean postoperative TG | | | | |
| ≤2 ng/ml | 1.01 (0.7–1.2) | | 1.05 (0.7–1.2) | |
| >2 ng/ml | 1.04 (0.9–1.5) | 0.6 | 1.00 (0.6–1.8) | 0.6 |
| RAI ablation | | | | |
| Yes | 0.35 (0.2–0.7) | | 0.30 (0.2–0.8) | |
| No | 1.09 (1.0–1.9) | <0.0001 | 1.00 (0.6–1.8) | <0.0001 |

I-131 radioactive iodine 131, RR relative risk, CI confidence interval, ETE extra-thyroidal extension, LVSI lymphovascular space invasion, TG thyroglobulin, RAI radioactive iodine

sclerosing variants) in our series, which is in agreement with few previously published studies of PMC [18–20].

Recent studies regarding PMC have reported that patients with multinodular goiter (MNG) and with lymphocytic or Hashimotos' thyroiditis are associated with better prognosis; however, we could not reproduce the same results. Reason could be (a) few cases of histopathological proven MNG (32.5 %); (b) lack of preoperative TFTs in MNG patients; and (c) few number of patients with lymphocytic/Hashimoto's thyroiditis (37.5 %) [21].

Further, present study showed the lymph node involvement and tumor size as the most significant independent risk factors for recurrence. Although we found tumor size > 0.5 cm seem to be associated with high recurrence rates, we were not able to identify a size threshold below which there was no lymph node involvement and no risk of recurrence; as in tumor of size ≤ 0.5 cm, 9.3 % lymph node metastasis were seen along with 2.5 % local and 1.3 % distant failures. This supports the hypothesis, that lymph node involvement status is higher in PMC of size > 0.8 cm, but is independent of tumor size [22]. Patients tolerated adjuvant RAI ablation very well with minimal toxicity. Failure of RAI ablation to decrease local or distant failure risk in N1a/b as compared to N0 disease is an indicator of underlying tumor burden in neck and this supports the idea of prophylactic central neck dissection during thyroidectomy [23]. However, still there is much debate over the prophylactic central neck dissection because of potential increased risk of hypoparathyroidism associated with central neck dissection [24].

Strengths of our study were; (a) reasonable sample size of Saudi patients with PMC, and (b) long term follow up period. Limitations of our study were; (a) retrospective data; (b) no intention to treat based analysis, and (c) lack of availability of preoperative clinical data, diagnostic methods (FNAC and radiology), tumor characteristics and baseline TFTs.

## Conclusions

In conclusion, among all PTC, 31.6 % of patients are diagnosed as PMC. Despite excellent DFS rates, a small proportion of patients with PMC develop recurrences after treatment. These recurrences not only badly affect physical health, but also mental and social health and overall quality of life. Based on our results we conclude that;

- High percentage of multifocality in our population of PMC favors near total or total thyroidectomy against lobectomy, which can be an option for unifocal PMC.
- Age > 45 years and gender were not found strong prognostic factors of DFS.
- Adjuvant RAI therapy improves DFS in PMC patients with aggressive histopathologic variants, multifocality, ETE, LVSI, tumor size (>0.5 cm in absence of other features) and lymph node involvement (≥150 mCi). In absence of N0 neck, there is significant difference of DFS in two doses (30 mCi vs. 100 mCi).

- Failure of RAI ablation to decrease risk in N1a/b supports prophylactic central neck dissection during thyroidectomy, however more trials are warranted.

## Abbreviations

DTC: Differentiated thyroid cancer; DFS: Disease free survival; DMC: Distant metastasis control; ETE: Extrathyroid extension; PMC: Papillary microcarcinoma; PTC: Papillary thyroid cancer; FTC: Follicular thyroid cancer; LVSI: Lymphovascular invasion; LR: Locoregional recurrence; LRC: Locoregional control; mCi: Millicurie; OS: Overall survival; RAI: Radioactive iodine-131; TG: Thyroglobulin; WBS: Whole body scintigraphy.

## Competing interests

The authors declared no potential conflicts of interest with respect to the research, authorship, or publication of this article.

## Authors' contribution

KAQ conceived the study. MAA, KAQ, AAH collected the data. MAT and YB performed the statistical analysis. NAJ and HF performed histopathological data collection and review. All authors read and approved the final manuscript.

## Author details

[1]Department of Otolaryngology-Head & Neck Surgery, College of Medicine, King Saud University, Riyadh, Saudi Arabia. [2]Radiation Oncology, Comprehensive Cancer Center, King Fahad Medical City, Riyadh 59046, Saudi Arabia. [3]Endocrinology and thyroid Oncology, King Fahad Medical City, Riyadh 59046, Saudi Arabia. [4]Radiation Oncology, NCI, Cairo University, Cairo, Egypt. [5]Histopathology, King Fahad Medical City, Riyadh 59046, Saudi Arabia. [6]Radiation Oncology, King AbdulAziz University, Riyadh 59046, Saudi Arabia.

## References

1. Jemal A, Siegel R, Ward E, Hao Y, Xu J, Thun MJ. Cancer statistics, 2009. CA Cancer J Clin. 2009;59:225–49.
2. Hussain F, Iqbal S, Mehmood A, Bazarbashi S, ElHassan T, Chaudhri N. Incidence of thyroid cancer in the Kingdom of Saudi Arabia, 2000–2010. Hematol Oncol Stem Cell Ther. 2013;6:58–64.
3. Cooper DS, Doherty GM, Haugen BR, Haugen BR, Kloos RT, Lee SL, et al. The american thyroid association guidelines taskforce. Management guidelines for patients with thyroid nodules and differentiated thyroid cancer. Thyroid. 2006;16:109–41.
4. Senchenkov A, Staren ED. Ultrasound in head and neck surgery: thyroid, parathyroid, and cervical lymph nodes. Surg Clin North Am. 2004;84:973–1000.
5. Lloyd R, De Lellis R, Heitz R, Eng C. World health organization classification of tumours: pathology and genetics of tumours of the endocrine organs Lyon. France: IARC Press International Agency for Research on Cancer; 2004.
6. Pellegriti G, Scollo C, Lumera G, Regalbuto C, Vigneri R, Belfiore A. Clinical behavior and outcome of papillary thyroid cancers smaller than 1.5 cm in diameter: study of 299 cases. J Clin Endo Metabol. 2004;89:3713–20.
7. Ito Y, Miyauchi A, Inoue H, Fukushima M, Kihara M, Higashiyama T, et al. An observational trial for papillary thyroid microcarcinoma in Japanese patients. World J Surg. 2010;34:28–35.
8. Ito Y, Miyauchi A, Kihara M, Higashiyama T, Kobayashi K, Miya A. Patient age is significantly related to the progression of papillary microcarcinoma of the thyroid under observation. Thyroid. 2014;24:27–34.
9. Yu XM, Wan Y, Sippel RS, Chen H. Should all papillary thyroid microcarcinomas be aggressively treated? An analysis of 18,445 cases. Ann Surg. 2011;254:653–60.
10. Kim HJ, Kim SW. Radioactive iodine ablation does not prevent recurrences in patients with papillary thyroid microcarcinoma. Clin Endocrinol (Oxf). 2013;79:445.
11. Mercante G, Frasoldati A, Pedroni C, Formisano D, Renna L, Piana S, et al. Prognostic factors affecting neck lymph node recurrence and distant metastasis in papillary microcarcinoma of the thyroid. Thyroid. 2009;19:707–16.
12. Besic N, Pilko G, Petric R, Hocevar M, Zgajnar J. Papillary thyroid microcarcinoma: prognostic factors and treatment. J Surg Oncol. 2008;97:221–5.
13. Ross DS, Litofsky D, Ain KB, Bigos T, Brierley JD, Cooper DS, et al. Recurrence after treatment of micropapillary thyroid cancer. Thyroid. 2009;19:1043–8.
14. McDougall IR, Camargo CA. Treatment of micropapillary carcinoma of the thyroid: where do we draw the line? Thyroid. 2007;17:1093–6.
15. Pelizzo MR, Merante Boschin I, Toniato A, Piotto A, Bernante P, Pagetta C, et al. Papillary thyroid microcarcinoma. Long-term outcome in 587 cases compared with published data. Minerva Chir. 2007;62:315–25.
16. Karatzas T, Vasileiadis I, Kapetanakis S, Karakostas E, Chrousos G, Kouraklis G. Risk factors contributing to the difference in prognosis for papillary versus micropapillary thyroid carcinoma. Am J Surg. 2013;206:586–93.
17. Creach KM, Siegel BA, Nussenbaum B, Grigsby PW. Radioactive iodine therapy decreases recurrence in thyroid papillary microcarcinoma. ISRN Endocrinol. 2012;2012:816386. doi:10.5402/2012/816386.
18. Bilimoria KY, Bentrem DJ, Ko CY, Stewart AK, Winchester DP, Talamonti MS, et al. Extent of surgery affects survival for papillary thyroid cancer. Ann Surg. 2007;246:375–81.
19. Bernstein J, Virk RK, Hui P, Prasad A, Westra WH, Tallini G, et al. Tall cell variant of papillary thyroid microcarcinoma: clinicopathologic features with BRAF (V600E) mutational analysis. Thyroid. 2013;23:1525–31.
20. Kazaure HS, Roman SA, Sosa JA. Aggressive variants of papillary thyroid cancer: incidence, characteristics and predictors of survival among 43,738 patients. Ann Surg Oncol. 2012;19:1874–80.
21. Koo JS, Hong S, Park CS. Diffuse sclerosing variant is a major subtype of papillary thyroid carcinoma in the young. Thyroid. 2009;19:1225–31.
22. Elisei R, Molinaro E, Agate L, Bottici V, Masserini L, Ceccarelli C, et al. Are the clinical and pathological features of differentiated thyroid carcinoma really changed over the last 35 years? Study on 4187 patients from a single Italian institution to answer this question. J Clin Endocrinol Metab. 2010;95:1516–27.
23. Ito Y, Higashiyama T, Takamura Y, Miya A, Kobayashi K, Matsuzuka F, et al. Risk factors for recurrence to the lymph node in papillary thyroid carcinoma patients without preoperatively detectable lateral node metastasis: validity of prophylactic modified radical neck dissection. World J Surg. 2007;31: 2085–91.
24. Wang TS, Cheung K, Farrokhyar F, Roman SA, Sosa JA. A meta-analysis of the effect of prophylactic central compartment neck dissection on locoregional recurrence rates in patients with papillary thyroid cancer. Ann Surg Oncol. 2013;20:3477–83.

# 10

# Transoral laser microsurgery for the treatment of oropharyngeal cancer

Jonathan C. Melong[1*], Matthew H. Rigby[1], Martin Bullock[2], Robert D. Hart[1], Jonathan R.B. Trites[1] and S. Mark Taylor[1]

## Abstract

**Objective:** The optimal treatment strategy for oropharyngeal squamous cell carcinoma is highly debated. However, growing evidence supports the use of minimally invasive techniques, such as transoral laser microsurgery (TLM), as a first-line treatment modality for these carcinomas. The purpose of our study was to assess the efficacy and safety of TLM for the treatment of primary and recurrent oropharyngeal carcinomas.

**Methods:** All patients with oropharyngeal carcinoma undergoing TLM at the QEII Health Sciences Centre in Halifax, Nova Scotia were identified within a prospective database monitoring TLM outcomes. Kaplan-Meier survival analysis was used to evaluate the following end points at 36 months: local control (LC), disease-specific survival (DSS), and disease-free survival (DFS). Safety endpoints included complications following surgery and long term morbidity related to TLM.

**Results:** Between 2003 and 2014, 39 patients with oropharyngeal carcinoma underwent TLM resection. Twenty-eight (72 %) patients had primary carcinoma, nine (23 %) were radiation/chemoradiation (RT/CRT) failures, and two (5 %) had second primaries following previous RT/CRT. Three patients had stage I disease, 8 stage II, 5 stage III, and 23 stage IV disease. HPV status was available for 26 patients, of which 23 (88 %) had HPV positive disease. Kaplan-Meier estimates of 36-month LC, DSS, and DFS for primary oropharyngeal carcinomas were 85.5 % (SE 10.6 %), 85.7 % (SE 13.2 %) and 77.7 % (SE 12.5 %) respectively. Thirty-six-month outcomes for RT/CRT failures were 66.76 % (SE 15.7 %) for LC and 55.6 % (SE 16.6 %) for DSS and DFS. Three patients developed complications following surgery.

**Conclusions:** Observed 36-month efficacy and safety outcomes support the use of TLM for the treatment of primary and recurrent oropharyngeal carcinoma.

**Keywords:** Transoral laser microsurgery, Minimally invasive surgery, Oropharyngeal carcinoma, Head and neck surgery, Head and neck cancer

## Introduction

The incidence of oropharyngeal squamous cell carcinoma (OSCC) has been increasing, largely because of increasing rates of Human Papilloma Virus (HPV) infection [1–4]. This is an important trend clinically as HPV positive OSCC is associated with a better prognosis and treatment outcome [5, 6]. In the past, the management of OSCC has largely been guided by treatments that minimized functional morbidities. Radiation/chemoradiation (RT/CRT) was often preferred because historically, surgical intervention involved open en bloc resection of the tumour with free flap reconstruction, resulting in significant compromise of surrounding structures and ultimately function. However, RT/CRT has been associated with significant acute and long term toxicities and decreased quality of life [7–10].

More recently, transoral laser microsurgery (TLM) has emerged as a minimally invasive, endoscopic surgical technique for the management of oropharyngeal and laryngeal carcinomas. Initially used for carefully selected early stage head and neck cancers, experience with TLM has expanded its use to include select advanced lesions [11, 12]. Contraindications to TLM include inadequate access to the primary site (e.g. trismus, large tongue base, prominent dentition, etc.), large vessel proximity or

* Correspondence: jonathan.melong@dal.ca
[1]Division of Otolaryngology - Head and Neck Surgery, Queen Elizabeth II Health Sciences Centre and Dalhousie University, Halifax, NS, Canada
Full list of author information is available at the end of the article

involvement (e.g. tumour adjacent to the carotid bulb or internal carotid, deep bilateral base of tongue invasion increasing the risk of damage to both lingual arteries, etc.), and oncologic contraindications including T4b cancers, unresectable neck disease or multiple distant metastases [13, 14]. Despite these limitations, TLM offers potential advantages over open surgery including shorter recovery time, fewer complications and better functional outcomes [15–17]. Similarly, preliminary studies have demonstrated TLM to have improved functional outcomes compared to RT/CRT, particularly with respect to swallowing function [18, 19]. Surgical intervention also offers the advantage of pathologic characterization of the tumour, helping to guide further management and treatment, an advantage that is not readily available with RT/CRT.

The purpose of this study was to evaluate the oncologic measures of TLM for OSCC at our center, adding to the growing evidence of support for the use of TLM as a first line treatment modality for these carcinomas.

## Methods
This was a prospective, cohort study based on a database monitoring all malignancies treated with TLM at the QEII Health Sciences Centre in Halifax, Nova Scotia. The collection of information within the database was approved by our institutional research ethics board. The database was created in 2005 and has been prospectively maintained since that time. Information prior to 2005 was collected retrospectively at the time of the creation of the database. Details regarding data collection and the information contained within the database have been described previously [20, 21].

Between January 2002 and December 2014, approximately 300 different patients with suspected upper aerodigestive tract malignancies were treated with TLM by the senior author at our centre. All cases of primary or recurrent OSCC treated with TLM were included in the current study. Exclusion criteria included malignancies in all other sites of the upper aerodigestive tract treated with TLM.

### TLM, neck dissection and adjuvant therapy
All patients in the cohort underwent TLM resection. At the time of resection, a FK Retractor and/or Bouchayer laryngoscope was used to obtain adequate tumour exposure. Once adequate exposure was obtained, tumours were excised with a $CO_2$ laser using a tumour-splitting approach. Margin status was determined at the time of surgery through frozen section analysis. Positive frozen margins were subsequently resected until negative margins were obtained. Following surgery, tissue submitted for intraoperative margin analysis was resubmitted for routine processing. The main resection specimen was also submitted in toto for pathological characterization of the tumor.

Neck dissections were done concurrently at the time of TLM resection. In keeping with current guidelines, all patients were considered for concurrent neck dissections unless they had previous radiation failure or had no evidence of clinical or radiologic neck disease [22]. The exception were patients who had previous radiation failure, but stopped radiation early because of side-effects or presented with new or recurrent neck disease for which a neck dissection was not previously done. Patients with primary tonsil carcinoma underwent ipsilateral neck dissections while patients with base of tongue carcinomas underwent bilateral neck dissections. External carotid branches were ligated at the time of the neck dissection, including ligation of lingual and facial arteries.

Adjuvant therapy was offered to patients who met one or more of the following criteria, unless there was a contraindication to therapy: advanced disease, multiple nodal involvement, extracapsular extension from involved lymph nodes, perineural invasion, or positive margins following TLM resection. This is in keeping with current evidence that demonstrates improved survival with adjuvant therapy in these select patients [22–25].

## Analysis
A descriptive analysis of demographics, morbidities, and outcomes was performed. HPV status was determined by p16 immunohistochemistry. HPV positive disease was defined by strong, diffuse nuclear and cytoplasmic positivity (>70 %) of tumor cells for the p16 marker. Smoking status was self-reported by patients and categorized into current, past or non-smoking status at the time of surgery. Margin status was determined by reviewing individual pathology reports for all patients in the cohort. Close margins were defined as any margin less than 5 mm.

All statistical testing was performed using an intention-to-treat analysis. Kaplan-Meier 36-month survival analysis was performed for the following end points: local control (LC), disease-free survival (DFS), and disease-specific survival (DSS). Local control was defined as local recurrence-free survival obtained with one TLM resection or with subsequent reresection(s) for positive or close margins. Disease-free survival was defined as no local or regional recurrence or presence of a new second primary oropharyngeal tumour. Cancers were defined as a second primary tumour if they occurred more than 5 years after the last received treatment or if they occurred on the contralateral side to a previously treated unilateral tumour that did not cross the midline.

## Results
Between 2002 and 2014, 39 patients (31 males and 8 females) with oropharyngeal carcinoma underwent TLM

resection (Table 1). The mean age of the cohort at the time of diagnosis was 59.6 years (range 32–80). Twenty-eight (72 %) patients had primary carcinoma, 9 (23 %) were RT/CRT failures, and 2 (5 %) had second primaries following previous RT/CRT. Three patients had stage I disease, 8 stage II, 5 stage III, and 23 stage IV. HPV status was available for 26 patients, of which 23 (88 %) had HPV positive disease. The mean time of follow-up was 23 months. Among patients with primary OSCC, 21 patients received adjuvant therapy; 14 received radiation therapy and seven received chemoradiation. Twenty-nine (75 %) patients underwent concurrent neck dissections at

**Table 1** Patient characteristics (n = 39)

| Characteristic | Number of patients (%) |
|---|---|
| Age, y | |
| Mean (Range) | 59.6 (32–80) |
| Sex | |
| Male | 31 (79.5 %) |
| Female | 8 (20.5 %) |
| Tumour subsite | |
| Base of tongue | 20 (51 %) |
| Tonsil | 19 (49 %) |
| Stage | |
| I | 3 (7.5 %) |
| II | 8 (20.5 %) |
| III | 5 (13 %) |
| IV | 23 (59 %) |
| T Stage | |
| T1 | 9 (23 %) |
| T2 | 23 (59 %) |
| T3 | 7 (18 %) |
| T4 | 0 (0 %) |
| N stage | |
| N0 | 13 (33 %) |
| N1 | 3 (8 %) |
| N2a | 5 (13 %) |
| N2b | 13 (33 %) |
| N2c | 2 (5 %) |
| N3 | 3 (8 %) |
| HPV status (n = 26) | |
| Positive | 23 (88.5 %) |
| Negative | 3 (11.5 %) |
| Smoking status (n = 37) | |
| Current smoker | 6 (16 %) |
| Past smoker | 20 (54 %) |
| Lifetime nonsmoker | 11 (30 %) |

the time of TLM resection. The average length of hospital stay was 3.8 days (range 2–10 days).

Three patients developed complications following TLM resection. One patient experienced significant postoperative bleeding requiring a blood transfusion 14 days postoperatively. The patient was taken to the OR for exploration, but no active site of bleeding could be identified. The bleeding resolved spontaneously and was later determined to be caused from a longstanding gastric ulcer. Two patients developed cardiovascular complications. One patient experienced a myocardial infarction following TLM reresection of a positive margin and another patient developed a pulmonary embolism 3 days postoperatively. All patients recovered from their complications.

Two patients required a gastrostomy tube (G-tube) postoperatively following initial TLM resection. One patient required a temporary G-tube (<2 months) following TLM resection for swallowing difficulties. The other patient required a long-term G-tube following postoperative CRT for a close margin. One and two year G-tube rates following initial TLM resection were 3 and 0 %, respectively. Three patients required G-tubes following salvage therapy for recurrences. One patient required a temporary G-tube (<6 months) following salvage radiation therapy for a local recurrence. Another patient, who underwent a radical neck dissection following recurrence of a neck mass, subsequently developed a hematoma postoperatively and required a tracheostomy and G-tube for breathing and swallowing difficulties. Finally, one patient who ultimately underwent a total laryngopharyngectomy for new primary disease, required a G-tube postoperatively after the development of a tracheoesophageal fistula. Of note, one patient developed mild velopharyngeal insufficiency postoperatively that improved overtime without intervention and another patient, who was a previous CRT failure with a preoperative G-tube, was able to have their G-tube successfully removed following TLM resection.

Five patients had temporary tracheostomies following TLM. Initially, this was done for all TLM resections for anticipated postoperative swelling. This practice was stopped after it was seen that most patients had minimal swelling postoperatively. All five patients had their tracheostomies removed prior to discharge. One and two year tracheostomy rates were 0 %.

There were eight cases of recurrence following TLM, including five local recurrences (two of which also had regional recurrence), two regional recurrences, and one case of metastasis. There was also one case of a new primary in a patient with a right tonsil OSCC who went on to develop a left piriform sinus OSCC following TLM. Recurrence was more common among RT/CRT failures compared to patients with new primary oropharyngeal carcinoma. Kaplan-Meier estimates of 36-month LC for new primary oropharyngeal carcinoma was 85.5 % (SE 10.6 %) compared to 66.76 % (SE 15.7 %) for RT/CRT failures (Fig. 1).

During follow-up, seven patients died from their disease. All four RT/CRT failures who developed recurrence died from their disease. Two of four patients with primary oropharyngeal carcinoma who developed recurrence died from their disease. One patient, who received TLM for a second primary following previous CRT, developed a new primary following TLM and despite undergoing a total laryngopharyngectomy, ultimately developed metastatic disease and died from their disease. Kaplan-Meier estimates of 36-month DSS and DFS for primary oropharyngeal carcinoma were 85.7 % (SE 13.2 %) and 77.7 % (SE 12.5 %) compared to 55.6 % (SE 16.6 %) and 55.6 % (SE 16.6 %) for RT/CRT failures (Fig. 2).

Adjuvant therapy was administered to 21 of 28 patients with new primary OSCC (Table 2). Fourteen patients received radiation therapy and seven received chemoradiation. The remaining seven patients received no postoperative therapy. Among patients who did not receive postoperative therapy, three developed recurrence. All three patients had stage III/IV oropharyngeal carcinoma and of these, two patients refused adjuvant therapy for personal reasons and one was not a candidate because of comorbid health conditions. No patients with stage I/II disease treated with TLM monotherapy developed recurrence. Among patients who received adjuvant therapy, one patient developed metastatic disease.

Salvage therapy was carried out in two of four cases of recurrence among patients with primary oropharyngeal carcinoma. One case of local recurrence was salvaged with radiation therapy and the patient currently remains disease free. The other case of regional recurrence was salvaged with a selective neck dissection, but unfortunately the patient went on to develop metastatic disease and died from their disease. Among the other two cases of recurrence, one patient developed metastatic disease for which further therapy was not indicated and the other patient refused further treatment after local recurrence. As previously mentioned, a total laryngopharyngectomy was carried out in a patient who developed a new primary following TLM, but the patient ultimately developed metastatic disease and died from their disease. No previous RT/CRT failures who developed recurrence received salvage therapy.

Four patients (10 %) had positive margins and one patient (3 %) had a close margin at the primary site following initial TLM resection (Table 3). Four patients, including the patient who had a close margin, had primary OSCCs and one patient was a previous RT failure. The previous RT failure subsequently underwent TLM reresection, but ultimately developed locoregional recurrence and died from their disease. Among the four patients with primary OSCCs, three received postoperative chemoradiation and one received postoperative radiation. Two of the three patients who received postoperative chemoradiation stopped their chemotherapy early because of side-effects. Of the patients who received adjuvant therapy, one developed metastatic disease and died from their disease. The other three patients remain disease free.

Twenty three patients had HPV positive disease and three patients had HPV negative disease. HPV status could not be determined in 13 patients. Among HPV positive patients, two developed recurrence. One patient

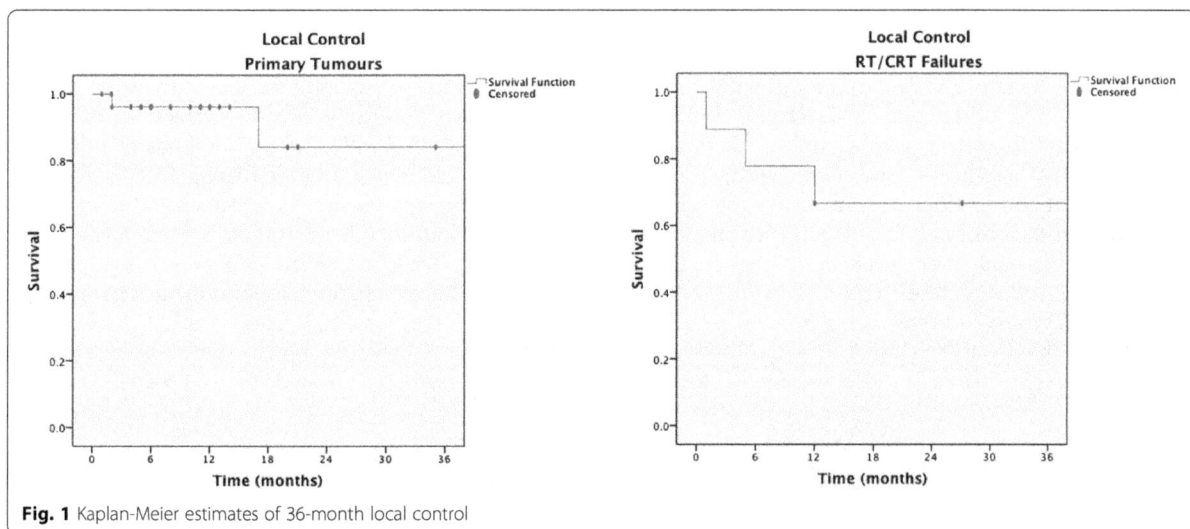

**Fig. 1** Kaplan-Meier estimates of 36-month local control

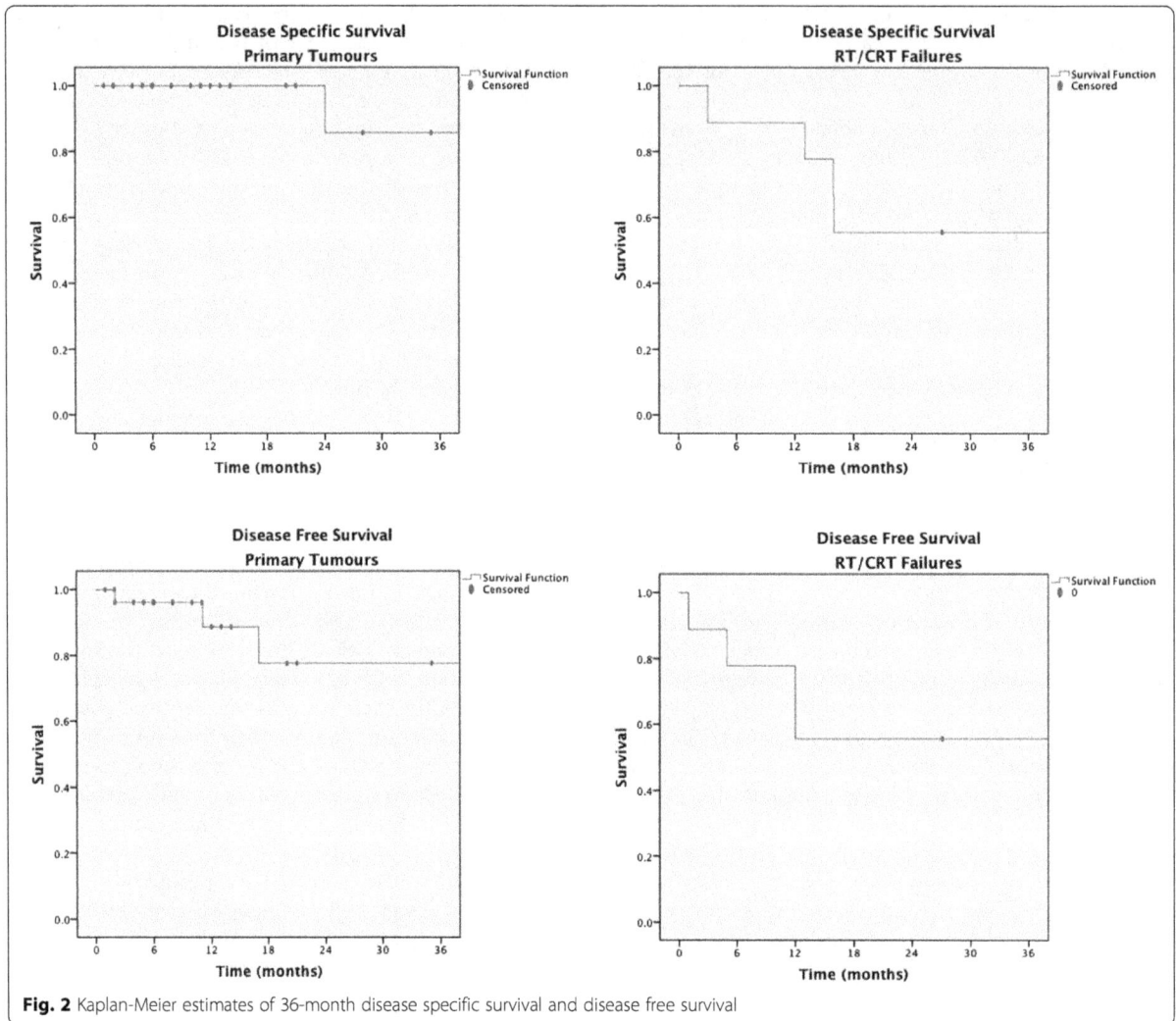

**Fig. 2** Kaplan-Meier estimates of 36-month disease specific survival and disease free survival

developed a local recurrence after initially refusing adjuvant radiation therapy and is currently awaiting further management. The other patient developed metastatic disease and died from their disease. Among the three patients with HPV negative disease, two developed recurrence. One patient developed recurrent regional disease and died from their disease. The other patient developed local recurrence and after receiving salvage radiation therapy, remains disease free.

## Discussion

Increasing evidence supports the use of transoral surgery as an effective, minimally invasive strategy for the treatment of OSCC. Currently, two transoral treatment modalities exist, TLM and transoral robotic surgery (TORS). Both transoral approaches have demonstrated excellent local control and overall survival for the treatment of primary OSCC, while minimizing functional compromise [11, 26–28]. Recent studies have also demonstrated TLM

**Table 2** Adjuvant therapy for new primary OSCC following TLM resection (n = 28)

| Adjunctive therapy | Number | Recurrence | New primary | Recurrence type | Laryngectomy | Death due to disease |
|---|---|---|---|---|---|---|
| None | 7 | 3 | 0 | 2 Local | 0 | 1 |
| | | | | 1 Regional | | |
| Radiation | 14 | 0 | 0 | 0 | 0 | 0 |
| Chemoradiation | 7 | 1 | 0 | 1 Metastatic | 0 | 1 |

**Table 3** Intraoperative disease control

|                  | Margins (−) | Margins (+) |
|------------------|-------------|-------------|
| Total            | 34          | 5           |
| Local recurrence | 3           | 0           |
| Locoregional     | 1           | 1           |
| Regional         | 2           | 0           |
| Metastatic       | 0           | 1           |
| New primary      | 1           | 0           |

and TORS to be effective as salvage therapy for recurrences in previous RT/CRT failures [29, 30]. This current study adds to the growing body of evidence, demonstrating TLM to have high rates of local control and overall survival for both primary and recurrent oropharyngeal cancers with excellent functional outcomes.

Eight patients in the cohort developed recurrence. This relatively high rate of recurrence can be expected based on the increased risk of recurrence among RT/CRT failures, which has been previously demonstrated to have a worse prognosis [31, 32]. Among the nine RT/CRT failures in the study, four developed recurrence. Despite these findings, TLM still demonstrated good local control and overall survival for RT/CRT failures when compared to other available salvage treatment modalities [31, 32].

Among patients with primary OSCC, recurrence was higher in patients who did not receive adjuvant therapy. This can be partly explained by the high rate of recurrence among patients with advanced disease who refused adjuvant therapy. In the current cohort, all three patients with advanced primary disease who did not receive adjuvant therapy following TLM, either because they refused or were not a candidate for RT/CRT, developed recurrence. There was no recurrence in patients with stage I/II primary disease who received TLM monotherapy. This is consistent with previous studies that have demonstrated TLM to be effective as a single treatment modality for early disease [33]. Although it is difficult to draw conclusions from small numbers, this study provides further evidence for the benefit of TLM as a single treatment modality for early disease and the potential benefit of postoperative adjuvant therapy in select patients with advanced disease.

In the current cohort, 4 patients had positive margins (10 %) and one patient (3 %) had a close margin at the primary site following initial TLM resection. This is comparable to other studies, which have demonstrated positive margin rates to be between 15 and 30 % [34]. Similar to the findings in other studies, patients with positive margins in the current cohort tended to have bulkier tumours (T2 or T3) and node positive disease [34]. One of the major advantages of TLM over other treatment modalities is the ability to perform reresection in the presence of positive margins. This is particularly beneficial for patients with previous RT/CRT failure, as treatment modalities for OSCC recurrence is limited. In the present study, only one patient with a positive margin underwent reresection. Unfortunately, the patient subsequently developed locoregional disease and died from their disease. The other three patients who had positive margins and one patient who had a close margin following initial TLM resection would also generally be considered for reresection. However, all four patients had advanced diseased and required postoperative adjuvant therapy. As pathology reports at our centre generally take several weeks to obtain, it was decided that RT/CRT should be initiated before final pathology results were obtained. This proved to be an effective approach as three of the four patients with positive/close margins who received adjuvant therapy currently remain disease free. However, in early disease TLM reresection alone could be considered, helping to avoid the acute and long term complications related to RT/CRT.

Previous studies have demonstrated HPV positive OSCCs to have a better prognosis and treatment outcome compared to HPV negative disease [5, 6]. This trend was reflected in our study where only 9 % (2/23) of patients with HPV positive disease developed a recurrence compared to 66 % (2/3) of patients with HPV negative disease. Unfortunately, status was unknown for 13 patients as p16 immunohistochemistry was only introduced and done routinely at our centre for OSCCs since 2009. Obviously with such a small number of HPV negative patients in our study, it is difficult to draw meaningful conclusions. However, the study does demonstrate TLM to be highly effective for the management of HPV positive disease.

One of the limitations of our study is the relatively limited period of follow-up for a large percentage of the cohort. Although the cohort included all patients undergoing TLM between 2002 and 2014, more than half of the patients underwent initial TLM resection from 2012 onward. As a result, statistical analysis was only adequately powered for follow-up at 3 years. Despite this limitation, the current study provides compelling evidence for the efficacy and safety of TLM for primary and recurrent OSCCs.

## Conclusion

The optimal treatment strategy for oropharyngeal carcinoma is highly debated. However, growing evidence supports the use of TLM as a safe and effective first-line treatment modality for OSCCs. This study provides further evidence for the use of TLM as a first-line treatment modality for primary and recurrent OSCCs, demonstrating excellent 3-year survival and functional outcomes.

## Abbreviations
OSCC: Oropharyngeal squamous cell carcinoma; HPV: Human Papilloma Virus; RT/CRT: Radiation/chemoradiation; TLM: Transoral laser microsurgery; TORS: Transoral robotic surgery; LC: Local control; DFS: Disease-free survival; DSS: Disease-specific survival.

## Competing interests
All authors declare that they have no competing interests.

## Author's contributions
JCM is the corresponding author and was involved in data acquisition, analysis and interpretation, and drafting of the manuscript. MHR was involved in data acquisition, analysis and interpretation and assisted with preparation and revision of the manuscript. MB was involved in tumour pathology characterization and assisted with revision of the manuscript. RDH and JRBT participated in data acquisition and assisted with revision of the manuscript. SMT was the research supervisor and assisted with primary data acquisition, analysis and interpretation, and assisted with preparation and revision of the manuscript. All authors have read and approved the final manuscript.

## Acknowledgements
Jonathan Melong held a summer studentship with funding provided by the DMRF Bergmann-Porter endowment.

## Author details
[1]Division of Otolaryngology - Head and Neck Surgery, Queen Elizabeth II Health Sciences Centre and Dalhousie University, Halifax, NS, Canada. [2]Division of Anatomical Pathology, Queen Elizabeth II Health Sciences Centre and Dalhousie University, Halifax, NS, Canada.

## References
1.  Nichols AC, Palma DA, Dhaliwal SS, Tan S, Theuer J, Chow W, et al. The epidemic of human papillomavirus and oropharyngeal cancer in a Canadian population. Curr Oncol. 2013;20(4):212–9.
2.  Habbous S, Chu KP, Qiu X, La Delfa A, Harland LT, Fadhel E, et al. The changing incidence of human papillomavirus-associated oropharyngeal cancer using multiple imputation from 2000 to 2010 at a Comprehensive Cancer Centre. Cancer Epidemiol. 2013;37(6):820–9.
3.  Ramqvist T, Dalianis T. Oropharyngeal cancer epidemic and human papillomavirus. Emerg Infect Dis. 2010;16(11):1671–7.
4.  Shack L, Lau HY, Huang L, Doll C, Hao D. Trends in the incidence of human papillomavirus-related noncervical and cervical cancers in Alberta, Canada: a population-based study. CMAJ Open. 2014;2(3):E127–32.
5.  Licitra L, Perrone F, Bossi P, Suardi S, Mariani L, Artusi R, et al. High-risk human papillomavirus affects prognosis in patients with surgically treated oropharyngeal squamous cell carcinoma. J Clin Oncol. 2006;24(36):5630–6.
6.  Nichols AC, Dhaliwal SS, Palma DA, Basmaji J, Chapeskie C, Dowthwaite S, et al. Does HPV type affect outcome in oropharyngeal cancer? J Otolaryngol Head Neck Surg. 2013;42:9.
7.  Broglie MA, Soltermann A, Haile SR, Röösli C, Huber GF, Schmid S, et al. Quality of life of oropharyngeal cancer patients with respect to treatment strategy and p16-positivity. Laryngoscope. 2013;123(1):164–70.
8.  Goepfert RP, Yom SS, Ryan WR, Cheung SW. Development of a chemoradiation therapy toxicity staging system for oropharyngeal carcinoma. Laryngoscope. 2015;125(4):869–76.
9.  Machtay M, Moughan J, Farach A, Martin-O'Meara E, Galvin J, Garden AS, et al. Hypopharyngeal dose is associated with severe late toxicity in locally advanced head-and-neck cancer: an RTOG analysis. Int J Radiat Oncol Biol Phys. 2012;84(4):983–9.
10. McBride SM, Parambi RJ, Jang JW, Goldsmith T, Busse PM, Chan AW. Intensity-modulated versus conventional radiation therapy for oropharyngeal carcinoma: long-term dysphagia and tumor control outcomes. Head Neck. 2014;36(4):492–8.
11. Haughey BH, Hinni ML, Salassa JR, Hayden RE, Grant DG, Rich JT, et al. Transoral laser microsurgery as primary treatment for advanced-stage oropharyngeal cancer: a United States multicenter study. Head Neck. 2011;33(12):1683–94.
12. Rich JT, Milov S, Lewis Jr JS, Thorstad WL, Adkins DR, Haughey BH. Transoral laser microsurgery (TLM) +/− adjuvant therapy for advanced stage oropharyngeal cancer: outcomes and prognostic factors. Laryngoscope. 2009;119(9):1709–19.
13. Hinni ML, Lott DG. Contemporary Transoral Surgery for Primary Head and Neck Cancer. San Diego, CA: Plural Publishing Inc, 2014: 86–94.
14. Weinstein GS, O'Malley BW Jr, Rinaldo A, Silver CE, Werner JA, Ferlito A. Understanding contraindications for transoral robotic surgery (TORS) for oropharyngeal cancer. Eur Arch Otorhinolaryngol. 2015;272(7):1551-2.
15. Mydlarz WK, Chan JY, Richmon JD. The role of surgery for HPV-associated head and neck cancer. Oral Oncol. 2014 Oct 30.
16. Sinha P, Hackman T, Nussenbaum B, Wu N, Lewis Jr JS, Haughey BH. Transoral laser microsurgery for oral squamous cell carcinoma: oncologic outcomes and prognostic factors. Head Neck. 2014;36(3):340–51.
17. Williams CE, Kinshuck AJ, Derbyshire SG, Upile N, Tandon S, Roland NJ, et al. Transoral laser resection versus lip-split mandibulotomy in the management of oropharyngeal squamous cell carcinoma (OPSCC): a case match study. Eur Arch Otorhinolaryngol. 2014;271(2):367–72.
18. Chen AM, Daly ME, Luu Q, Donald PJ, Farwell DG. Comparison of functional outcomes and quality of life between transoral surgery and definitive chemoradiotherapy for oropharyngeal cancer. Head Neck. 2015;37(3):381–5.
19. Huang SH, Hansen A, Rathod S, O'Sullivan B. Primary surgery versus (chemo)radiotherapy in oropharyngeal cancer: the radiation oncologist's and medical oncologist's perspectives. Curr Opin Otolaryngol Head Neck Surg. 2015;23(2):139–47.
20. Taylor SM, Rigby MH. Endoscopic treatment of Cis-T2 glottic cancer with a CO2 laser: 2-year survival analysis of 36 cases. J Otolaryngol Head Neck Surg. 2008;37:582–5.
21. Rigby MH, Taylor SM. Endoscopic treatment of Cis-T2 glottic cancer with a CO(2) laser: preliminary results from a Canadian centre. J Otolaryngol. 2007;36:106–10.
22. National Comprehensive Cancer Network Practice Guidelines in Oncology-v.2.2013, Head and Neck Cancers, Cancer of the Oropharynx. 2013.
23. Cooper JS, Zhang Q, Pajak TF, Forastiere AA, Jacobs J, Saxman SB, et al. Long-term follow-up of the RTOG 9501/intergroup phase III trial: postoperative concurrent radiation therapy and chemotherapy in high-risk squamous cell carcinoma of the head and neck. Int J Radiat Oncol Biol Phys. 2012;84(5):1198–205.
24. Zhang H, Dziegielewski PT, Biron VL, Szudek J, Al-Qahatani KH, O'Connell DA, et al. Survival outcomes of patients with advanced oral cavity squamous cell carcinoma treated with multimodal therapy: a multi-institutional analysis. J Otolaryngol Head Neck Surg. 2013;42:30.
25. Patel SH, Hinni ML, Hayden RE, Wong WW, Dueck AC, Zarka MA, et al. Transoral laser microsurgery followed by radiation therapy for oropharyngeal tumors: the Mayo Clinic Arizona experience. Head Neck. 2014;36(2):220–5.
26. Grant DG, Salassa JR, Hinni ML, Pearson BW, Perry WC. Carcinoma of the tongue base treated by transoral laser microsurgery, part one: Untreated tumors, a prospective analysis of oncologic and functional outcomes. Laryngoscope. 2006;116(12):2150–5.
27. Hinni ML, Nagel T, Howard B. Oropharyngeal cancer treatment: the role of transoral surgery. Curr Opin Otolaryngol Head Neck Surg. 2015;23(2):132–8.
28. Kelly K, Johnson-Obaseki S, Lumingu J, Corsten M. Oncologic, functional and surgical outcomes of primary Transoral Robotic Surgery for early squamous cell cancer of the oropharynx: a systematic review. Oral Oncol. 2014;50(8):696–703.
29. Reynolds LF, Rigby MH, Trites J, Hart R, Taylor SM. Outcomes of transoral laser microsurgery for recurrent head and neck cancer. J Laryngol Otol. 2013;127(10):982–6.
30. White H, Ford S, Bush B, Holsinger FC, Moore E, Ghanem T, et al. Salvage surgery for recurrent cancers of the oropharynx: comparing TORS with standard open surgical approaches. JAMA Otolaryngol Head Neck Surg. 2013;139(8):773–8.
31. Omura G, Saito Y, Ando M, Kobayashi K, Ebihara Y, Yamasoba T, et al. Salvage surgery for local residual or recurrent pharyngeal cancer after radiotherapy or chemoradiotherapy. Laryngoscope. 2014;124(9):2075–80.
32. Zafereo ME, Hanasono MM, Rosenthal DI, Sturgis EM, Lewin JS, Roberts DB, et al. The role of salvage surgery in patients with recurrent squamous cell carcinoma of the oropharynx. Cancer. 2009;115(24):5723–33.

33.  Grant DG, Hinni ML, Salassa JR, Perry WC, Hayden RE, Casler JD. Oropharyngeal cancer: a case for single modality treatment with transoral laser microsurgery. Arch Otolaryngol Head Neck Surg. 2009;135(12):1225–30.
34.  Zevallos JP, Mitra N, Swisher-McClure S. Patterns of care and perioperative outcomes in transoral endoscopic surgery for oropharyngeal squamous cell carcinoma. Head Neck. 2014 Oct 28. [Epub ahead of print]

# 11

# Serum microRNA profiling to distinguish papillary thyroid cancer from benign thyroid masses

M. Elise R. Graham[1], Robert D. Hart[1], Susan Douglas[2], Fawaz M. Makki[1], Devanand Pinto[2], Angela L. Butler[1], Martin Bullock[3], Matthew H. Rigby[1], Jonathan R. B. Trites[1], S. Mark Taylor[1] and Rama Singh[2*]

## Abstract

**Objectives:** Papillary thyroid cancer (PTC) is increasing in incidence. Fine needle aspiration is the gold standard for diagnosis, but results can be indeterminate. Identifying tissue and serum biomarkers, like microRNA, is therefore desirable. We sought to identify miRNA that is differentially expressed in the serum of patients with PTC.

**Methods:** Serum miRNA was quantified in 31 female thyroidectomy patients: 13 with benign disease and 18 with PTC. qPCR results were compared for significant fold-changes in 175 miRNAs, against a pooled control.

**Results:** 128 miRNA qualified for analysis. There were identifiable fold-changes in miRNA levels between benign and control, and between PTC and control. There were statistically significant fold changes in the level of four miRNAs between benign and PTC: hsa-miR-146a-5p and hsa-miR-199b-3p were down-regulated, while hsa-let7b-5p and hsa-miR-10a-5p were up-regulated.

**Conclusions:** MicroRNA is differentially expressed in the serum of patients with PTC. Serum miRNA has the potential to aid in thyroid cancer diagnosis.

**Keywords:** Papillary thyroid cancer, MicroRNA, Serum testing, Biomarkers

## Background

Papillary thyroid carcinoma (PTC) accounts for up to 90 % of thyroid carcinomas, yet distinguishing carcinoma from benign thyroid conditions such as follicular adenomas, cysts and goiter can be difficult [1]. Thirty percent of fine needle aspirate specimens from thyroid nodules are indeterminate, and up to 75 % of patients undergo a hemithyroidectomy for benign disease unnecessarily [2–5]. As the incidence of PTC increases, along with the detection of incidental thyroid nodules on CT and ultrasound, research into the development of more sophisticated means of diagnosis is needed.

Recent research on the development of such diagnostic tools has focused on determining thyroid carcinoma gene expression profiles to identify markers of benign or malignant pathology [6]. Such markers, traditionally tested in tumor tissue, have been used to stratify indeterminate fine needle aspiration results to those more likely to be PTC versus benign nodules. Examples of potential markers that appear to be consistently up-regulated in PTC tissue samples are chitinase 3 like-1 (YKL-40), galectin-3 (Gal-3), cytokeratin 19 (CK19), tissue inhibitor of metalloproteinases-1 (TIMP-1) and angiopoetin-1 (Ang –1) [7–10].

An alternative to tumor tissue sampling is serum-based diagnostic testing. Serum testing would potentially allow for minimally invasive, safe and repeatable diagnosis, requiring less technical skill for collection. Although the feasibility of potential blood-based diagnostic testing has been shown [11], no biomarkers have been identified that reliably reflect elevated tumor tissue levels.

MicroRNAs (miRNAs) are non-coding RNA molecules involved in the regulation of gene expression [12]. miRNAs bind to messenger RNA (mRNA) and promote their degradation or prevent their translation into proteins. Over 2000 miRNA have been identified in the human genome,

* Correspondence: rama.singh@nrc-cnrc.gc.ca
Robert D. Hart and Rama Singh are co-senior authors on this manuscript
[2]NRC Human Health Therapeutics, Oxford Street, Halifax, NS, Canada
Full list of author information is available at the end of the article

and more are being identified at a rapid rate [13]. The first miRNA was incidentally identified in 1993; however, its function as a positive and negative bioregulator was not recognized until the early 2000s [14, 15]. Deregulation of miRNA has been associated with a number of diseases, including malignancies such as chronic lymphocytic leukemia, colon cancer, glioblastoma and astrocytoma [16–19]. Traditionally, miRNAs have been detected in tissue specimens; however, recent studies have also shown that miRNAs remains relatively stable and detectable in blood samples [20, 21].

Numerous independent studies have identified miRNA expression profiles in differentiated thyroid carcinoma tissue, suggesting they may play a role in the development and progression of this carcinoma. miRNA profiles identified in thyroid cancer have included miRNA-221, −222 and -181b [22, 23]. It is possible that these unique miRNA may allow for improved diagnosis, prognosis and monitoring response to treatment in thyroid carcinoma.

The objective of this study was to identify potential miRNA serum markers in patients with PTC. We hypothesized that, given the stability of miRNA in serum compared to traditional biomarkers, patients with PTC would show a measureable change in the select miRNA levels relative to patients with benign lesions.

## Materials and methods
### Patient sampling
This study was approved by the Capital Health Research Ethics Board and informed consent was obtained from all participants.

Blood samples (approximately 15 mL) were collected in EDTA tubes from patients at the time of intravenous catheter placement in the operating room, prior to the administration of any anesthetic. A dedicated research nurse prepared serum samples from whole blood by centrifugation to separate serum from other blood components. Serum was aliquoted into 1.5 mL Eppendorf tubes, which were de-identified, barcoded and stored at −80 °C for future use. This process generated a biobank of 205 samples. From these, 45 samples (26 PTC and 19 benign) were randomly selected from female patients with thyroid masses greater than 1 cm. Separate RNA extractions were performed on three aliquots of a commercially available serum samples from a pool of twenty healthy individuals (Precision Biologics, Dartmouth, NS, Canada) for use as controls. These samples were screened for the presence of hemolyzed red cells using the Nano-Drop™ 1000 spectrophotometer (NanoDrop Products, Wilmington, DE, USA) to detect optical density at 415 nm. Samples with evidence of hemolysis were excluded prior to further analysis, leaving 31 samples (13 benign, 18 PTC) (Table 1).

**Table 1** Sample selection

|  | # of samples | Female | Tumor >1 cm | Passed hemolysis |
|---|---|---|---|---|
| Benign | 118 | 87 | 19 | 13 |
| PTC | 87 | 50 | 26 | 18 |
| Control | 3 | - | - | 3 |

Serum sample collection. Control samples came from a commercially available pooled serum sample of 20 healthy individuals

### RNA isolation
Total RNA was extracted from 200 µL serum using the miRNeasy® Mini Kit (Qiagen, Mississauga, ON, Canada) as described by the manufacturer. A mixture containing 1.25 µg/mL of MS2 bacteriophage RNA, and RNA spike-ins was added to the serum. RNA was purified on an RNeasy® Mini spin column (Qiagen), eluted in 50 µL of RNase-free water, and stored at −80 °C.

### Sample quality control using spike-ins
To ensure that the quality of the input RNA was sufficiently high for effective reverse transcription (RT), cDNA synthesis and amplification, two types of RNA spike-ins were used. RNA isolation controls (UniSp2 and UniSp4) were added to the sample prior to purification and used to detect differences in extraction efficiency and the presence of inhibitors. The cDNA synthesis control (UniSp6) was added in the RT reaction to evaluate cDNA synthesis.

### Reverse Transcription (RT) and RT-qPCR
For quality assessment, qPCR assays for miRNA-103, −191, −23a, −30c, and −451 were performed. These miRNAs are expressed at a predictable level in the majority of sample types and are used to evaluate baseline miRNA content in the samples. A second hemolysis test was performed at this time using two of these microRNA: miR-451, which is increased in hemolyzed red blood cells compared to miR-23a, which is relatively stable in serum and plasma. A difference in Ct values (miR-23a minus miR-451) <8.0 qualified samples for analysis. Negative controls excluding template from the RT reaction were performed and profiled with the samples. Total RNA (2 µL) was reverse transcribed in 10 µL reactions using the miRCURY LNA™ Universal RT microRNA PCR, Polyadenylation and cDNA synthesis kit (Exiqon, Woburn, MA, USA). Each RT was performed in duplicate, including an artificial RNA spike-in (UniSp6). cDNA was diluted 50-fold and assayed in 10 µL qPCR reactions according to the protocol for miR-CURY LNA™ Universal RT microRNA PCR (Exiqon).

miRNAs were profiled using the microRNA Ready-to-Use PCR human serum/plasma panel containing 175 miRNAs plus controls (Exiqon). 5 µL RNA was reverse transcribed in 25 µL reactions and assayed as described above. Each microRNA was assayed once by qPCR and negative controls excluding template from the RT reaction were included. PCR was performed in a LightCycler® 480 Real-Time PCR System

(Roche Applied Science, Laval, QC, Canada) in 384-well plates. The amplification curves were analyzed using the Roche LC software, both for determination of expression values (2nd derivative Ct method) and for melting curve analysis.

### Data analysis and statistics

The raw data was extracted from the LightCycler 480 software. For quality control samples, an average Ct was calculated for the duplicate RTs, and evaluation of expression levels was performed based on raw Ct-values. The amplification efficiency was calculated using algorithms similar to the LinReg software [24]. All assays were inspected for distinct melting curves to ensure that the Tm was within the known specifications for the assay.

Statistics (limma expression analysis, including t-tests and false-discovery rates) were done on the R platform using the HTqPCR package [25]. Features where values were missing in more than 50 % of samples from any group (PTC, benign, control) and features where the negative controls were within 5 Ct values of the experimental Ct values were removed from the analysis. Data for microRNAs that were present in all 31 samples were normalized using norm rank-invariant normalization because it yielded the lowest standard deviations in the control replicates. For differential expression analysis, features with standard deviation >0.5 in the control group were removed. Random forest analysis was performed in the R platform using the random Forest package [26] and the ROCR package [27].

Gene targets for differentially expressed microRNAs were identified using a microRNA target prediction and annotation database (mirDB) using a prediction score of ≥80 (www.mirDB.org).

### Results

The consistent levels of all assays using RNA spike-ins (Uni-Sp2, Uni-Sp4 and Uni-Sp6) show that the RNA extraction as well as RT efficiency was similar for all samples, and that both RT and qPCR were successful. The baseline level, which is derived from the no-template control RT reaction, also shows that none of the samples contain inhibitors. Quality assessment of all positive and negative controls using qPCR assays for the commonly expressed miR-103, −191, −23a, −30c, and −451 showed Ct values between 22–24 for the positive control and ~40 for the negative control, indicating that the RT reaction worked well. The expression levels for all of the tested samples for these miRNAs were comparable to each other and to what is seen for other samples of similar types. Furthermore, the difference in Ct between miR-23a and miR-451 are 8.0 or lower in all samples, indicating minimal signs of hemolysis. Based on these quality control data we proceeded with the miR-panel profiling of all passed samples.

On average, 136 miRNAs were detected per sample and 128 miRNAs qualified for analysis, of which 64 were detected in all 31 samples profiled. After rank invariant normalization followed by Random Forest, t-Test and limma statistical analyses, two miRNAs (hsa-miR-150-5p and hsa-miR-342-3p) were down-regulated and two (hsa-let7b-5p and hsa-miR-191-5p) were up-regulated in benign vs. control samples (Fig. 1a; $p < 0.001$, FDR <5 %). For PTC vs. control samples, one additional microRNA (hsa-miR-146a-5p) was down-regulated and one additional microRNA was up-regulated (hsa-miR-93-5p) (Fig. 1b; $p < 0.001$, FDR <1 %). Importantly, between PTC and benign samples, there was statistically significant down-regulation of hsa-miR-146a-5p and hsa-miR-199b-3p, and up-regulation of hsa-let7b-5p and hsa-miR-10a-5p (Fig. 1c, $p < 0.05$), although the false discovery rate was high (50 %) in this comparison. Random Forest analysis produced a classifier consisting of 11 microRNAs (Fig. 2a), of which miRNAs hsa-miR-10a-5p, hsa-miR-146a-5p and hsa-miR-199b-3p were the most informative. Using this classifier, an Area Under the Curve (AUC) of 0.851 was obtained (Fig. 2b). Results of the limma and t-Test analysis are shown in Table 2.

We performed additional statistical testing by adjusting the p-values for multiple comparisons. The miRNA differences between control and benign samples were statistically significant (adjusted $p < 0.05$ for all miRNA), as were the comparison between PTC and control. When this additional statistical analysis was performed, the difference in miRNA between benign and malignant miRNA was no longer significant ($p > 0.05$).

By searching miRDB with the 11 microRNAs in the classifier, 186 unique gene targets were identified. These targets were mostly associated with metabolic process (GO:0008152, 100 targets), cellular process (GO:0009987, 70 targets) and cell communication (GO:0007154, 54 targets) (Fig. 3). Six microRNAs were down-regulated (hsa-miR-146a-5p, −199-3p, −376a-3p, 339-5p, 28-3p, and let-7d-3p), which would result in enhanced expression of the target genes. Five microRNAs were up-regulated (hsa-miR-375, −10b-5p, −10a-5p, −505-3p, and -let7b -5p), which would result in repression of the target genes.

### Discussion

This study identified that the serum of patients with benign thyroid tumors showed statistically significant down-regulation of miR-150-5p and miR-342-3p, and up-regulation of miR-let7b-5p and miR-191-5p compared to controls. The serum of patients with PTC also showed deregulation of these miRNA, with additional down-regulation of miR-146a-5p and up-regulation of miR-93-5p. Most importantly, there was statistically significant down-regulation of miR-146a-5p and miR-

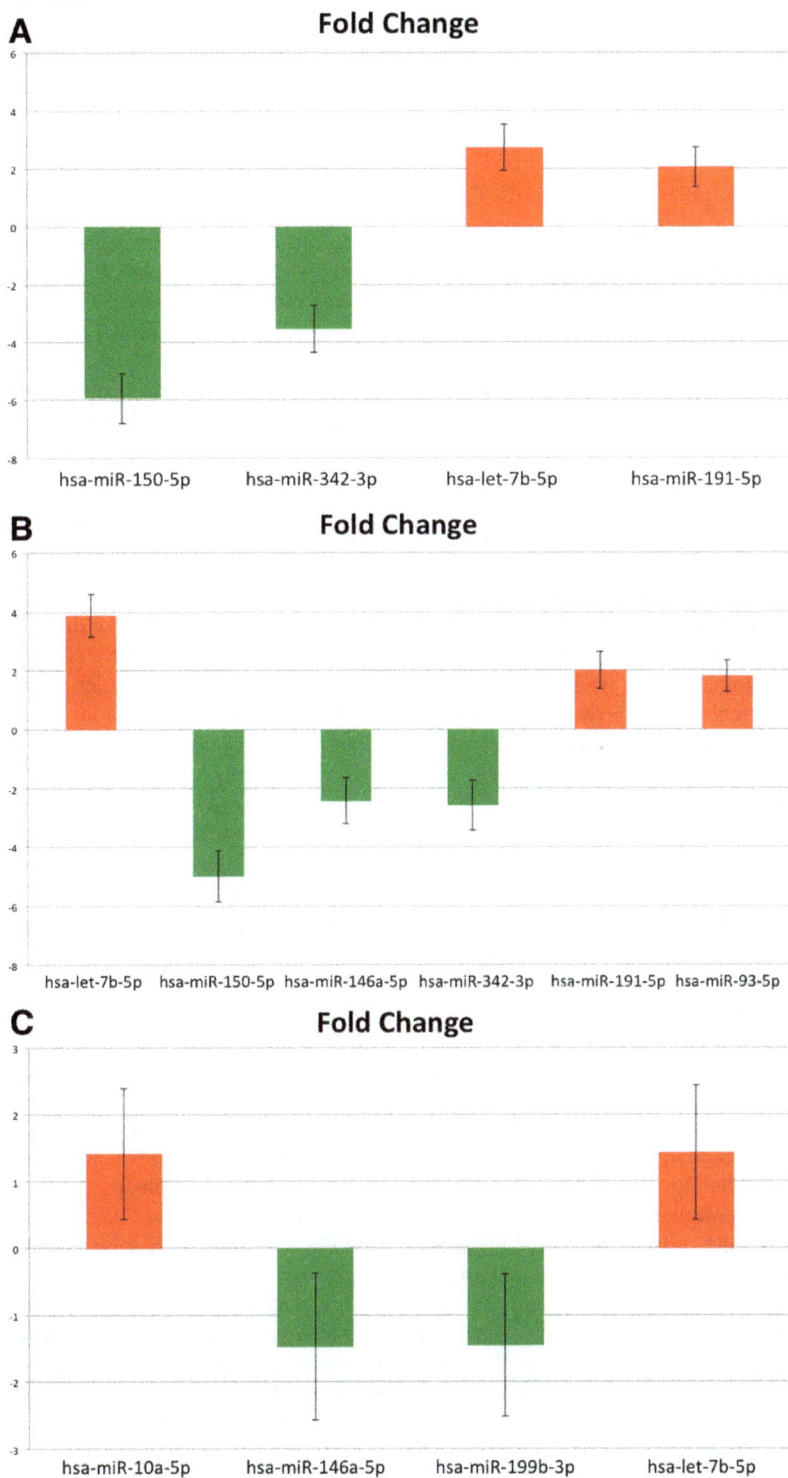

**Fig. 1** (See legend on next page.)

(See figure on previous page.)
**Fig. 1 a** Fold change in benign vs. control samples. Significant fold-changes were demonstrated in expression of four miRNAs between benign and control samples. **b** Fold change in PTC vs. control samples. Significant fold changes were demonstrated in expression of six miRNAs between PTC and control serum. Four of these were common to the benign vs. PTC comparison. **c** Fold change in PTC vs. benign samples. Statistically significant up-regulation of hsa-miR-10a-5p and hsa-let-7b-5p was seen between the serum of PTC vs. Benign patients, and statistically significant down-regulation of hsa-miR-146a-5p and hsa-miR-199b-3p. MicroRNAs hsa-miR-10-5p, hsa-miR-146a-5p and has-miR-199b-3 were also the most important hits in the Random Forest analysis

199b-3p and up-regulation of let7b-5p and miR-10a-5p when comparing PTC serum to that of patients with benign tumors using limma and t-tests. These are the standard tests used in miRNA literature. Unfortunately, these differences between miRNA between benign and PTC patients did not reach significance with the addition of adjusted p-value for multiple comparators.

The differences in expression levels between the control group and both the benign and PTC groups were the greatest, with average fold changes of 3.5 and 3.0 respectively. However, the average fold change between miRNAs that were differentially regulated between the patients with PTC and those with benign thyroid tumors was only 1.5. The practical impact of this modest difference is a relatively high false discovery rate of 50 %. In other words, two of the four miRNA are likely false positives. Therefore, this panel of miRNAs would require further validation in an independent cohort of patients.

Random Forest plots are used for classification and regression to create predictive models for the variable importance of large numbers of variables. A perfect predictor would have an area under the curve (AUC) of 1, whereas a predictor with an AUC of 0.5 has a predictive value no better than chance. The AUC in the Random Forest plot in PTC versus benign using a set of the 11 most informative miRNA was 0.851. These miRNA target genes were confirmed to be involved in metabolic and cellular processes and cell communication (Fig. 3).

Numerous studies have identified tissue miRNAs involved in PTC tumorigenesis. The majority of these compare PTC tissue to normal thyroid tissue – either from comparative controls or from adjacent "normal" thyroid tissue. He *et al.* were among the first to identify up-regulation of miRNA 146b, 221 and 222 in 20 patients with PTC [28]. miRNA-146b is closely related to miRNA-146a, which was identified in our study. MiR-146a is a known tumor suppressor and its down-regulation appears to enhance tumorigenesis. It plays a role in the classical NF-κB signal transduction pathway in PTC by modulating expression of protein kinase C epsilon (PKCε) and Ras/Raf-1 signaling. It also targets TRAF6 (mirDB score 100) and IRAK1 (mirDB score 87), which form part of a negative feedback loop in NF-κB signaling [29]. Pallate *et al.* also identified the down-regulation of miRNA-181b in PTC tissue, corroborating the results of He's group [30]. Tetzlaff *et al.* compared PTC tissue to multinodular goiter using formalin fixed paraffin embedded

tissue for analysis rather than fresh frozen tissue, and identified 13 up-regulated and 26 down-regulated miRNAs, including those stated above [31].

The let7 family of miRNA was the second group to be identified during the early study of miRNA [32]. Let7b-5p was up-regulated in our study, both in benign and malignant tumors, and exhibited a statistically significant increase when they were compared. It is often significantly up-regulated in various cancers and exerts its effects by enhancing expression of oncogenes such as Ras, c-Myc, cyclin D and HMG [33–35]. Elevated let-7b expression in PTC may have a similar effect on these genes [36–38].

The most significant limitation of our study was its small sample size (13 benign, 18 PTC and 3 controls), limiting our statistical power. This pilot study does have the potential to guide future research into these and other miRNAs to aid in the diagnosis of PTC.

Our study only included the PTC subtype of thyroid carcinoma. Although the diagnostic accuracy for anaplastic and medullary carcinoma is greater on cytopathology alone, follicular carcinoma still remains in the differential diagnosis in non-diagnostic FNA. A limited number of studies have published data on tissue miRNAs in FTC patients. The incidence of FTC is significantly less than that of PTC, therefore obtaining sufficient numbers for meaningful data analysis is more difficult [39, 40].

Although the application of tissue tumor markers such as miRNA and gene profiling may potentially improve diagnostic accuracy, these must be obtained by FNA biopsy and therefore remain invasive, unpleasant and inconvenient for patients. This study suggests miRNA in serum is stable enough for detection, supporting previous evidence to this effect. This would potentially provide clinicians with a novel, non-invasive method to improve diagnostic accuracy while avoiding discomfort to the patients. Serum miRNA for diagnosis would be particularly useful in patients with multinodular goiter. In these patients, there are often numerous thyroid nodules >15 mm and it can be difficult to select which nodules should be biopsied [41]. Serum-based testing would allow thyroid malignancy to be identified much more simply in these patients. A previous study suggests Canadian wait times for thyroid surgery are inappropriately long [42, 43]. Preoperative risk stratification for malignancy will help manage the limited operative time

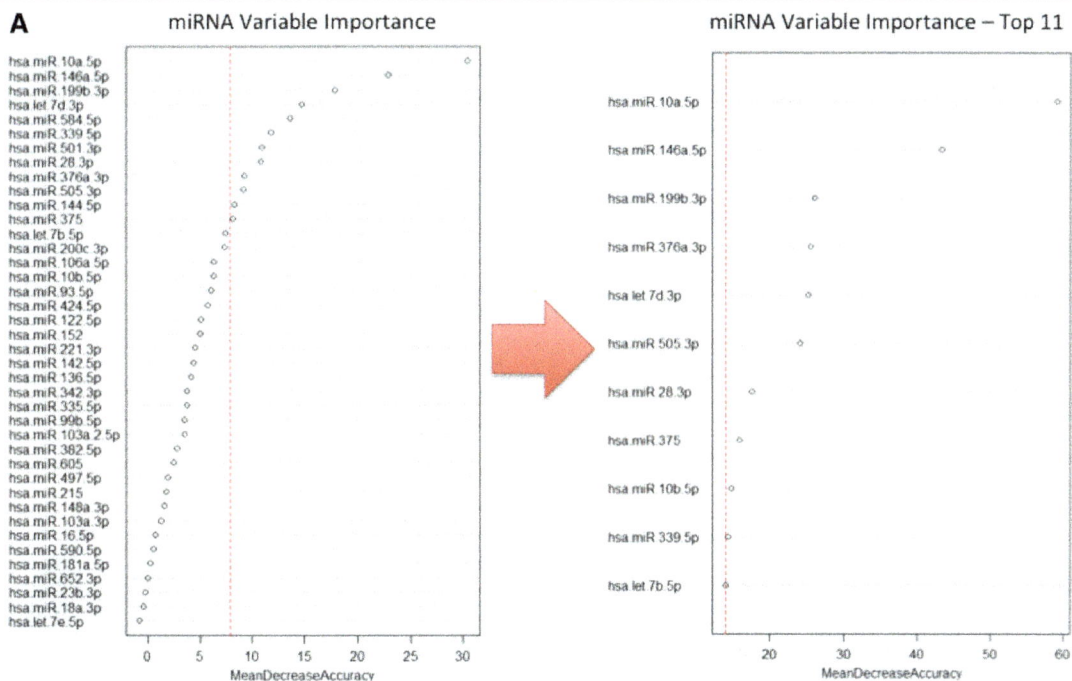

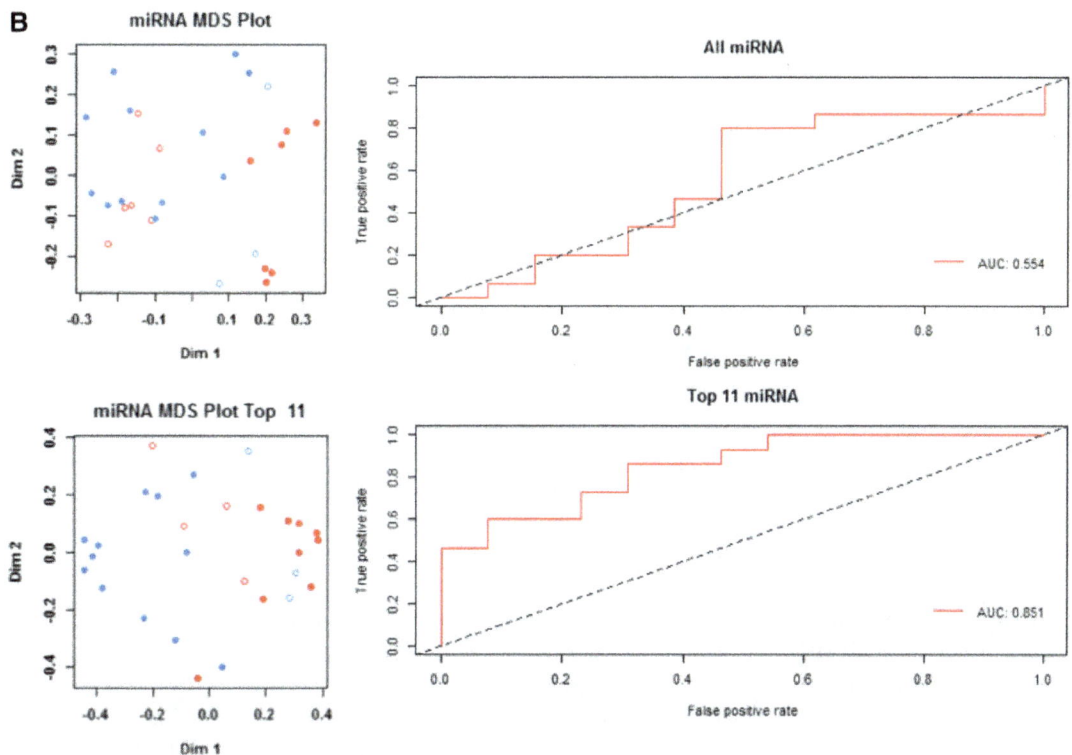

Fig. 2 a Random Forest analysis classifier of 11 microRNAs. The top three miRNAs in this classifier (hsa-miR-10a-5p, hsa-miR-146a-5p and hsa-miR-199b-3p) were consistent with those identified in the limma and *t*-test statistics. b Random Forest Area Under the Curve. AUC using all miRNAs and the 11-miRNA random forest classifier was 0.554 and 0.851, respectively. Red circles represent benign patients, blue represent PTC patients, filled represent correct classification, and open represent incorrect classification

**Table 2** Limma statistics and fold change

| MiRNA | p-value | adj. p.Value | t-Test | Mean target Ct | Mean calibrator Ct | ddCT | Fold change |
|---|---|---|---|---|---|---|---|
| Benign vs. Control[a] | | | | | | | |
| hsa-miR-150-5p | <0.001 | <0.001 | 6.2 | 30.35 | 27.79 | 2.6 | −5.9 |
| hsa-miR-342-3p | <0.001 | <0.01 | 4.8 | 32.34 | 30.51 | 1.8 | −3.5 |
| hsa-let-7b-5p | <0.001 | 0.01 | −4.0 | 29.92 | 31.36 | −1.4 | 2.7 |
| hsa-miR-191-5p | 0.001 | 0.04 | −3.5 | 31.73 | 32.76 | −1.0 | 2.0 |
| PTC vs. Control[b] | | | | | | | |
| hsa-let-7b-5p | <0.001 | <0.001 | −5.6 | 29.40 | 31.36 | −2.0 | 3.9 |
| hsa-miR-150-5p | <0.001 | <0.001 | 5.7 | 30.11 | 27.79 | 2.3 | −5.0 |
| hsa-miR-146a-5p | <0.001 | 0.02 | 3.7 | 33.49 | 32.21 | 1.3 | −2.4 |
| hsa-miR-342-3p | <0.001 | 0.03 | 3.7 | 31.88 | 30.51 | 1.4 | −2.6 |
| hsa-miR-191-5p | <0.001 | 0.03 | −3.5 | 31.75 | 32.76 | −1.0 | 2.0 |
| hsa-miR-93-5p | <0.001 | 0.03 | −3.5 | 28.68 | 29.53 | −0.85 | 1.8 |
| PTC vs. Benign[c] | | | | | | | |
| hsa-miR-10a-5p | <0.01 | 0.5 | −3.1 | 35.45 | 35.95 | −0.50 | 1.4 |
| hsa-miR-146a-5p | 0.01 | 0.5 | 2.7 | 33.49 | 32.93 | 0.56 | −1.5 |
| hsa-miR-199b-3p | 0.01 | 0.5 | 2.7 | 33.33 | 32.79 | 0.54 | −1.5 |
| hsa-let-7b-5p | 0.02 | 0.5 | −2.4 | 29.40 | 29.92 | −0.51 | 1.4 |

Fold-changes and significance of changes by t-Test/Limma. ddCT = delta delta CT – measure of relative expression quantification (comparative cycle threshold)
Adjusted p-value accounts for multiple comparisons
[a]False discovery rate (FDR) <5 %
[b]FDR <1 %
[c]FDR <50 %

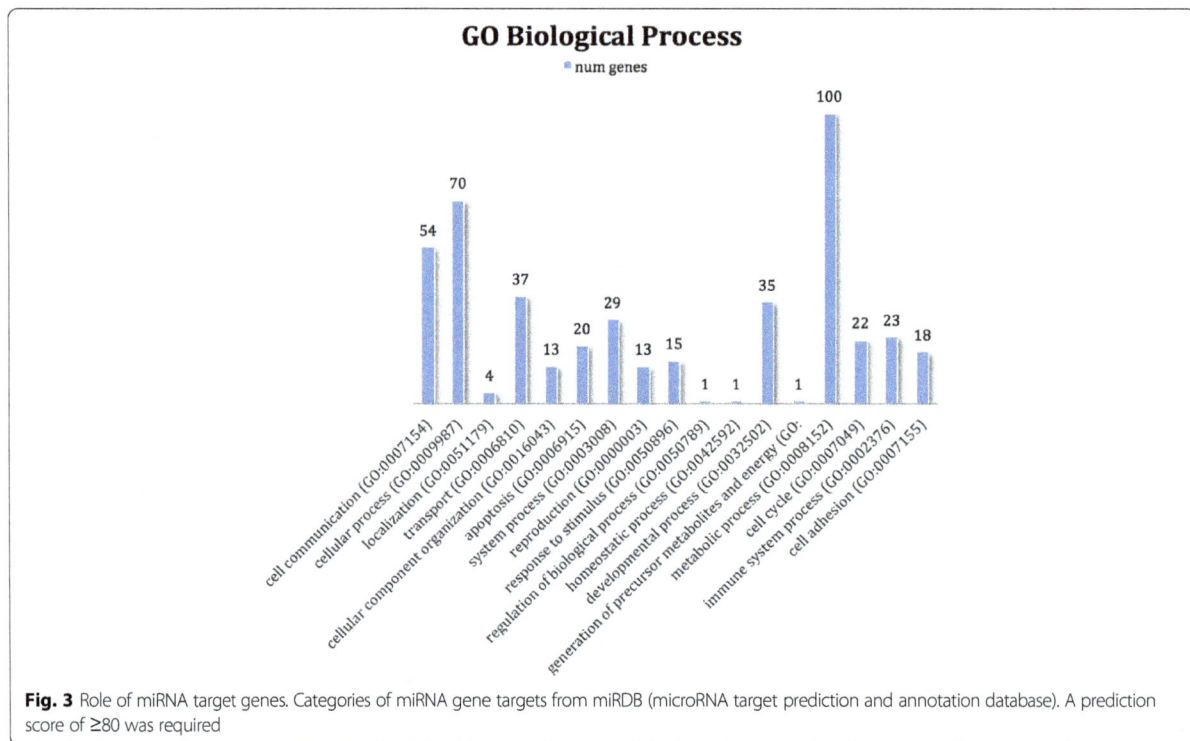

**Fig. 3** Role of miRNA target genes. Categories of miRNA gene targets from miRDB (microRNA target prediction and annotation database). A prediction score of ≥80 was required

available in our Canadian health care system to expedite care for those more likely to have malignancy.

Serum-based testing in cancer is gaining in popularity as its potential feasibility is recognized. By March 2015, more than 10 papers on this topic had been published in a diversity of tumor types. These include non-small cell lung carcinoma [44, 45], hepatocellular carcinoma [46], ovarian cancer [47], and others. Studies in thyroid cancer have been limited to date. A study by Yu *et al.* in 2012 was the first to examine serum miRNAs in PTC and identified three that were significantly up-regulated in Chinese patients with PTC relative to benign and control patients [48]. This study was limited in that it only aimed to detect 5-fold-changes or more, and only looked for those miRNA that were up-regulated in sera from patients with PTC relative to those with benign disease. A second study in Caucasian patients identified a single miRNA as being significantly up-regulated and one down-regulated in PTC compared to benign sera [49]. These targets, however, were different than the miRNAs identified in the study focusing on Chinese patients.

The previous studies have failed to tightly stratify patients based on clinical characteristics, which can have a significant effect on miRNA expression profiles, although this has not universally been found to be the case [50]. Each study has identified different miRNAs that are differentially expressed in sera of patients with PTC. The populations have all been quite disparate from one another. We have chosen to include exclusively female patients with tumors >1 cm in order to more tightly control differences in baseline miRNA profiles. Nonetheless, the differences in miRNA expression identified between studies suggests a need for a large-scale, tightly controlled study which would serve as a baseline for studies in other populations with different clinical characteristics.

Clinical application of miRNAs may extend to disease monitoring and prognostication. The prognosis of patients with PTC is generally good, with a 10-year survival of 85 % [51]. Some thyroid tumors, such as the tall cell variant, can present aggressively. miRNA detection may identify important molecular information that may determine tumor clinicopathological characteristics and predict aggressiveness of disease and patients at risk of poorer outcomes, and future studies are planned to stratify based on histological subtypes. A previous study has already shown promise in detecting serum miRNAs that may be increased in recurrent PTC [50]. Future miRNA research may even aid in management of PTC patients, given the role of miRNA in cell proliferation, differentiation and apoptosis.

## Conclusion

This study identifies four microRNAs that exhibit statistically significant changes when comparing the serum of patients with PTC to those with benign nodules. These results demonstrate the potential for serum-based miRNA assays to improve diagnostic accuracy of PTC.

### Competing interests

The authors have no financial disclosure or conflicts of interest. This material has not previously been published and is not currently under evaluation in any other peer-reviewed publication.

### Authors' contributions

MERG participated in sample preparation, specimen processing, assisted in bench-top analysis, data compilation and analysis, and drafted the manuscript. RDH was involved in study design, subject recruitment, specimen collection and processing and manuscript preparation. FM submitted the ethics proposal and assisted in specimen collection and processing. RS supervised miRNA analysis and assisted in study design, sample stratification and GQ, data analysis and preparation of the manuscript. DP was involved in study design, statistical analysis and manuscript preparation. AB assisted in manuscript preparation. MB was responsible for specimen preparation and was involved in study design. MHR assisted in statistical analysis and manuscript preparation. JRBT and SMT assisted in subject recruitment, specimen collection, and study design. SD was involved in study design and manuscript preparation. All authors read and approved the final manuscript.

### Acknowledgements

The authors would like to acknowledge Susanne Penny and Andrew Leslie, project bioinformaticians, for their work in statistical analysis. This project was funded by the Dalhousie Department of Surgery Seed Grant and the National Research Council of Canada (NRC).

### Author details

[1]Division of Otolaryngology, Queen Elizabeth II Health Sciences Centre and Dalhousie University, Halifax, NS, Canada. [2]NRC Human Health Therapeutics, Oxford Street, Halifax, NS, Canada. [3]Division of Anatomical Pathology, Queen Elizabeth II Health Sciences Centre and Dalhousie University, Halifax, NS, Canada.

### References

1. Chappell H, Mery L, Pritwish D, Dryer D, Ellison L, MacIntyre M, Marrett L, Wier HK: Canadian Cancer Society's steering committee on cancer statistics. In *Book Canadian Cancer Society's steering committee on cancer statistics* (Editor ed.^eds.). City: Canadian Cancer Society; 2012
2. Hartl DM, Travagli JP. The updated american thyroid association guidelines for management of thyroid nodules and differentiated thyroid cancer: a surgical perspective. Thyroid. 2009;19(11):1149–51.
3. Wiseman SM, Baliski C, Irvine R, Anderson D, Wilkins G, Filipenko D, et al. Hemithyroidectomy: the optimal initial surgical approach for individuals undergoing surgery for a cytological diagnosis of follicular neoplasm. Ann Surg Oncol. 2006;13:425–32.
4. Isaac A, Jeffery CC, Seikaly H, Al-Marzouki H, Harris JR, O'Connell DA. Predictors of non-diagnostic cytology in surgeon-performed ultrasound guided fine needle aspiration of thyroid nodules. Isaac et al. J Otolaryngol Head Neck Surgery. 2014;43:48. http://www.journalotohns.com/content/43/1/48.
5. Williams BA, Bullock MJ, Trites JR, Taylor SM, Hart RD. Rates of thyroid malignancy by FNA diagnostic criteria. J Otolaryngol Head Neck Surgery. 2013;42:61. http://www.journalotohns.com/content/42/1/61.
6. Yip L. Molecular diagnostic testing and the indeterminate thyroid nodule. Curr Opin Oncol. 2014;26:8–13.
7. Park YJ, Kwak SH, Kim DC, Kim H, Choe G, Park Do J, et al. Diagnostic value of galectin-3, HBME-1, cytokeratin 19, high molecular weight cytokeratin, cyclin D1 and p27(kip1) in the differential diagnosis of thyroid nodules. J Korean Med Sci. 2007;22:621–8.
8. Jarzab B, Wiench M, Fujarewicz K, Simek K, Jarzab M, Oczko-Wojciechowska M, et al. Gene expression profile of papillary thyroid cancer: sources of variability and diagnostic implications. Cancer Res. 2005;65:1587–97.
9. Shi Y, Parhar RS, Zou M, Hammami MM, Akhtar M, Lum ZP, et al. Tissue inhibitor of metalloproteinases-1 (TIMP-1) mRNA is elevated in advanced stages of thyroid carcinoma. Br J Cancer. 1999;79:1234–9.

10. Hsueh C, Lin JD, Wu IC, Chao TC, Yu JS, Liou MJ, et al. Vascular endothelial growth factors and angiopoietins in presentations and prognosis of papillary thyroid carcinoma. J Surg Oncol. 2011;103:395–9.

11. Makki FM, Taylor SM, Shahnavaz A, Leslie A, Gallant J, Douglas S, et al. Serum biomarkers of papillary thyroid cancer. Otolaryngol Head Neck Surg. 2013;42:16.

12. He L, Hannon GJ. MicroRNAs: Small RNAs with big roles in gene regulation. Nat Rev Genet. 2004;5:522–31.

13. Friedlander MR, Lizano E, Houben AJS, Bezdan D, Báñez Coronel M, Kudla G, et al. Evidence for the biogenesis of more than 1000 novel human microRNAs. Genome Biol. 2014;15:R57. doi:10.1186/gb-2014-15-4-r57.

14. Lee RC, Feinbaum RL, Ambros V. The C. elegans heterochronic gene lin-4 encodes small RNAs with antisense complementarity to lin-14. Cell. 1993;75(5):843–54.

15. Cuellar TL, McManus MT. MicroRNAs and endocrine biology. J Endocrinol. 2005;187(3):327–32.

16. Mraz M, Pospisilova S. MicroRNAs in chronic lymphocytic leukemia: From causality to associations and back. Expert Rev Hematol. 2012;5(6):579–81.

17. He L, Thomson JM, Hemann MT, Hernando-Monge E, Mu D, Goodson S, et al. A microRNA polycistron as a potential human oncogene. Nature. 2005;435(7043):828–33.

18. Mraz M, Pospisilova S, Malinova K, Slapak I, Mayer J. MicroRNAs in chronic lymphocytic leukemia pathogenesis and disease subtypes. Leuk Lymphoma. 2009;50(3):506–9. doi:10.1080/10428190902763517.

19. Moller H, Rasmussen A, Anderson H, Johensen K, Henriksen M, Duroux M. A systemic review of microRNA in glioblastoma multiforme: micromodulators in the mesenchymal mode of migration and invasion. Mol Neurobio. 2013;47:131–44.

20. Blondal T, Jensby Nielsen S, Baker A, Andreasen D, Mouritzen P, Wrang Teilum M, et al. Assessing sample and miRNA profile quality in serum and plasma or other biofluids. Methods. 2013;59:81–6.

21. Cortez M, Calin G. MicroRNA identification in plasma and serum: a new tool to diagnose and monitor diseases. Expert Opin Biol Ther. 2009;9:703–11.

22. Li X, Abdel-Mageed A, Mondal D, Kandil E. MicroRNA expression profiles in differentiated thyroid cancer, a review. Int J Clin Exp Med. 2013;6:74–80.

23. Chapelle A, Jazdzewski K. MicroRNAs in thyroid cancer. J Clin Endocrinol Metabl. 2011;96:3326–36.

24. Ruijter JM, Ramakers C, Hoogaars WMH, Karlen Y, Bakker O, van den Hoff MJB, et al. Amplification efficiency: linking baseline and bias in the analysis of quantitative PCR data. Nucleic Acids Res. 2009;37(6):e45.

25. Dvinge H, Bertone P. HTqPCR: High-throughput analysis and visualization of quantitative real-time PCR data in R. Bioinformatics. 2009;25(24):3325.

26. Liaw A, Wiener M. Classification and regression by randomForest. R News. 2002;2(3):18–22.

27. Sing T, Sander O, Beerenwinkel N, Lengauer T. ROCR: visualizing classifier performance in R. Bioinformatics. 2005;21(20):7881.

28. He H, Jazdzewski K, Li W, Liyanarachchi S, Nagy R, Volinia S, et al. The role of microRNA genes in papillary thyroid carcinoma. Proc Natl Acad Sci U S A. 2005;102:19075–80.

29. Jazdzewski K, Liyanarachchi S, Swierniak M, Pachucki J, Ringel MD, Jarzab B, et al. Polymorphic mature microRNAs from passenger strand of pre-miR-146a contribute to thyroid cancer. Proc Natl Acad Sci U S A. 2009;106:1502–5.

30. Pallante P, Visone R, Ferracin M, Ferraro A, Berlingieri MT, Troncone G, et al. MicroRNA deregulation in human thyroid papillary carcinomas. Endocr Relat Cancer. 2006;13:497–508.

31. Tetzlaff MT, Liu A, Xu X, Master SR, Baldwin DA, Tobias JW, et al. Differential expression of miRNAs in papillary thyroid carcinoma compared to multinodular goiter using formalin fixed paraffin embedded tissues. Endocr Pathol. 2007;18:163–73.

32. Ambros V. MicroRNAs: tiny regulators with great potential. Cell. 2001;107(7):823–6.

33. Ricarte-Filho JC, Fuziwara CS, Yamashita AS, Rezende E, Da Silva MJ, Kimura ET. Effects of let-7 microRNA on cell growth and differentiation of papillary thyroid cancer. Transl Oncol. 2009;2(4):236–41.

34. Esquela-Kerscher A, Slack FJ. Oncomirs - microRNAs with a role in cancer. Nat Rev Cancer. 2006;6:259–69.

35. Ruzzo A, Canestrari E, Galluccio N, Santini D, Vincenzi B, Tonini G, et al. Role of KRAS let-7 LCS6 SNP in metastatic colorectal cancer patients. Ann Oncol. 2010;22(1):234–5.

36. Osada H, Takahashi T. Review Article: let-7 and miR-17-92: Small-sized major players in lung cancer development. Cancer Sci. 2010;102(1):9–17.

37. Nie K, Zhang T, Allawi H, Gomez M, Liu Y, Chadburn A, et al. Epigenetic down-regulation of the tumor suppressor gene PRDM1/blimp-1 in diffuse large B cell lymphomas : a potential role of the MicroRNA Let-7. Am J Pathol. 2010;177(3):1470–9.

38. Lee ST, Chu K, Oh HJ, Im WS, Lim JY, Kim SK, et al. Let-7 microRNA inhibits the proliferation of human glioblastoma cells. J Neurooncol. 2010;102(1):19–24.

39. Rossing M, Borup R, Henao R, Winther O, Vikesaa J, Niazi O, et al. Down-regulation of microRNAs controlling tumourigenic factors in follicular thyroid carcinoma. J Mol Endocrinol. 2012;48:11–23.

40. Weber F, Teresi RE, Broelsch CE, Frilling A, Eng C. A limited set of human MicroRNA is deregulated in follicular thyroid carcinoma. J Clin Endocrinol Metab. 2006;91:3584–91.

41. Luo J, Mcmanus C, Chen H, Sippel RS. Are there predictors of malignancy in patients with multinodular goiter? J Surg Res. 2012;174:209–10.

42. Brake MK, Moore P, Taylor SM, Trites J, Murray S, Hart R. Expectantly waiting: a survey of thyroid surgery wait times among Canadian Otolaryngologists. J Otolaryngol Head Neck Surgery. 2013;42:47. http://www.journalotohns.com/content/42/1/47.

43. Merdad M, Eskander A, De Almeida J, Freeman J, Rotstein L, Ezzat S, et al. Current management of papillary thyroid microcarcinoma in Canada. J Otolaryngol Head Neck Surgery. 2014;43:32. http://www.journalotohns.com/content/43/1/32.

44. Singh RK, Bethune DC, Xu Z, Douglas SE. Role of microRNAs in progression and recurrence of early-stage lung adenocarcinoma. Pulm Res Respir Med. 2015;2(1):52–62.

45. Wang RJ, Zheng YH, Wang P, Zhang JZ. Serum miR-125a-5p, miR-145 and miR-146a as diagnostic biomarkers in non-small cell lung cancer. Int J Clin Exp Pathol. 2015;8(1):765–71.

46. He S, Zhang DC, Wei C. MicroRNAs as biomarkers for hepatocellular carcinoma diagnosis and prognosis. Clin Res Hepatol Gastroenterol 2015; http://dx.doi.org/10.1016/j.clinre.2015.01.006.

47. Liang H, Jiang Z, Xie G, Lu Y. Serum microRNA-145 as a novel biomarker in human ovarian cancer. Tumor Biol. doi:10.1007/s13277-015-3191-y. Published online February 27, 2015.

48. Yu S, Liu Y, Wang J, Guo Z, Zhang Q, Yu F, et al. Circulating microRNA profiles as potential biomarkers for diagnosis of papillary thyroid carcinoma. J Clin Endocrinol Metab. 2012;97(6):2084–92.

49. Cantara S, Pilli T, Sebastiani G, Cevenini G, Busonero G, Cardinale S, et al. Circulating miRNA 95 and miRNA190 are sensitive markers for the differential diagnosis or thyroid nodules in a Caucasian population. J Clin Endocrinol Metab. 2014;99(11):4190–8.

50. Lee JC, Zhao JT, Clifton-Bligh RJ, Gill A, Gundara JS, Ip JC, et al. MicroRNA-222 and micro-RNA-146b are tissue and circulating biomarkers of recurrent papillary thyroid cancer. Cancer. 2013; doi:10.1002/cncr.28254.

51. Busaidy NL, Cabanillas ME. Differentiated thyroid cancer: management of patients with radioiodine nonresponsive disease. J Thyroid Res. 2012;2012:618985.

# 12

# Endoscopic Dacryocystorhinostomy (DCR): a comparative study between powered and non-powered technique

Islam Herzallah[1], Bassam Alzuraiqi[2], Naif Bawazeer[3], Osama Marglani[3], Ameen Alherabi[3,8*], Sherif K. Mohamed[4], Khalid Al-Qahtani[5], Talal Al-Khatib[6] and Abdullah Alghamdi[7]

## Abstract

**Background:** Dacrocystorhinostomy (DCR) is an operation used to treat nasolacrimal duct obstruction. Essentially there are two approaches: external and endoscopic. Several modalities are used in endoscopic DCR; all aiming to improve success rate, reduce complications, and shorten operative time. Both kerrison punch and drill are widely used in endoscopic DCR with non-conclusive knowledge about differences in operative details as well as on the outcome. The aim of this study is to compare between powered (drill) and non-powered (kerrison punch) DCR to clarify the superiority of one over the other.

**Methods:** A retrospective chart review of 59 patients who underwent endoscopic DCR procedure at our institution from June 2013 until July 2014 (34 kerrison punch and 32 powered drill). Operative details, surgical outcome and complications were compared between both groups.

**Results:** A total of 66 endoscopic DCRs were performed on 59 patients. Procedure success rate among kerrison punch group was 87.88 % vs. 90.9 % in powered drill group ($p = 0.827$), while complications for both groups were statistical not significant ($p = 0.91$). The mean operating time among kerrison punch group was significantly lower than in powered drill group (75 min vs. 125 min, $p = 0.0001$).

**Conclusion:** Kerrison punch showed significant reduction in operating time when compared to powered drill for endoscopic DCR. No statistically significant difference was found between both groups regarding procedures' success rate and complication.

**Keywords:** Kerrison, Drill, Endoscopic Dacryocystorhinostomy, DCR

## Background

Epiphora due to nasolacrimal duct obstruction is a common clinical problem that can be caused by functional or anatomical abnormality. An anatomical obstruction could be at any point along the lacrimal excretory system and could be congenital or acquired. The primary acquired nasolacrimal duct obstruction is believed to occur due to chronic inflammatory process resulting in fibrosis, stenosis, and closure of the duct ostium [1]. This can be managed surgically by dacryocystorhinostomy (DCR), which is used to create a fistula that bypasses the obstruction and restores the tear flow. The operative approach could be external or an endoscopic approach. External DCR was the gold standard method even after the endoscopic approach had been described, because of limited technology at that time with a success rate ranging between 80 and 100 % [2]. However, improvements of visualization & instrumentation technology made the endoscopic DCR gain its popularity. In addition, endoscopic DCR has several advantages over external DCR including: no external incision, shorter recovery time, maintenance of the lacrimal pumping mechanism and lower postoperative morbidity [3].

Several modalities and adjuncts such as Kerrison punch, powered drill, and lasers have been described in endoscopic DCR with the aim of improving operative technique

* Correspondence: herabi@hotmail.com
[3]Department of Otolaryngology-Head & Neck Surgery, Umm Al-Qura University, Makkah, Saudi Arabia
[8]P.O.Box 41405, Jeddah 21521, Saudi Arabia
Full list of author information is available at the end of the article

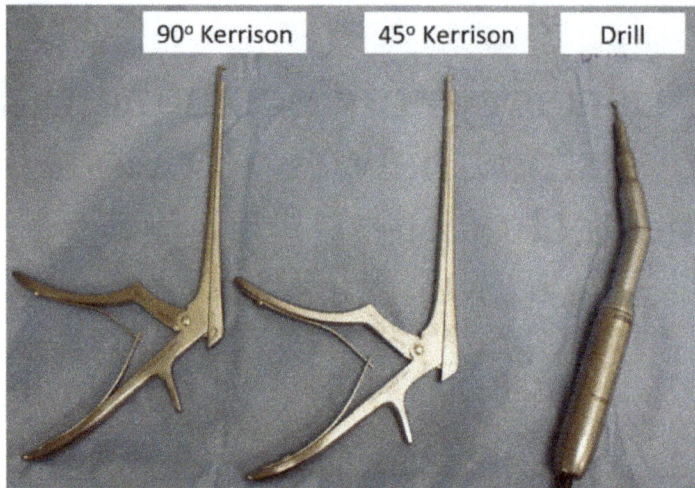

**Fig. 1** Instruments compared in this study; namely 90°, 45° kerrison punch, and powered drill

and success rate [2]. However, the variety of tools used in endoscopic DCR made it difficult to determine the best approach, and thus a comparison between some of the available techniques seems to be important to know the advantages and disadvantages. Both kerrison punch and powered drill are widely used in endoscopic DCR with slowly expanding knowledge about the differences in operative details as well as in the surgical outcome [4]. Our objective is to compare those two modalities and try to clarify the superiority of one technique over the other.

## Methods

### Study design

A retrospective review was conducted after creation and development of an electronic DCR DATABASE using Microsoft© Access 2012 (Microsoft Corporation) on all patients underwent endoscopic DCR procedure at our institution from July 2013 until June 2014. Appropriate patients' demographics, diagnoses, radiological evaluation, surgical details, complications, and outcomes were included. Exclusion criteria were posttraumatic lacrimal obstruction, congenital cases, cases with combined other sino-nasal procedures (e.g. septoplasty, turbinate procedures, sinus surgery), cases were both drill & kerisson used together, and cases with follow up less than three months. Institutional review board approval of the study protocol was obtained prior to initiation of the study.

### Surgical technique

All patients received a standard preoperative assessment including history & physical examination, endoscopic evaluation, and CT scan of paranasal sinuses to exclude possible sinonasal pathologies. Diagnosis of nasolacrimal

duct obstruction was made by classical symptomatic presentation along with fluorescein dye test, and syringing test.

All operations were performed under general anesthesia. Endoscopic DCR was done using a standard surgical technique. For the Osteotomy part of the surgery, two different instruments were used to remove the bone of the maxillary frontal process. In the first group, the powered drill was used; while in the second group the kerisson punch was utilized to get sufficient exposure of the lacrimal sac, see Fig. 1. Once the drill or the kerisson was used, no instrument conversion was allowed. Standard silicone stent was used to stent the lacrimal canaliculi. Operating time represents the duration from lateral nasal mucosal incision till the stent is secured. All surgeries were

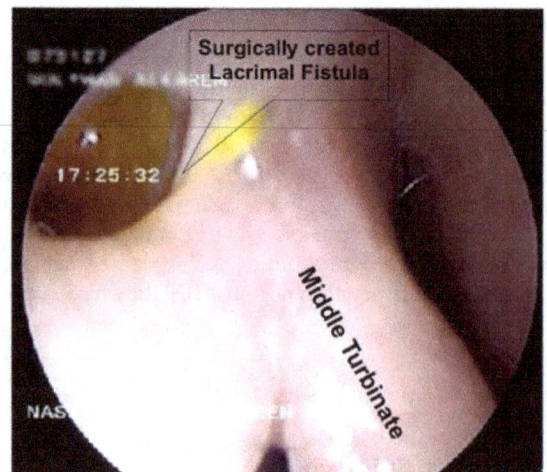

**Fig. 2** Three months post operative endoscopic examination showing positive fluorescein test and patent lacrimal fistula

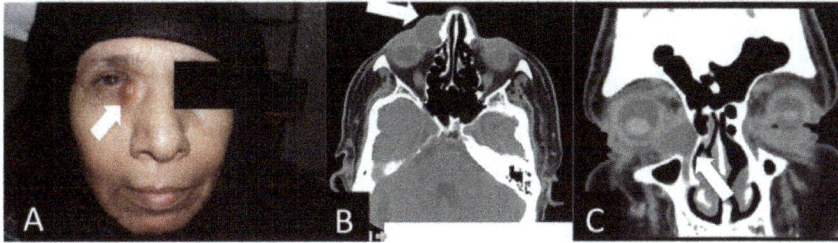

**Fig. 3** Preoperative diagnosis. **a** A Clinical photo of a patient with right eye dacrocele. **b** CT Axial cut showing medial canthus dacrocele. **c** CT Coronal cut showing the same finding

performed; or under direct supervision, of the two senior surgeons with comparable experience and training (O.M & A.A). Postoperatively, outpatient standardized follow up were scheduled at one week then 1, 3, 6, & 12 months. Further follow up was individualized as per patient cases especially those requiring the other side to be done. Three criteria were used to judge success of the operation: the patient expressed improvement of the epiphora, a positive fluorescein test, and patent fistula during endoscopic examination [5] see Fig. 2.

Data were analyzed using SPSS software® (version 16). The Independent two-sample $t$-test was used to assess significance between variables and a value of $P < 0.05$ was taken as statistically significant with a confidence interval level of 95 %.

## Results

A total of 66 endoscopic DCRs were performed on 59 patients. Forty patients were women and 19 were men, with a mean age of 45 years (range 13–96 years). All 59 patients were local residents without any significant racial difference. Thirty-one cases were done in the right eye and 35 in the left eye. The original diagnosis of primary DCRs (59 cases) was acute, recurrent acute, chronic dacryocystitis, and dacroceles in 44 cases; and functional idiopathic epiphora in 15 patients. All patients failed syringing and fluorescein testing. No surgery

was done during the acute phase. See Fig. 3 for an example of a case of dacrocele and Fig. 4 for a case if acute dacrocystitis. Eight cases were revision DCR; of which 4 cases were in each group. Thirty-two cases were done using powered drill technique and 34 utilizing kerrison punch. Postoperative follow-up had a mean duration of 8.2 (range = 3–24) months both groups. The mean time for stent removal was 9.5 weeks for both groups; see Table 1 for complete patients demographics.

The overall success rate was 89.39 %. The success rate for powered drill group was 90.91 %, compared with 87.88 % for kerrison punch group. The mean operating time of surgery in the powered drill group was 125 min compared to 75 min in the kerrison punch group; see Table 2.

Reported intraoperative and postoperative complications were all minor and included: intranasal synechiae in two cases, stent accidental fall out in five cases and eye/cheek bruise in three cases, and nostril burn in three cases. The overall minor complication rate was 18 % and there was no record of any major complications. Comparing the two groups it was not statistically significant ($p = 0.53$). Looking into nostril burn alone was also not statistically significant but showed a trend ($p = 0.1$); see Table 3.

## Discussion

External DCR was considered superior procedure compared to the endoscopic approach classically, but in the

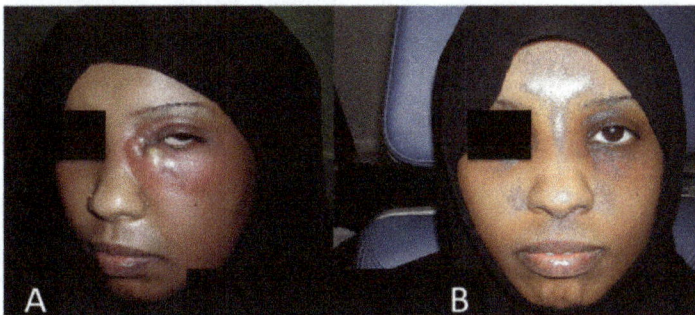

**Fig. 4** Preoperative diagnosis. **a** A Clinical photo of a patient with left eye acute dacrocystitis. **b** Same patient after medical treatment

**Table 1** Patients demographics & descriptive statistics

| | | Overall | | Instrument used | | | |
|---|---|---|---|---|---|---|---|
| | | | | Drill | | Kerrison punch | |
| Age | Range | 13–96 Years | | 13–96 Years | | 16–75 Years | |
| | Mean | 45 | | 48 | | 41 | |
| Gender | Male | 19 | 32.20 % | 11 | 34.40 % | 8 | 29.60 % |
| | Female | 40 | 67.80 % | 21 | 65.60 % | 19 | 70.40 % |
| Eye affected | Right | 31 | 47 % | 17 | 53.13 % | 14 | 41.20 % |
| | Left | 35 | 53 % | 15 | 46.87 % | 20 | 58.80 % |
| Stent removal | Range | 0–48 Weeks | | 0–48 weeks | | 1–20 Weeks | |
| | Mean | 9.5 | | 12 | | 8 | |
| Follow up | Range | 3–24 Months | | 3–24 Months | | 3–19 Months | |
| | Mean | 8.2 | | 7.03 | | 9.93 | |

last years there were significant improvements in the technique of endoscopic DCR [3, 6]. These improvements are the result of evolution in surgical instruments, improvement in endoscopic equipment and growing surgical experience [3].

Osteotomy and creation of the bony lacrimal window is a crucial step during endoscopic DCR; a previous study reported that sometimes only 2 % of the original stoma created intra-operatively will remain patent after healing process; but found no statistically valid correlation between the size of the bony opening and the final size of the healed intranasal ostium [7]. Creation of a large bony stoma does not mean successful procedure since minimization of intra-operative tissue damage and postoperative scarring is another key point for success [7, 8]. Other literature, however, showed a relationship between the size of the bony ostium created during DCR surgery and the outcome of the procedure [2, 4, 6, 9]. The creation of the bony window can be achieved by many technical variations including powered drill, kerrison bone punch, radio-surgical electrodes, and lasers. Each instrument has been well described in literature with different results and consequences, but comparison between those instruments and surgical outcome is still non conclusive.

The value of non-traumatic procedure is an emerging concept in endoscopic DCR. The main idea of this concept is to avoid using instruments and tools that might

**Table 2** Procedure success and operating time according to the equipment of endoscopic DCR

| | | Overall | Powered drill | Kerrison punch | $p$ value |
|---|---|---|---|---|---|
| | | | ($n = 32$) | ($n = 34$) | |
| Success rate | | 89.39 % | 90.91 % | 87.88 % | 0.827 |
| Operating time (Minutes) | Range | 24–210 | 24–210 | 30–125 | 0.0001 |
| | Mean | 99.75 | 125 | 75 | |

**Table 3** Minor complications of endoscopic DCR

| | Drill | | Kerrison punch | | |
|---|---|---|---|---|---|
| | ($n = 32$) | | ($n = 34$) | | |
| | n | % | n | % | |
| Intranasal synechiae | 1 | 1.5 | 1 | 1.5 | $P = 0.53$ |
| Stent fell out | 2 | 3 | 3 | 4.5 | |
| Eye/Cheek bruise | 2 | 3 | 1 | 1.5 | |
| Nostril burn | 2 | 3 | 0 | 0 | |
| Total | 7 | 10.5 | 5 | 7.5 | |

increases the tissue trauma within the surgical field [10]. Trauma could be in form of excessive mechanical force as when using powered drill or can be transmitted heats from cautery and laser assisted instruments. While using powered drill, temperature could reach up to 70 °C at the tip during drilling with possibility of causing local edema and tissue reaction in the postoperative period [11, 12]. Avoiding trauma in this narrow anatomical site will increase chances of first-intention healing process with less formation of scarring and granulation tissue, which ultimately may reduce risk of closure of previously surgically opened lacrimal sac and soft tissue window [4]. In addition, presence of the drill's rotating shaft within narrow surgical corridor may add some risk to damage nearby tissue [3]. Other disadvantages of powered drills or other high techniques instruments include the possibility of damage to orbital wall or lamina papyracea leading to orbital fat prolapse or penetration to the ethmoidal sinus or skull base with CSF leakage [11]. Nevertheless, with

**Table 4** Comparison between success rates of our study and previous similar studies

| Author | Country | Instrument used | Success rate (%) |
|---|---|---|---|
| Ben Simon, et al. [2] | USA | Kerrison punch | 84 |
| Gurler, et al. [3] | | Drill | 88.9 |
| Wormald [6] | Australia | Drill | 95.7 |
| Kim, et al. [8] | Korea | Kerrison punch | 90.5 |
| Codere, et al. [10] | Canada | Kerrison punch | 98 |
| Graz-Cabrerizo, et al. [13] | Spain | Kerrison punch | 83 |
| Naraghi, et al. [14] | Iran | Kerrison punch | 95 |
| Agarwal [15] | India | Kerrison punch | 94 (100 % with Revisions) |
| Yoshida, et al. [16] | Japan | Drill | 93.6 |
| Saratziotis, et al. [17] | Greece | Drill | 97.8 |
| Jin, et al. [18] | Korea | Drill | 96 |
| Razavi, et al. [20] | Iran | Kerrison punch | 96 |
| Current study | Saudi Arabia | Kerrison punch | 87.88 |
| | | Drill | 90.91 |

favorable result of non-traumatic endoscopic DCR in theory, published results in the literature showed comparable outcome for drill and punch endoscopic DCR [13–18].

The use of advanced tools like drills is not necessary to increase the success rate for endoscopic DCR in general [8]. Our current study showed similar result, where procedure success rate among kerrison punch group was 87.88 % vs. 90.91 % in the powered drill group ($p = 0.82$); see Table 4 for a summary of some previous studies success rates.

Operating time is a valuable factor in health care economics, ranges approximately from 750 to 2200 dollars per hour operating time in USA & Europe [19–23]. In addition, less operating time may accomplish increased surgical efficiency, volume of performed cases, and reduction of patient's waiting list, especially in high volume setting centres [19–22]. Our results showed that there is a statistically significant difference between operating time for endoscopic DCR using the drill compared with kerrison punch. Powered drill need more time for setup, irrigation during drilling, and suctioning after that to remove generated bony dust, with meticulous use to prevent any injure to surrounding vital structures [24].

Our overall rate of minor complication (18 %) between the powered versus non powered group showed no statistical difference and was generally similar to some previous studies on endoscopic DCR [2, 8, 13]. A recent article from Germany by Horn et al. reported a minor complication rate of 10 % [25]. Rahman et al. reported a minor complication rate of 23.8 % [26]. Despite meticulous work with the drill, we observed two cases with minor nostril burn indicating a requirement of more carefulness in handling the drill [3, 27, 28].

The limitations of this study are mainly the retrospective design of the study and the moderately small sample size.

## Conclusion

No significant difference was found between the powered and the non powered groups in terms of success rate and complications. Non-powered kerrison punch showed significant reduction in operating time compared to powered drill for endoscopic DCR. Larger prospective studies are advisable before any generalization can be made.

### Competing interests
The authors declare that they have no competing interests.

### Authors' contributions
All authors read and approved the final manuscript.

### Acknowledgement
We would like to thank Dr. Omar Abu Soliman, Dr. Fares Alhgamdi, Dr. Haneen Alharbi, Dr. Ahmad Khawandanah, Dr. Salem Al-Otaibi, and Dr. Abdullah Shalabi, from Umm Al-Qura university for their help in data collection and entry.

### Disclosure of Benefit
Authors have no conflict of interests and the work was not supported or funded by any drug company.

### Author details
[1]Department of Otolaryngology, Zagazig University, Zagazig, Egypt. [2]Department of Otolaryngology-Head & Neck Surgery, King Abdullah Medical City, Makkah, Saudi Arabia. [3]Department of Otolaryngology-Head & Neck Surgery, Umm Al-Qura University, Makkah, Saudi Arabia. [4]Department of Otolaryngology, Ain Shams University, Cairo, Egypt. [5]Department of Otolaryngology-Head and Neck Surgery, King Saud University, Riyadh, Saudi Arabia. [6]Department of Otolaryngology-Head & Neck Surgery, King Abdulaziz University, Jeddah, Saudi Arabia. [7]Department of Ophthalmology, Umm Al-Qura University, Makkah, Saudi Arabia. [8]P.O.Box 41405, Jeddah 21521, Saudi Arabia.

### References
1.  Önerci M. Dacryocystorhinostomy; Diagnosis and treatment of nasolacrimal canal obstructions. Rhinology. 2002;40(2):49–65.
2.  Ben Simon GJ, Joseph J, Lee S, Schwarcz RM, McCann JD, Goldberg RA. External versus endoscopic dacryocystorhinostomy for acquired nasolacrimal duct obstruction in a tertiary referral center. Ophthalmology. 2005;112(8):1463–8.
3.  Gurler B, San I. Long-term follow-up outcomes of non laser intranasal endoscopic dacryocystorhinostomy: how suitable and useful are conventional surgical instruments? Eur J Ophthalmol. 2004;14(6):453–60.
4.  Wormald PJ, A. A. F. P. S. Angelo Tsirbas FRACO. Powered endoscopic dacryocystorhinostomy. The Lacrimal System. Springer New York; 2006. 223–235.
5.  Anijeet D, Dolan L, Macewen CJ. Endonasal versus external dacryocystorhinostomy for nasolacrimal duct obstruction. Cochrane Database Syst Rev. 2011;1:CD007097.
6.  Wormald PJ. Powered endonasal dacryocystorhinostomy. Laryngoscope. 2002;112:69–71.
7.  Linberg JV, Anderson RL, Bumsted RM, Barreras R. Study of intranasal ostium external dacryocystorhinostomy. Arch Ophthalmol. 1982;100(11):1758–62.
8.  Kim SY, Paik JS, Jung SK, Cho WK, Yang SW. No thermal tool using methods in endoscopic dacryocystorhinostomy: no cautery, no drill, no illuminator, no more tears. Eur Arch Otorhinolaryngol. 2013;270(10):2677-82.
9.  Welham RA, Wulc AE. Management of unsuccessful lacrimal surgery. Br J Ophthalmol. 1987;71:152–7.
10. Codère F, Denton P, Corona J. Endonasal dacryocystorhinostomy: a modified technique with preservation of the nasal and lacrimal mucosa. Ophthalmic Plast Reconstr Surg. 2010;26(3):161–4.
11. Badilla J, Dolman PJ. Cerebrospinal fluid leaks complicating orbital or oculoplastic surgery. Arch Ophthalmol. 2007;125(12):1631.
12. Chang DJ. The No "Drill" Technique of Anterior Clinoidectomy: A Cranial Base Approach to the Paraclinoid and Parasellar Region. Neurosurgery. 2009;64(3):ons96–ons106.
13. Gras-Cabrerizo JR, Montserrat-Gili JR, León-Vintró X, Lopez-Vilas M, Rodríguez-Álvarez F, Bonafonte-Royo S, et al. Endonasal endoscopic scalpel-forceps dacryocystorhinostomy vs endocanalicular diode laser dacryocystorhinostomy. Eur J Ophthalmol. 2013;23(1):7–12.
14. Naraghi M, Tabatabaii Mohammadi SZ, Sontou AF, Farajzadeh Deroee A, Boroojerdi M. Endonasal endoscopic dacryocystorhinostomy: how to achieve optimal results with simple punch technique. Eur Arch Otorhinolaryngol. 2012;269(5):1445–9.
15. Agarwal S. Endoscopic dacryocystorhinostomy for acquired nasolacrimal duct obstruction. J Laryngol Otol. 2009;123(11):1226–8.
16. Yoshida N, Kanazawa H, Shinnabe A, Iino Y. Powered endoscopic dacryocystorhinostomy with radiowave instruments: surgical outcome according to obstruction level. Eur Arch Otorhinolaryngol. 2013;270(2):579–84.
17. Saratziotis A, Emanuelli E, Gouveris H, Babighian G. Endoscopic dacryocystorhinostomy for acquired nasolacrimal duct obstruction: creating a window with a drill without use of mucosal flaps. Acta Otolaryngol. 2009;129(9):992–5.
18. Jin H-R, Yeon J-Y, Choi M-Y. Endoscopic dacryocystorhinostomy: creation of a large marsupialized lacrimal sac. J Korean Med Sci. 2006;21(4):719–23.
19. Etzioni DA, Liu JH, Maggard MA, Ko CY. The aging population and its impact on the surgery workforce. Ann Surg. 2003;238(2):170.

20. Balakrishnan K, Goico B, Arjmand EM. Applying cost accounting to operating room staffing in otolaryngology: time-driven activity-based costing. Otolaryngol Head Neck Surg. 2015;152(4):684–90.

21. Raft J, Millet F, Meistelman C. Example of cost calculations for an operating room and a post-anaesthesia care unit. Anaesth, Crit Care Pain Med. 2015;34(4):211–5.

22. Tabib CH, Bahler CD, Hardacker TJ, Ball KM, Sundaram CP. Reducing Operating Room Costs Through Real-Time Cost Information Feedback: A Pilot Study. J Endourol. 2015;29(8):963–8.

23. Tsai M. The true cost of operating room time. Arch Surg. 2011;146(7):886.

24. Razavi ME, Noorollahian M, Eslampoor A. Non-endoscopic mechanical endonasal dacryocystorhinostomy. J Ophthalmic Vision Res. 2011;6(3):219.

25. Horn IS, Tittmann M, Fischer M, Otto M, Dietz A, Mozet C. Endonasal nasolacrimal duct surgery: a comparative study of two techniques. Eur Arch Otorhinolaryngol. 2014;271(7):1923–31.

26. Rahman SH, Tarafder KH, Ahmed MS, Saha KL, Tariq A. Endoscopic dacryocystorhinostomy. Mymensingh Med J. 2011;20(1):28–32.

27. Marr JE, Drake-Lee A, Willshaw HE. Management of childhood epiphora. Br J Ophthalmol. 2005;89:1123–6.

28. Fayet, Bruno, Emmanuel Racy, Michael Assouline. Complications of standardized endonasal dacryocystorhinostomy with unciformectomy. Ophthalmology, 2004;111(4):837-45.

# 13

# Face and content validity of a virtual-reality simulator for myringotomy with tube placement

Caiwen Huang[1], Horace Cheng[2], Yves Bureau[4,5], Sumit K. Agrawal[1,2,6*†] and Hanif M. Ladak[1,2,3,5*†]

## Abstract

**Background:** Myringotomy with tube insertion can be challenging for junior Otolaryngology residents as it is one of the first microscopic procedures they encounter. The Western myringotomy simulator was developed to allow trainees to practice microscope positioning, myringotomy, and tube placement. This virtual-reality simulator is viewed in stereoscopic 3D, and a haptic device is used to manipulate the digital ear model and surgical tools.

**Objective:** To assess the face and content validity of the Western myringotomy simulator.

**Methods:** The myringotomy simulator was integrated with new modules to allow speculum placement, manipulation of an operative microscope, and insertion of the ventilation tube through a deformable tympanic membrane. A questionnaire was developed in consultation with instructing surgeons. Fourteen face validity questions focused on the anatomy of the ear, simulation of the operative microscope, appearance and movement of the surgical instruments, deformation and cutting of the eardrum, and myringotomy tube insertion. Six content validity questions focused on training potential on surgical tasks such as speculum placement, microscope positioning, tool navigation, ear anatomy, myringotomy creation and tube insertion. A total of 12 participants from the Department of Otolaryngology—Head and Neck Surgery were recruited for the study. Prior to completing the questionnaire, participants were oriented to the simulator and given unlimited time to practice until they were comfortable with all of its aspects.

**Results:** Responses to 12 of the 14 questions on face validity were predominantly positive. One issue of concern was with contact modeling related to tube insertion into the eardrum, and the second was with the movement of the blade and forceps. The former could be resolved by using a higher resolution digital model for the eardrum to improve contact localization. The latter could be resolved by using a higher fidelity haptic device. With regard to content validity, 64 % of the responses were positive, 21 % were neutral, and 15 % were negative.

**Conclusions:** The Western myringotomy simulator appears to have sufficient face and content validity. Further development with automated metrics and skills transference testing is planned.

**Keywords:** Myringotomy, Education, Simulator, Virtual reality, Face validity

* Correspondence: Sumit.Agrawal@lhsc.on.ca; hladak@uwo.ca
†Equal contributors
[1]Department of Electrical and Computer Engineering, Western University, London, ON, Canada
Full list of author information is available at the end of the article

## Introduction

Myringotomy with tube insertion is one of the most common procedures in Otolaryngology—Head & Neck Surgery, and is encountered by residents throughout their training. Despite the fact that it is a ubiquitous procedure, the instruction of junior trainees, who often have little experience in microscopic procedures, is often challenging. Montague et al. [1] have analyzed surgical errors through video analysis of actual procedures and note that the 4 most frequently occurring errors in order from most to least occurring include (1) failure to perform a unidirectional myringotomy, (2) making multiple attempts to place the tube, (3) making multiple attempts to complete the myringotomy, and (4) setting the microscope magnification too high. More serious intraoperative complications can also occur including external auditory canal lacerations, medial displacement of tubes into the middle ear, and vascular injuries [2–4]. Although surgical residents can eventually perform standard cases well, they often struggle with narrow canals, retracted tympanic membranes, T-tubes, and procedures performed under local anaesthestic. The goal of simulation is to decrease the learning curve prior to entering the operating, minimize complications in patients, and provide the ability to practice difficult cases.

Several physical models have been described in the literature to provide practice without potential harm to patients [5–9]. Generally, these consist of a tube to mimic the ear canal with a synthetic membrane attached to one end to represent the eardrum. These models do not appear to have gained general acceptance in residency programs, presumably because they are not able to represent anatomical variability easily and the mechanical properties of the materials used do not mimic that of the actual tissues.

Compared with physical models, simulators based on virtual-reality (VR) technologies have the ability to simulate difficult anatomy, model various pathologies, provide automated feedback, and even allow trainees to practice on patient-specific models generated from CT/MRI scans. VR-based simulators have been applied in Otolaryngology, especially for endoscopic sinus surgery [10–14] and for temporal bone drilling [15–18].

In VR simulators, the trainee interacts with realistic 3D digital models of anatomical structures and views them using 3D displays. Simulated tissues can be operated upon using digital representations of actual surgical tools that can be moved in the workspace using devices such as a haptic arm. The sensation of contact force between a digital surgical tool and simulated tissue can be computed and applied to the trainee's hand via the haptic arm.

The Auditory Biophysics Laboratory at Western University has developed and reported on several aspects of VR-based myringotomy simulation. A blade navigation software system [19, 20] and a system for real-time deformation and cutting of the tympanic membrane [21] were implemented on different software platforms as separate training modules. These versions of the simulator were not integrated and they did not include speculum placement, operating microscope controls for positioning/zooming, or tube insertion through the myringotomy.

As recently reported [22], the Western myringotomy simulator has integrated the previous modules into a common software platform. Moreover, new software modules have been added to allow the user to adjust their surgical view through positioning and tilting of the virtual speculum and operative microscope, and to allow insertion of a ventilation tube into the myringotomy created in a deformable tympanic membrane. The goal is to further expand this simulator in the future to allow trainees to raise tympanomeatal flaps andto eventually perform tympanoplasty/ossiculoplasty on patient-specific anatomy.

In order for training simulators to be accepted into a residency curriculum, a variety of validation studies need to be conducted starting with face validity and culminating in the demonstration that skills acquired in the VR environment transfer to the OR (operating room) environment. Face validity refers to the degree to which a simulation appears like the real situation [23] and content validity measures whether the simulator would be appropriate or useful in training [24, 25]. Although face validity has previously been established for individual software modules [19–21], validation testing has not been performed on the current integrated system, which simulates the entire procedure from microscope positioning to ventilation tube insertion [22].

The objective of this paper is to determine the face and content validity of the new integrated Western myringotomy simulator.

## Methods
### Simulator

An overview of the major features of the simulator is given here; in-depth technical details on the system can be found in a previous publication [22]. The simulator consists of 3 major components: the simulation software, a display system, and a haptic arm as shown in Fig. 1. The simulation software was developed in the Auditory Biophysics Laboratory at Western University [19–22]. The simulator runs on a Z420 Hewitt-Packard personal computer, equipped with an Intel(R) Xeon E5-1620 processor (Intel Corp., Sanata Clara, CA) and a NVIDIA Quadro 4000 graphics card (NVIDIA Corp., Santa Clara, CA). The system is capable of real-time rendering of the 3D digital models of the ear, surgical tools, and tympanic membrane as shown in Fig. 2a. The simulator can import various ear canal and tympanic membrane models,

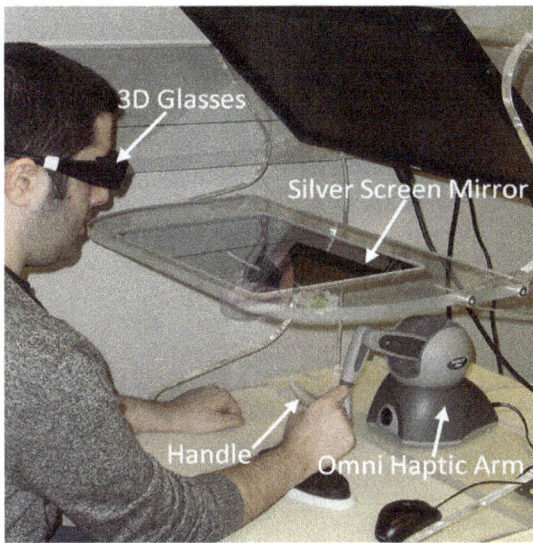

**Fig. 1** Simulator set up. A user is shown using the Western myringotomy simulator. By moving the handle of the haptic arm, the user controls the movement of a virtual myringotomy blade and forceps. The virtual ear and tools floating under the silver screen mirror are an artistic rendering of what the user would see through the 3D glasses

however for the purposes of this study, a normal pediatric ear canal and tympanic membrane was used. The system also incorporates multi-point collision detection to monitor for all interactions between the virtual tools and virtual ear and performs real-time deformation and tissue cutting as required. The software displays the models and all interactions on a silver screen mirror that is part of the DevinSense Display 300 system (DevinSense Display Solutions, Sundbyberg, Sweden). When the screen is viewed using active 3D glasses (Nvidia Corp., Santa Clara, CA) provided with the DevinSense system, the 3D digital scene consisting of the virtual ear and tools appears to exist in the space below the silver screen mirror. The display in this region is correctly co-located with the haptic arm (Omni haptic arm, Geomagic, Inc., Morrisville, NC) so movements of the haptic arm appear to occur in the same space as the 3D scene. Using the haptic arm, the user can move the virtual surgical tools. Currently, a single haptic arm is used to control the various instruments, however a second haptic arm could be added to simultaneously manipulate multiple instruments (e.g. speculum and myringotomy blade).

The haptic arm can be used to position and rotate the virtual speculum, position and tilt the microscope, and adjust magnification to obtain different views of the operative site as shown in Fig. 2b. The user can then create

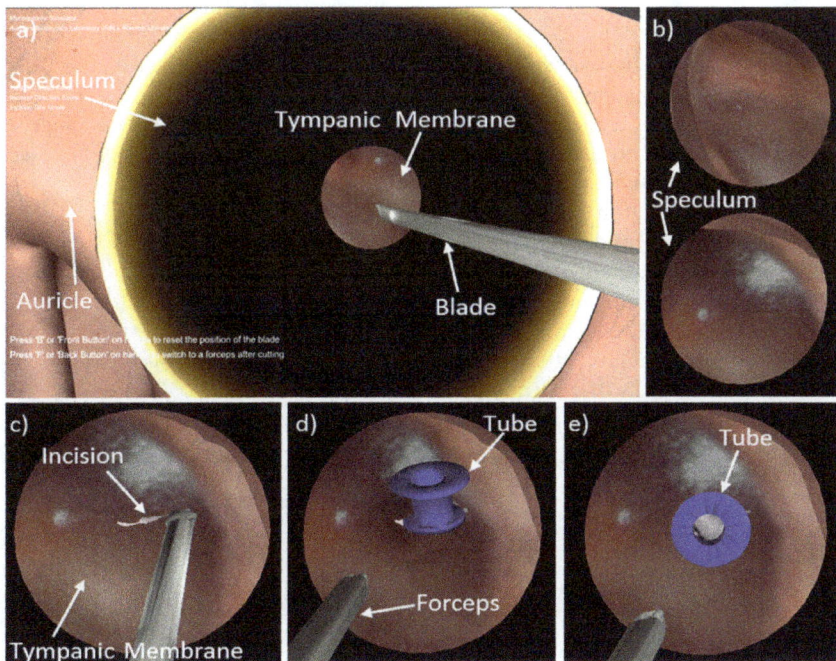

**Fig. 2** Simulator scene shown in 2D. The actual scene would be viewed by the user in stereoscopic 3D. **a)** View of the speculum and myringotomy blade. **b)** Magnified views of the tympanic membrane through the speculum (represented by the black circle). The view changes depending on the (i) magnification and (ii) position and tilt of the speculum and microscope. **c)** Myringotomy **d)** Tube insertion and splaying of the incision. **e)** Tube in final position with middle ear visible through the lumen of the tube

a myringotomy as shown in Fig. 2c using a virtual myringotomy blade; the position and orientation of the blade are controlled by moving the handle of the haptic arm. A tube may be inserted using virtual forceps, which is also controlled by the user using the haptic device [Fig. 2d]. The opening and closing of the forceps can be toggled using a button on the haptic arm. During tube insertion, the eardrum deforms and the incision splays as the tube enters the myringotomy. The tube may also be repositioned with various instruments until it is in its final position [Fig. 2e].

## Participants

Research ethics board approval was obtained from Western University (#105239) and participants were contacted via telephone or electronic mail. All participants were recruited from the Department of Otolaryngology - Head & Neck Surgery, Western University. A total of 12 subjects agreed to participate, which included seven junior Otolaryngology residents (postgraduate years 1 to 3) and five senior Otolaryngologists who routinely performed ventilation tube insertions in their practice. These groups were chosen to reflect the target group of the simulator (junior residents) as well as experts in the field (Otolaryngologists). The participants did not have any previous exposure to myringotomy simulation.

## Protocol

All participants were initially given an orientation session which consisted of: 1) an information sheet outlining the software features of the simulator, 2) a demonstration video of how to perform a myringotomy and tube insertion using the simulator controls, and 3) a live demonstration of the simulator and haptic arm. The same graduate student and surgical resident performed the orientation session for each participant, and a standardized script was used to ensure consistency. The participants were specifically asked to perform the tasks listed in Table 1 so that they could comment on all the various aspects of the simulator. Finally, the participants were given an unlimited period of time to use the

simulator until they felt comfortable completing the face and content validity questionnaires.

## Questionnaire

Previously, we had tested individual software modules focusing on blade navigation [19], haptics [20] and tympanic membrane deformation and cutting [21]. Since this new simulator [22] refined each of these components, including the graphical representations of the ear and virtual tools, and included new features such as microscope handling, speculum positioning and tube insertion, the Myringotomy Surgery Simulation Scale (MS$^3$) used in previous publications [20, 21] was modified to include these features. The questionnaire was divided into three sections (A, B, and C) with a total of 20 questions. Section A included 14 questions focusing on face validity as listed in Table 2. The appearance and realism of the surgical instruments; anatomy of the auricle, ear canal and eardrum; movement of surgical instruments; deformation and cutting of the eardrum; tube insertion and 3D microscopic view of the scene were assessed.

Section B included six questions focusing on content validity as listed in Table 3. These questions were used to determine training potential on specific surgical tasks.

In Sections A and B, study participants were asked to answer each question using a 7-point Likert scale, an equal appearing interval measurement. The scale had values of "1"—Strongly Disagree, 2—"Mostly Disagree", 3—"Disagree", 4—"Neither Agree/Disagree", 5—"Agree", 6—"Mostly Agree" and 7—"Strongly Agree".

In Section C, a free-form comment area was provided for each participant to provide feedback to elaborate on

**Table 1** Tasks involved in the face validity study

| Tasks | Description |
|---|---|
| Speculum adjustment | Rotate and tilt the speculum to obtain view of tympanic membrane |
| Microscope manipulation | Translate and rotate the microscope to obtain a proper view |
| Blade navigation | Navigate surgical blade through the external auditory canal |
| Myringotomy | Make an incision in the tympanic membrane |
| Ventilation tube insertion | Insert ventilation tube into the myringotomy using forceps |

**Table 2** Questions in Section A for face validity

| No. | Question: Rate whether the following aspects of the simulator are realistic |
|---|---|
| 1 | Visual appearance of the auricle and ear canal |
| 2 | Visual appearance of the speculum |
| 3 | Movement of the speculum |
| 4 | Movement of the microscope/camera |
| 5 | Zoom of the microscope/camera |
| 6 | Visual appearance of the eardrum |
| 7 | Movement of the eardrum when physically contacted |
| 8 | Visual appearance of the myringotomy blade |
| 9 | Visual appearance and splay of the myringotomy |
| 10 | Visual appearance of the forceps |
| 11 | Movement and stability of the myringotomy blade and forceps |
| 12 | Visual representation of the tube |
| 13 | Movement of the tube within the myringotomy |
| 14 | Three-dimensional microscopic view of the scene based on light rendering, shadows, and 3D goggles |

**Table 3** Questions in Section B for training potential

| No | Question: Do you feel that the simulator would be useful in teaching Otolaryngology trainees the following skills |
|----|------|
| 15 | Speculum placement |
| 16 | Microscope positioning |
| 17 | Tool navigation |
| 18 | Ear canal and eardrum anatomy |
| 19 | Myringotomy creation |
| 20 | Tube insertion |

previous questions and to address issues not covered in Sections A and B.

## Statistical analysis

The responses were initially divided by group (junior resident or practising Otolaryngologist), and the median, quartiles, minimum, and maximum response values were computed for each question. The sample size was maximized to include all eligible participants at a single academic institution. For each question, the Mann–Whitney $U$-test was used to test the significance of the differences in responses between the two groups. A frequency distribution histogram was plotted to investigate the number of favourable responses (score $\geq 5$), neutral responses (score $= 4$), and negative responses (score $\leq 3$) to each question. All data were computed and analysed using the SPSS statistical software (SPSS Inc, Chicago, IL). The significance was set at p < .05 and the Holm-Bonferroni method was used to correct for multiple comparisons.

## Results

### Demographics

The first group was comprised of seven junior Otolaryngology residents in postgraduate years 1 to 3. They were all familiar with the operating microscope and the procedure, however they were in the active phase of learning with each resident having performed fewer than 20 myringotomy and tube insertions in training. The second group had five fellowship trained Otolaryngologists who routinely performed myringotomy and tube insertions in their practice. Each member of this group had performed at least 200 procedures since completing their fellowship.

### Comparison of groups

The mean response and confidence interval for each question in Section A (face validity) and Section B (content validity) are summarized in Fig. 3. Application of the Mann–Whitney $U$-test indicates no statistically significant differences between residents and senior Otolaryngologists once the Holm-Bonferroni correction was applied. However, the largest differences between the groups were seen in Question 13 ($U = 5.5$, $p = 0.043$) and Question 20 ($U = 7$, $p = 0.097$), which related to the movement of the tube within the myringotomy.

### Face and content validity

Given that mean responses were not different at the $p = .05$ level, the results for the two groups were pooled when analyzing face and content validity. The responses to the questionnaires were categorized as positive (score $\geq 5$), neutral (score $= 4$) or negative (score $\leq 3$).

### Face validity

The realism of the simulator was investigated through the 14 questions in Section A of the questionnaire. As can be seen in Fig. 4, the number of positive responses exceeds the number of neutral and negative responses except in the case of Questions 9 and 11. Question 9 focuses on the realism of the visual appearance and splay of the myringotomy, whereas Question 11 focuses on

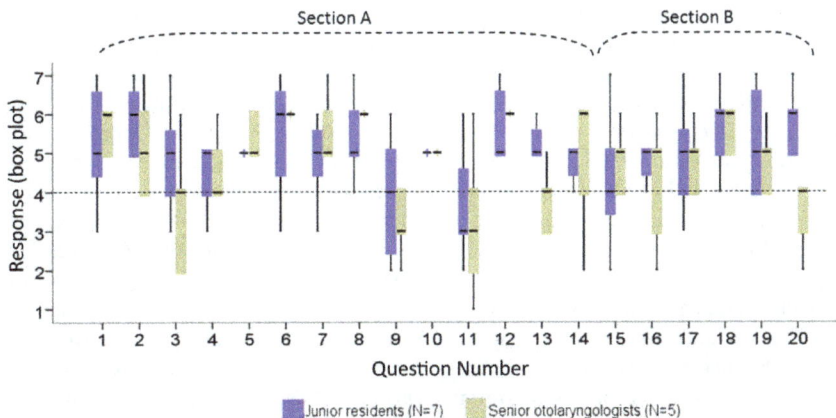

**Fig. 3** Box plot of the Likert item responses for the two groups of participants. Face validity was assessed in Questions 1–14, and content validity was assessed in Questions 15–20. A response of 4 is neutral, and higher values are more favourable than lower values

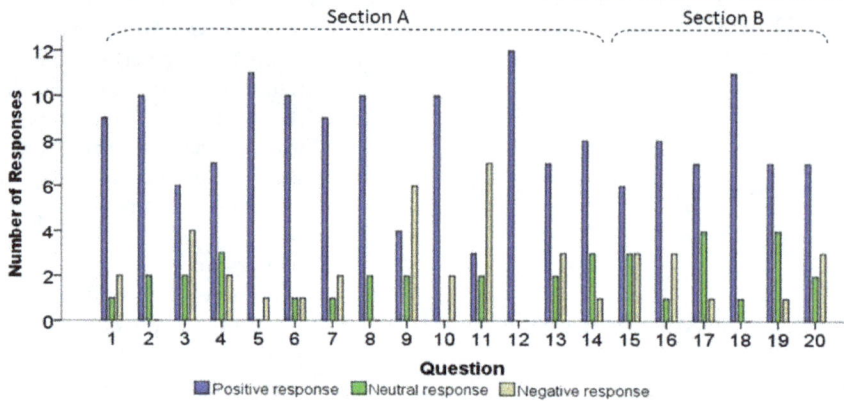

**Fig. 4** Total number of positive, neutral and negative responses to each question, pooling responses of junior residents and of senior Otolaryngologists. The blue bar indicates the number of positive responses (score ≥ 5), the green bar is the number of neutral responses (score = 4), and the beige bar indicates the number of negative responses (score ≤ 3)

the realism of the movement and stability of the myringotomy blade and forceps. Overall, when the 14 questions over 12 participants (168 total responses) were considered, there were 116 (69.0 %) positive responses, 21 (12.5 %) neutral responses, and 31 (18.5 %) negative responses.

### Content validity

The training potential of the simulator was tested through 6 questions in Section B of the questionnaire. As shown in Fig. 4, the number of positive responses was greater than the number of negative responses for each question in this section. Among the total 72 responses (6 questions x 12 participants), 46 (63.9 %) were positive, 15 (20.8 %) were neutral, and 11 (15.3 %) were negative.

### Discussion

The MS3 scale used in this study had to be developed at our institution as no other validated measure was available to assess a virtual-reality myringotomy simulator. This questionnaire has not been externally validated by other centres, however content validity was assessed by a group of experts during the development of the questionnaire. In addition, previous publications [20, 21] did demonstrate reliability of the MS3 with a strong correlation across raters. The MS3 was also correlated against a visual analogue scale measuring the same construct, thus providing a measure of concurrent validity [21].

The lack of statistically significant differences in mean responses between residents and senior Otolaryngologists to Questions 1 to 20 suggests that even with limited exposure to the actual procedure of myringotomy with tube insertion, junior residents had similar assessments of the realism and utility of the simulator as those experienced in the OR.

The only differences between the groups approaching significance were in Questions 13 and 20, which pertained the movement of the tube within the myringotomy. Senior Otolaryngologists perceived the simulated tube movement to be less realistic than did residents. Similarly, Question 9 in the pooled responses dealt with the splay of the myringotomy, and this had a higher number of negative responses overall. From the written comments in Section C of the questionnaire, it appears that splaying (i.e., spreading) of the virtual eardrum when it is contacted by the virtual blade is realistic, and this was also the case in our previous report [21]; however, splaying is less realistic during tube insertion when the virtual tube contacts the eardrum and causes it to spread.

This difference could be explained by a design decisions made during the development of the tube insertion module. First, although the tympanic membrane has real-time deformation, the physics of the interaction between the edges of the myringotomy and a ventilation tube is quite complex. In order to detect contact with the tube, the tympanic membrane is represented as a discrete collection of spatially distributed points as shown in Fig. 5. Collision detection is performed at each of these discrete contact points. When the spatial density of points is high (i.e. the points are close together) the location of contact can be calculated with more precision than when the spatial density is lower. Unfortunately, multi-point collision detection is computationally intensive, therefore the rendering speed decreases rapidly as the spatial density and precision is increased. The particular choice of density in the simulator was chosen to permit animations to occur at a realistic pace on an inexpensive personal computer, however this negatively affected the precision of the tympanic membrane splay in response to the tube.

Second, the physics of tympanic membrane 'tearing' with large forces and displacements during tube insertion

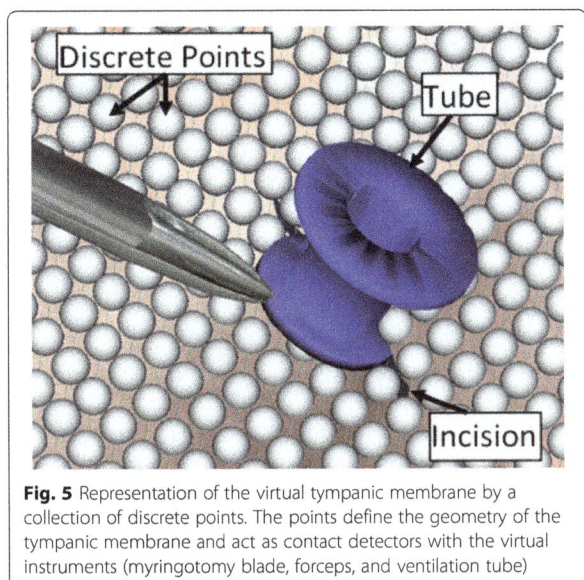

**Fig. 5** Representation of the virtual tympanic membrane by a collection of discrete points. The points define the geometry of the tympanic membrane and act as contact detectors with the virtual instruments (myringotomy blade, forceps, and ventilation tube)

are difficult to model in real-time. To overcome this, pre-programmed animations were used based on the length of incision, the trajectory of the tube, and the contact between the flange of the tube and the myringotomy. Although this significantly reduced computation time, Question 13 revealed that this lack of realism was noted by the experts and not the residents. This could be explained by the fact that senior surgeons would have had much more experience knowing how the ventilation tube *should* slide into the incision, therefore they were able to notice the subtle differences more than the junior trainees still learning the procedure. On average, Otolaryngologists' rankings fell between "Disagree" to "Neither Agree/Disagree", suggesting that slight improvements to the tube insertion simulation could make this aspect more acceptable.

Question 11 was the only other question with a higher proportion of negative responses, and this pertained to the movement and stability of the blade and forceps. Section C clarified this finding as concerns were raised about the limited range of motion of the haptic device and that the friction of the device affected the movements of the virtual blade and forceps. The haptic arm used in this study is a low-cost device that is suitable for design of a prototypical simulator. The device can easily be swapped for a higher fidelity device with greater range of motion and substantially reduced friction (e.g., Geomagic Phantom Premium device from Geomagic, Inc., Morrisville, NC), albeit at greater financial cost. Utilizing the higher fidelity device may result in acceptable range of motion and unnoticeable friction. A second concern with the device was the feel of the handle of the haptic arm when it was used to control the blade and forceps (Fig. 1). As the handle is thick, it feels

unnatural compared to holding an actual surgical tool. We have implemented approaches described in the literature to replace the haptic arm handle with actual surgical tools to improve the feel and realism of the simulation [26]. The goal in this hybrid simulator would be have one haptic arm attached to a myringotomy blade or forceps, and have the second haptic arm attached to a real speculum to maximize realism.

Face and content validity are only initial steps in validation, and they do not ensure that a simulator will be useful in training residents [24, 25]. Future development on the Western myringotomy simulator will address concerns raised in this study. Refinement and optimization of the tube insertion and tympanic membrane splay may help to increase the realism of the simulator, but it is unclear if increased fidelity will actually result in additional skills transference [27]. In order to determine the construct validity of the simulator, automated metrics including time, length and direction of incision, collisions, magnification, etc. have been incorporated into the simulator. A separate study will examine if these metrics are capable of distinguishing experts from residents, and a skills transference study will be needed to determine if the simulator can result in better operating room performance. A multi-centred study will be considered at that time to maximize sample size and feedback from different centres.

The authors hope that by using standardized libraries while programming the simulator, and the ability of the simulator to run on low-cost hardware, will allow easy adoption by Otolaryngology training programs and allow other groups to make modifications as needed.

## Conclusion

The Western myringotomy simulator has a number of new features including microscope handling, speculum positioning and ventilation tube insertion. The simulator has good face and content validity, except with respect to splaying of the myringotomy during tube insertion and with respect to the haptic arm. These issues are currently being addressed with further refinements and adaptations. Automated metrics have been developed and they will be used to assess for construct validity of the simulator. Although the entire myringotomy and ventilation tube insertion can now be simulated, a skills transference study is needed to establish training efficacy and clinical impact.

**Competing interests**
The authors declare that they have no competing interests.

**Authors' contributions**
CH, SKA and HML developed the myringotomy simulator. CH, HC, SKA and HML designed the face validity study. CH, SKA, and HC collected the data. CH and YB analyzed the data. SKA and HML reviewed the analysis results.

CH, YB, SKA and HML wrote the manuscript. SKA and HML were primary supervisors for CH and HC. All authors read and approved the final manuscript.

**Authors' information**
HML and SKA were co-senior authors on this study.

**Acknowledgements**
The authors would like to thank the Natural Sciences and Engineering Research Council of Canada (NSERC), Medtronic of Canada Ltd., and the Ontario Research Fund (ORF) for financial support of this project.

**Author details**
[1]Department of Electrical and Computer Engineering, Western University, London, ON, Canada. [2]Department of Otolaryngology – Head and Neck Surgery, Schulich School of Medicine and Dentistry, Western University, London, ON, Canada. [3]Biomedical Engineering Graduate Program, Western University, London, ON, Canada. [4]Lawson Health Research Institute, London, ON, Canada. [5]Department of Medical Biophysics, Western University, London, ON, Canada. [6]London Health Sciences Centre, Room B1-333, University Hospital, 339 Windermere Rd., London N6A 5A5ON, Canada.

**References**
1.  Montague M, Lee MSW, Hussain SSM. Human error identification: an analysis of myringotomy and ventilation tube insertion. Arch Otolaryngol Head Neck Surg. 2004;130:1153–7.
2.  Brodish BN, Woolley AL. Major vascular injuries in children undergoing myringotomy for tube placement. Am J Otolaryngol. 1999;20:46–50.
3.  Kumar M, Khan AM, Davis S. Medial displacement of grommets: an unwanted sequel of grommet insertion. J Laryngol Otol. 2000;114:448–9.
4.  Groblewski JC, Harley EH. Medial migration of tympanostomy tubes: an overlooked complication. Int J Pediatr Otorhinolaryngol. 2006;70:1707–14.
5.  Walker T, Duvvi S, Kumar BN. The wigan grommet trainer. Clin Otolaryngol. 2006;31:349–50.
6.  Duijvestein M, Borgstein J. The bradford grommet trainer. Clin Otolaryngol. 2006;31:163.
7.  Leong A, Kundu S, Martinez-Devesa P, Aldren C. Artificial ear: a training tool for grommet insertion and manual dexterity. ORL. 2006;68:115–7.
8.  Hong P, Webb AN, Corsten G, Balderston J, Haworth R, Ritchie K, et al. An anatomically sound surgical simulation model for myringotomy and tympanostomy tube insertion. Int J Pediatr Otorhinolaryngol. 2008;78:522–9.
9.  Volsky PG, Hughley BB, Peirce SM, Kesser BW. Construct validity of a simulator for myringotomy with ventilation tube insertion. Otolaryngology - Head and Neck Surg. 2009;141:603–8.
10. Weghorst S, Airola C, Oppenheimer P, Edmond CV, Patience T, Heskamp D, et al. Validation of the madigan ESS simulator. Stud Health Technol Informat. 1998;50:399–405.
11. Anil SM, Kato Y, Hayakawa M, Yoshida K, Nagahisha S, Kanno T. Virtual 3-dimensional preoperative planning with the Dextroscope for excision of a 4th ventricular ependymoma. Minim Invasive Neurosurg. 2007;50:65–70.
12. Audette M, Delingette H, Fuchs A, Astley O, Chinzei K. A topologically faithful, tissue-guided, spatially varying meshing strategy for computing patient-specific head models for endoscopic pituitary surgery simulation. Stud Health Technol Inform. 2006;119:22–7.
13. Tolsdorff B, Pommert A, Höhne KH, Petersik A, Pflesser B, Tiede U, et al. Virtual reality: a new paranasal sinus surgery simulator. Laryngoscope. 2010;120:420–6.
14. Varshney R, Frenkiel S, Nguyen LHP, Young M, Del Maestro R, Zeitouni A, et al. The McGill simulator for endoscopic sinus surgery (MSESS): a validation study. J Otolaryngol Head Neck Surg. 2014;43:40.
15. Wiet GJ, Stredney D, Kerwin T, Hittle B, Fernandez SA, Abdel-Rasoul M, et al. Virtual temporal bone dissection system: development and testing. Laryngoscope. 2012;122 Suppl 1:S1–S12.
16. Morris D, Sewell C, Barbagli F, Salisbury K, Blevins NH, Girod S. Visuohaptic simulation of bone surgery for training and evaluation. IEEE Comput Graph Appl. 2006;26:48–57.
17. Sewell C, Morris D, Blevins NH, Dutta S, Agrawal S, Barbagli F, et al. Providing metrics and performance feedback in a surgical simulator. Comput Aided Surg. 2008;13:63–81.
18. Arora A, Khemani S, Tolley N, Singh A, Budge J, Varela DA, et al. Face and content validation of a virtual reality temporal bone simulator. Otolaryngol Head Neck Surg. 2012;146:497–503.
19. Wheeler B, Doyle PC, Chandarana S, Agrawal S, Husein M, Ladak HM. Interactive computer-based simulator for training in blade navigation and targeting in myringotomy. Comput Meth Programs Biomed. 2010;98:130–9.
20. Sowerby LJ, Rehal G, Husein M, Doyle PC, Agrawal S, Ladak HM. Development and face validity testing of a three-dimensional myringotomy simulator with haptic feedback. J Otolaryngol Head Neck Surg. 2010;39:122–9.
21. Ho AK, Alsaffar H, Doyle PC, Ladak HM, Agrawal SK. Virtual reality myringotomy simulation with real-time deformation: development and validity testing. Laryngoscope. 2012;122:1844–51.
22. Huang C, Agrawal SK, Ladak HM. Virtual-reality simulator for training in myringotomy with tube placement. BC: Vancouver; 2014. Proceedings of the 37th Canadian medical and biological engineering conference: 20–23 May 2014.
23. Carter FJ, Schijven MP, Aggarwal R, Grantcharov T, Francis NK, Hanna GB, et al. Consensus guidelines for validation of virtual reality surgical simulators. Surg Endosc. 2005;19:1523–32.
24. Gallagher AG, Ritter EM, Satava RM. Fundamental principles of validation, and reliability rigorous science for the assessment of surgical education and training. Surg Endosc. 2003;17:1525–9.
25. Schout BM, Hendrikx AJ, Scheele F, Bemelmans BL, Scherpbier AJ. Validation and implementation of surgical simulators: a critical review of present, past, and future. Surg Endosc. 2010;24:536–46.
26. Coles TR, John NW, Sofia G, Gould DA, Caldwell DG. Modification of commercial force feedback hardware for needle insertion simulation. Stud Health Technol Inform. 2011;163:135–7. MMVR18 – Medicine Meets Virtual Reality 2011 Poster: 8–12 February 2011; Newport Beach, CA.
27. Hamstra SJ, Brydges R, Hatala R, Zendejas B, Cook DA. Reconsidering fidelity in simulation-based training. Acad Med. 2014;89:387–92.

# 14

# Optimal detection of hypothyroidism in early stage laryngeal cancer treated with radiotherapy

Graeme B. Mulholland[1] ⓘ, Han Zhang[1], Nhu-Tram A. Nguyen[2], Nicholas Tkacyzk[3], Hadi Seikaly[1], Daniel O'Connell[1], Vincent L. Biron[1] and Jeffrey R. Harris[1]*

## Abstract

**Background:** Hypothyroidism following radiation therapy (RT) for treatment of Head and Neck Cancer (HNC) is a common occurrence. Rates of hypothyroidism following RT for Early Stage Laryngeal Squamous Cell Carcinoma (ES-LSCC) are among the highest. Although routine screening for hypothyroidism is recommended; its optimal schedule has not yet been established. We aim to determine the prevalence and optimal timing of testing for hypothyroidism in ES-LSCC treated with RT.

**Method:** We conducted a population-based cohort study. Data was extracted from a prospective provincial head and neck cancer database. Demographic, survival data, and pre- and post-treatment thyroid stimulating hormone (TSH) levels were obtained for patients diagnosed with ES-LSCC from 2008–2012. Inclusion criteria consisted of patients diagnosed clinically with ES-LSCC (T1 or 2, N0, M0) treated with curative intent. Patients were excluded if there was a history of hypothyroidism before the treatment or any previous history of head and neck cancers.

**Results:** Ninety-five patients were included in this study. Mean age was 66.1 years (range: 44.0–88.0 years) and 82.3 % of patients were male. Glottis was the most common subsite at 77.9 % and the average follow-up was 40 months (Range: 12–56 months). Five-year overall survival generated using the Kaplan-Meier method was 79 %. Incidence of hypothyroidism after RT was found to be 46.9 %. The greatest frequency of developing hypothyroidism was at 12 months.

**Conclusions:** We found a high prevalence of hypothyroidism for ES-LSCC treated with RT, with the highest rate at 12 months. Consequently, we recommend possible routine screening for hypothyroidism using TSH level starting at 12 months. To our knowledge, this is the first study to suggest the optimal timing for the detection of hypothyroidism.

**Keywords:** Hypothyroidism, Early stage laryngeal squamous cell carcinoma, Radiation therapy

## Introduction

Head and neck cancer (HNC) encompasses 3 % of total malignancies in North America, with a large proportion presenting as laryngeal squamous cell carcinoma (LSCC) [1]. One thousand and fifty cases were diagnosed alone in Canada in 2014 [2]. Treatment for early stage LSCC (ES-LSCC) has traditionally utilized single modality regimes consisting of either radiation therapy (RT) or surgical resection [3, 4]. Due to increasing advances in radiation planning over the past decade using computerized tomography based image planning, many cancer treatment centers including ours have adopted RT as the preferred method of treatment for ES-LSCC [5].

Despite improvements in RT therapy, its effects on the thyroid gland remains significant, as it is located in very close proximity to the target of treatment [6, 7]. Hypothyroidism as the result of radiation induced fibrosis and compromise of thyroid vascularity is still a common unnoticed complication after treatment of LSCC with a frequency of 14–36 % [8]. The most common signs and symptoms of hypothyroidism present as dry skin, cold sensitivity, fatigue, muscle cramps, voice changes, and constipation [9]. Left untreated hypothyroidism is associated

* Correspondence: Jeffrey.Harris@albertahealthservices.ca
Poliquin Residents' Competition, 69th Annual General Meeting of the Canadian Society of Otolaryngology—Head & Neck Surgery, Winnipeg MB, June 6, 2015.
Presented by Dr. Graeme B. Mulholland.
[1]Division of Otolaryngology-Head and Neck Surgery, University of Alberta Hospital, 1E4.29 WMC, 8440 – 112 Street, Edmonton, AB T6G 2B7, Canada
Full list of author information is available at the end of the article

with increased total low-density lipoprotein cholesterol and cardiac morbidity including mortality and atherosclerotic events [10]. As a result of these risks, the NCCN guidelines recognise the risk of developing hypothyroidism in association with treatments for LSCC and recommend screening every 6 to 12 months following treatment [11]. However, to our knowledge there has been no conclusive evidence looking at the optimal time in screening for hypothyroidism for ES-LSCC treated with RT. Therefore, we sought to investigate the ideal time of testing for hypothyroidism in patients with ES-LSCC treated with RT defined as the point in time where the test is associated with the highest frequency. We also evaluated the incidence of hypothyroidism in this patient population within Alberta, Canada.

## Method

Ethics approval was granted by the University of Alberta's Health Research Ethics Board (HREB) and the Alberta Cancer Board.

### Patients

Inclusion criteria were defined as: residents of Alberta greater than 18 years of age, with biopsy-proven early stage (T1 or T2, N0) LSCC (based on the 7th Edition of the AJCC TNM Staging Manual) [12]. All treated using primary RT with curative intent in Alberta.

Exclusion criteria were defined as: patients with previous HNC with or without treatment, a diagnosis of hypothyroidism prior to radiation treatment or incomplete data sets from chart review.

### Data collection

All patients diagnosed with ES-LSCC meeting inclusion criteria from January 1, 2008 to December 31, 2012 were included in the study. Demographic, survival and clinicopathologic data was obtained initially through the Alberta Cancer Registry (ACR) by a data analyst. The ACR is a population-based registry established in 1942 that records and maintains data of all new cancer cases, their treatments, and resulting deaths in the province of Alberta in a longitudinal and prospective fashion [13]. A review of outpatient, inpatient, and cancer clinic records was then performed for quality assurance and to extract relevant patient, tumour, lab values (pre-treatment albumin and pre and post-treatment thyroid stimulating hormone (TSH) levels), treatment, follow-up, as well as survival data Charlson Comorbidity Index (CCI) scores, which were not included in the ACR database, were calculated using relevant comorbidities taken from chart review [14]. Date of diagnosis was defined as the date of pathologically confirmed ES-LSCC.

### Staging

Staging of the tumours was clinical and according to the seventh edition of the American Joint Committee on Cancer (AJCC) TNM staging manual [12].

### Treatment

All patients underwent radiation therapy (RT) for curative intent. Patients receiving RT or CRT for distant metastases or palliation were not included. Intensity-modulated or 3-D conformal RT were utilized with dosing between 60.75 and 70 Gy, using 2 Gy per fraction, depending on the T-status [11].

### Outcomes

The primary outcome was set as the optimal time of testing for the elevation of TSH after treatment of ES-LSCC defined as the point in time where the testing is the most sensitive. The time interval to the initial elevation of TSH after treatment of ES-LSCC with RT was calculated for every patient. This was defined as the time from completion of RT until the first elevated TSH. The secondary outcome was the incidence of hypothyroidism after treatment of ES-LSCC with RT.

### Hypothyroidism

All included patients had pre-treatment TSH values. Patients were then screened for elevated TSH levels at 3–6 month intervals starting at 3 months until 30 months. Hypothyroidism was defined as an elevated TSH value based on the reference value given for each type of TSH test (TSH only (0.20–4.00 mU/L) or Progressive TSH (0.30–4.00 mU/L).

### Follow-up

All patients were followed at regional cancer treatment centers at regular intervals following treatment. Our cut off time point was February 1st, 2015. Patients who were suspected to have disease recurrence underwent a metastatic workup including appropriate imaging, endoscopy and biopsy as per standard of care.

### Statistical analysis

Baseline characteristics were compared using standard modes of comparison. Continuous data was analyzed using analysis of variance (ANOVA). Categorical data was compared using the chi-squared test. Univariate analysis was performed to determine the prevalence of hypothyroidism and the optimal timing of the elevation of TSH. Analyses were performed using SPSS Statistics 20.0 (SPSS Inc, Chicago, IL).

## Results

One hundred and sixty two patients were diagnosed with ES-LSCC in Alberta from 2008 to 2013. Of these,

67 patients were excluded: 11 for insufficient data points, 8 patients were treated with primary surgery and 48 patients had an elevated TSH prior to the start of RT treatment. Exclusion criteria were then applied to inclusion criteria, leading to a final data set of 95 patients for analysis.

Figure 1 represents overall and disease-free survival for our ES-LSCC data set. Five-year overall and disease-free survivals were 79 and 81 % respectively.

Table 1 contains patient demographic and tumour subsites information. The average age was 66.1 years (range: 41.0–88.0 years) with a strong male predominance (82.3 %). Glottis was the most common tumor subsite (77.9 %), followed by subglottis (14.7 %). A minority of cases were represented by supraglottis and transglottis subsites at 4.2 and 3.2 % respectively.

Tables 2 shows TSH specific data. Forty five (46.9 %) of patients had elevated TSH during the period of follow up. In addition, 27 patients were found to have a TSH greater than 10.00 mU/L. Figure 2 shows the breakdown in terms of time to elevated TSH. The majority of patients (42 %) had elevated TSH at the 12-month interval.

Seventy six of 95 (80.0 %) and 79 of 95 patients (83.2 %) received TSH testing within the first 15 and 18 months following initiation of RT. Of the 19 patients not receiving TSH testing during the first 15 months following treatment 6 patients presented with elevated TSH values upon first TSH testing. Figure 3 illustrates the distribution and frequency of TSH screening. Testing started at 3 month and was continued through 30 months after completion of RT treatments. The

**Table 1** Patient characteristics

| Variable | N |
|---|---|
| n | 95 |
| Mean Age (range), years | 66.1 (41.0–88.0) |
| Gender, no. (%) | |
| Male | 79 (82.3) |
| Female | 16 (16.7) |
| Mean CCI (range) | 2.8 (0.0–13.0) |
| Tumour Subsite, no. (%) | |
| Glottis | 74 (77.9) |
| Subglottis | 14 (14.7) |
| Supraglottis | 4 (4.2) |
| Transglottic | 3 (3.2) |
| T-Stage, no. (%) | |
| 1 | 59 (61.4) |
| 2 | 37 (38.6) |

*CCI* Charlson comorbidity index

majority of TSH testing took place within the first 21 months. For TSH levels tested at 3, 6, 9, 12, 15, 18 and 21 months the frequency of patients tested was greater than 50 % for all intervals (56.8, 66.3, 60.0, 67.4, 66.3, 60.0 and 56.8 %) respectively. From 24 to 30 months between 36.8 and 42.1 % of patients received TSH screening. A standard error calculation was performed for this data with a value of 0.44. The single greatest screening interval was at 12 months, where 67.4 % of patients had TSH testing. The lowest screening interval was at 24 months with 36.8 % of patients tested.

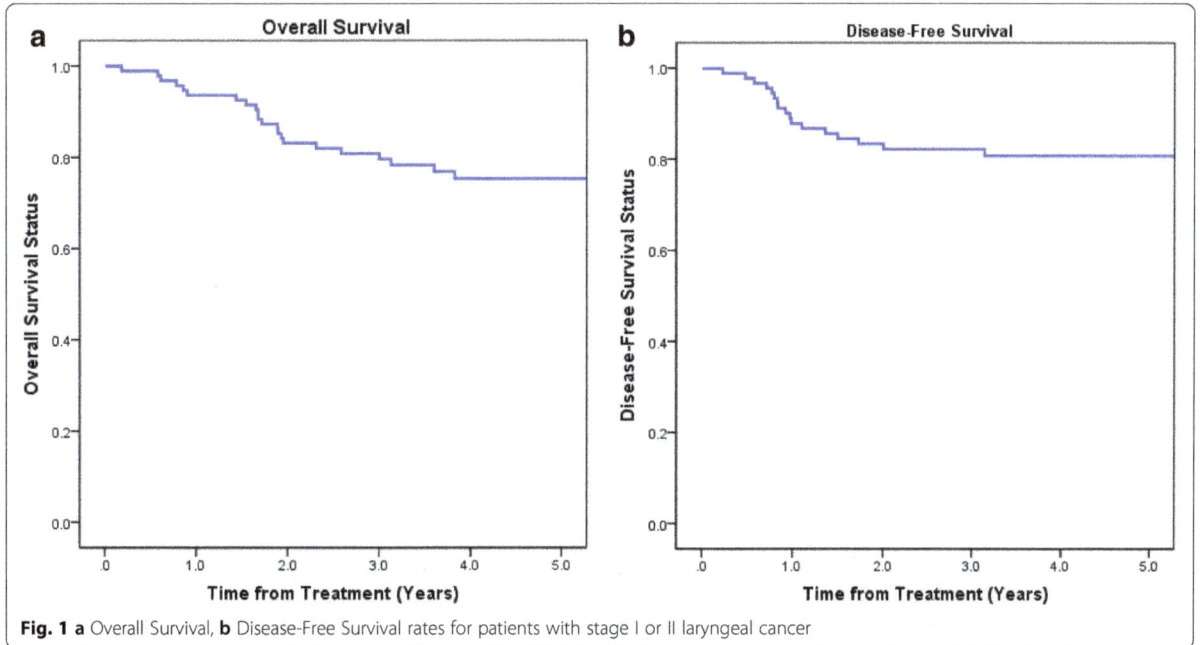

**Fig. 1 a** Overall Survival, **b** Disease-Free Survival rates for patients with stage I or II laryngeal cancer

**Table 2** Hypothyroidism variables

| Variable | N |
| --- | --- |
| Elevated TSH, no. (%) | 45 (46.9) |
| Mean Peak TSH (range), mIU/mL | 16.9 (4.0–55.9) |
| Number of Patients TSH > 10 mU/L | 27 |

*TSH* Thyroid stimulating hormone

## Discussion

It is well established that treatment of HNC using RT, chemotherapy or surgery increases the risk of developing hypothyroidism. Based on the literature, compared to other treatments modalities for ES-LSCC, RT is associated with the greatest risk, 48 % at 5 years and 67 % at 8 years following treatment [15]. Its pathophysiology is not completely understood, but most likely involves damage to thyroid vasculature. Additional theories specific to RT involve direct micro and macrovascular damage, fibrosis of the thyroid capsule which may limit compensatory thyroid enlargement and even the formation of induced antithyroglobulin antibodies [7]. The risk of developing hypothyroidism becomes greater the closer the anatomical relationship between the treated tissue and thyroid tissue [16]. Despite this high incidence, no study has looked at hypothyroidism in patients who receive single modality therapy with RT for ES-

LSCC. As such, there are currently no standardised post treatment hypothyroidism screening recommendations specifically for this patient population.

The literature has yielded multiple studies investigating the effects of RT in the treatment of HNC and LSCC within a heterogeneous patient population. Two of the most relevant studies are discussed. A systematic review published in 2011 by Boomsma et al. [17] looking at the incidence of hypothyroidism in all presentations of HNC treated with RT cited rates of subclinical hypothyroidism from 23 to 53 % at median follow up times of 2.4 to 6.1 years post RT. They found that hypothyroidism developed at a median interval of 1.4 to 1.8 years after treatment. The paper suggests that the development of subclinical hypothyroidism found at median follow up times should act as an indicator for the duration of TSH monitoring following treatment. However, no follow up regime or optimal time to initiate screening was suggested. The study by Kumar et al. [18] is the best example of a population similar to the one we examined. They looked at all curative treatment modalities including RT, surgery as well as chemoradiotherapy (CRT) for ES-LSCC and found rates of subclinical hypothyroidism at 24 % and symptomatic hypothyroidism at 6 %. Unfortunately, they were unable to provide information related to timing of onset of hypothyroidism post RT.

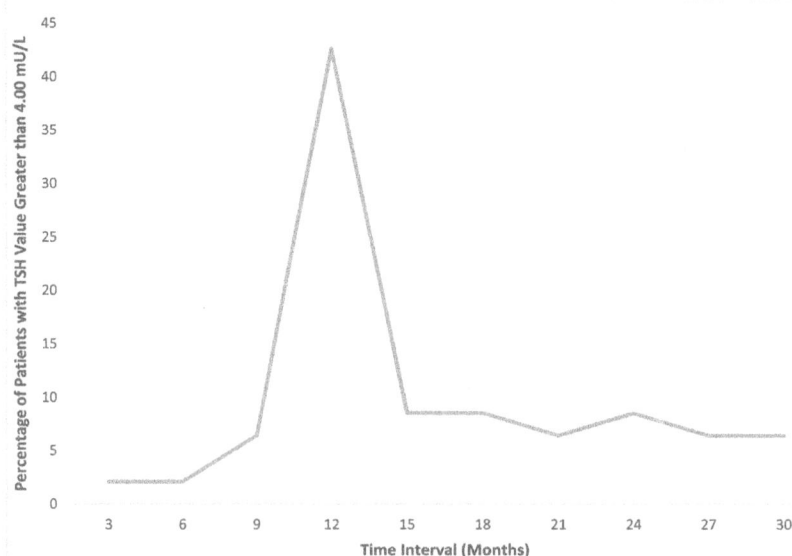

*Elevated TSH measurements where based on values for individual TSH test used. Two variations of TSH testing were used.

TSH Only reference range (0.20-4.00 mU/L)

Progressive TSH reference range (0.30-4.00 mU/L)

**Fig. 2** Patients with TSH Greater than 4.00 mU/L by Time of Presentation

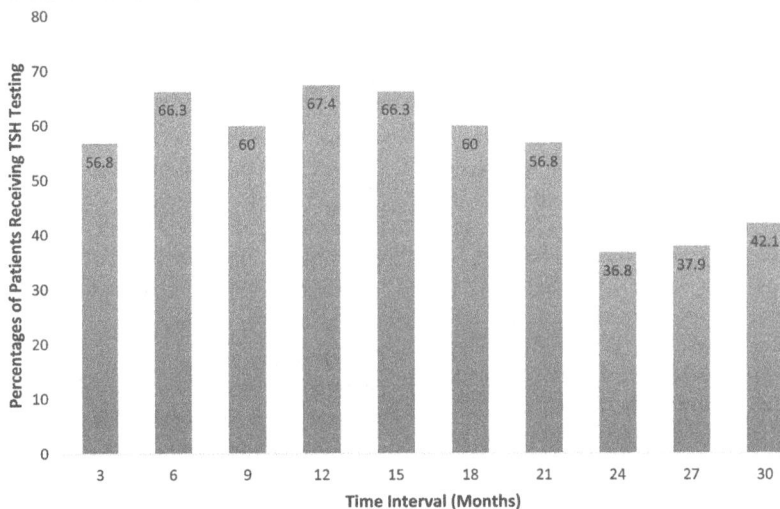

Standard error: 0.44

**Fig. 3** Percentage of Patients Receiving TSH Testing at Given Time Intervals

Information in relation to the length of follow up was also insufficient as a result of limited access to patient TSH results and follow up clinical information. In comparison, we found 46.9 % of our study group developed elevated TSH following treatment with RT. This is most commonly observed at the 12 month mark with 89.4 % of patients whom developed and elevated TSH at or after this time point.

Screening for hypothyroidism with TSH is reliant on a normal functioning hypothalamic–pituitary–thyroid axis. The use of TSH is cheap, reliable and sensitive to fluctuations in thyroxine (T4) levels [9]. Our study used TSH as a marker for hypothyroidism, identifying cases of thyroid gland dysfunction. Subclinical hypothyroidism (mild thyroid gland failure) is defined as persistently elevated TSH with normal thyroxine (T4) levels over a period of at least 3 months. Overt hypothyroidism relies on a persistently elevated TSH with low T4 levels [19]. Prolonged elevation of TSH levels correlate with significant long term sequelae. Increased total low-density lipoprotein cholesterol and cardiac morbidity including mortality and atherosclerotic events are among the most severe [10]. Therefore, thyroid hormone replacement therapy is recommended in all cases where TSH is > than 10 mIU/L [9]. Given the strong correlation between TSH values and significant long term sequelae, at our institution, the use of TSH alone suffices in determining need for treatment as well as for use as a maker of thyroid dysfunction.

Utilizing TSH ensured sufficient data for collection and ease of comparison from one institution to another. Reference ranges for elevated TSH varied depending on institution or type of test (progressive TSH or TSH only). All elevated TSH tests were categorized as hypothyroidism as measured by reference ranges for each test. We obtained mean peak TSH values of 16.9 mIU/L (4.0–55.9 mIU/L) in our population indicating a need for thyroxine replacement to avoid long term sequelae. Status and treatment of clinical versus sublinical hypothyroidism was beyond the scope of our study. Within our patient cohort, access to TSH information was more reliable than T3/T4 which was not routinely done as part of the hypothyroidism work up. Additionally, a protocol for treating subclinical versus clinical hypothyroidism is still not well defined. From the literature, a study looking at presentations of subclinical versus biochemical hypothyroidism in 2 randomized controlled trials by Murthy et al. [20] examined 122 patients affected by head and neck cancers treated with 3D conformational RT. They measured TSH and T4 levels every 3 to 6 months following completdraw ion of treatment. Patients with elevated TSH alone were deemed subclinical hypothyroidism and patients with elevated TSH and low T4 levels were classified as biochemical hypothyroidism. Hypothyroidism presented in 55 % of patients at a median follows up of 44 months, of these 39.3 % subclinical and 15.7 % biochemical. As described by the author, the decision to treat patient was not based on T4, rather treatment initiation was based on presentation with symptoms of hypothyroidism or prolonged elevation of TSH. This is in keeping with the literature. A TSH level greater or equal to 10 mIU/L for a period longer than 3 months is deemed significant enough to initiate thyroid hormone replacement therapy in order to obviate long term consequences. Therefore for our own population of ES-LSCC treated with RT, TSH was utilized alone as the cut-off point to avoid long term sequelae.

Based on our results, the optimal time to initiating screening for hypothyroidism is at 12 months. We observed a significant peak at this time point represented by 20 cases (42.6 %). The earliest elevated TSH was noted at 3 month in a minority of cases (2.1 %). It should be noted the majority of patients presented with elevation of TSH at or after 12 months (87.3 %). The incidence of elevated TSH in the Albertan ES-LSCC population was 45 patents (46.9 %). We found evidence that thyroid function worsens with time, the mean peak TSH was observed at 26.6 months with an average TSH value of 16.9 mIU/L. The delay in presentation in peak TSH is likely explained by a combination of factors. Thyroid stimulating hormone values greater than 4 mIU/L and less than 10 mIU/L are indeterminate in terms of initiating treatment [9]. The onset of hypothyroidism following RT is insidious and increases significantly with time following treatment [15]. Likely, the development of TSH level greater than 10mIU/L appeared more frequently at a greater duration of time following RT. Also, time for treatment optimization and patient compliance with treatment (routinely elevated TSH levels do not produce symptomatology) may contribute to the delay in peak TSH values. Given that our study indicates a peak TSH a later time point than the first observed elevation of TSH and that the risk of developing hypothyroidism increases with time following treatment. This may reinforce the need for lifelong TSH screening. Not only to pick up hypothyroidism initially but to titrate treatments appropriately.

Limitations of the study are acknowledged. The prospectively collected, retrospectively reviewed population-based design of the study did not allow for controls. No set protocol for TSH screening following RT is in place throughout Alberta. Although patients generally receive screening in an every 6–12 month fashion the number of screening events are at the discretion of the family physician, radiation or surgical oncologist. The majority of screening took place between 3 and 21 months. At each of these time intervals greater than 50 % of patients received screening (Fig. 3), a good indication that although no explicit screening regime is implemented, the majority of patients received routine investigation for hypothyroidism. Screening tapered after 21 months with between 36.8 and 42.1 % patients being screened between 24 and 30 months. Additionally, we were only able to consistently access TSH results, consequently without T4 results we were unable to definitively classify patients into categories of subclinical versus overt hypothyroidism. Even without T4 information available TSH information was able to indicate the need for

treatment in our ES-LSCC population. Our study also lacked fields of RT therapy for individual patients, while this may have led to confounding of data, all patients were staged at T1/2 and N0 with standardized curative RT protocol as per the Division of Radiation Oncology at the Cross Cancer Institute, University of Alberta. Given these limitations a multi-institutional, prospectively planned study utilizing a set hypothyroidism screening regime—including TSH and T4 monitoring at set time intervals—would be useful to determine whether hypothyroid screening protocols affect patient outcomes.

## Conclusion

Hypothyroidism in patients with ES-LSCC treated with curative RT is common. This population-based study suggests that optimal timing for screening for hypothyroidism using TSH is at 12 months' time. Future prospective studies to develop screening protocols for hypothyroidism in patients with ES-LSCC treated with curative RT should be undertaken.

### Competing interests

The authors declare that they have no competing interests.

### Authors' contributions

GBM, HZ and NT carried out data collection and drafted the manuscript. HZ performed statistical analysis. GBM, HZ and NAN participated in the design of the study and draft of the manuscript. JRH conceived of the study, and participated in its design and coordination and helped to draft the manuscript. All authors read and approved the final manuscript.

### Author details

[1]Division of Otolaryngology-Head and Neck Surgery, University of Alberta Hospital, 1E4.29 WMC, 8440 – 112 Street, Edmonton, AB T6G 2B7, Canada. [2]Division of Radiation Oncology, McMaster University, Hamilton, Canada. [3]Northern Ontario School of Medicine, Sudbury, Canada.

### References

1. Siegel RL, Miller KD, Jemal A. Cancer statistics, 2015. CA Cancer J Clin. 2015;65(1):5–29.
2. Canadian Cancer Society statistics. 2013. Available at: http://www.cancer.ca/en/cancer-information/cancer-type/laryngeal/statistics/?region=ab (accessed on February, 2015).
3. Makki FM, Williams B, Rajaraman M, Hart RD, Trites J, Brown T, et al. Current practice patterns in the management of glottic cancer in canada: results of a national survey. J Otolaryngol Head Neck Surg. 2011;40(3):205–10.
4. Taylor SM, Kerr P, Fung K, Aneeshkumar MK, Wilke D, Jiang Y, et al. Treatment of T1b glottic SCC: Laser vs. radiation—a canadian multicenter study. J Otolaryngol Head Neck Surg. 2013;42:22-0216-42-22.
5. Chera BS, Amdur RJ, Morris CG, Kirwan JM, Mendenhall WM. T1N0 to T2N0 squamous cell carcinoma of the glottic larynx treated with definitive radiotherapy. Int J Radiat Oncol Biol Phys. 2010;78(2):461–6.
6. Gupta T, Agarwal J, Jain S, Phurailatpam R, Kannan S, Ghosh-Laskar S, et al. Three-dimensional conformal radiotherapy (3D-CRT) versus intensity modulated radiation therapy (IMRT) in squamous cell carcinoma of the head and neck: a randomized controlled trial. Radiother Oncol. 2012;104:343.
7. Miller MC, Agrawal A. Hypothyroidism in postradiation head and neck cancer patients: incidence, complications, and management. Curr Opin Otolaryngol Head Neck Surg. 2009;17(2):111–5.

8. Kumpulainen EJ, Hirvikoski PP, Virtaniemi JA, Johansson RT, Simonen PM, Terävä MT, et al. Hypothyroidism after radiotherapy for laryngeal cancer. Radiother Oncol. 2000;57(1):97–101.

9. Garber JR, Cobin RH, Gharib H, Hennessey JV, Klein I, Mechanick JI, et al. Clinical practice guidelines for hypothyroidism in adults: cosponsored by the American Association of Clinical Endocrinologists and the American Thyroid Association. Endocr Pract. 2012;18:988–1028.

10. Surks MI, Ortiz E, Daniels GH, Sawin CT, Col NF, Cobin RH, et al. Subclinical thyroid disease: scientific review and guidelines for diagnosis and management. JAMA. 2004;291:228–38.

11. Pfister DG, Spencer S, Brizel DM, Burtness BA, Busse PM, Caudell JJ et al. NCCN Clinical Practice Guidelines in Oncology (NCCN Guidelines) Head and Neck Cancers. 2nd ed. Washington, PA: National Comprehensive Cancer Network; 2014.

12. Edge SB. AJCC cancer staging handbook: from the AJCC cancer staging manual. 7th ed. New York: Springer; 2010.

13. Alberta Heath Services. Cancer Available at: http://www.albertahealth services.ca/2171.asp (accessed March 1, 2013).

14. Charlson ME, Pompei P, Ales KL, MacKenzie CR. A new method of classifying prognostic comorbidity in longitudinal studies: development and validation. J Chronic Dis. 1987;40:373–83.

15. Mercado G, Adelstein DJ, Saxton JP, Secic M, Larto MA, Lavertu P. Hypothyroidism: a frequent event after radiotherapy and after radiotherapy with chemotherapy for patients with head and neck carcinoma. Cancer. 2001;92(11):2892–7.

16. Sinard RJ, Tobin EJ, Mazzaferri EL, Hodgson SE, Young DC, Kunz AL, et al. Hypothyroidism after treatment for nonthyroid head and neck cancer. Arch Otolaryngol Head Neck Surg. 2000;126(5):652–7.

17. Boomsma MJ, Bijl HP, Langendijk JA. Radiation-induced hypothyroidism in head and neck cancer patients: a systematic review. Radiother Oncol. 2011;99(1):1–5.

18. Kumar S, Moorthy R, Dhanasekar G, Thompson S, Griffiths H. The incidence of thyroid dysfunction following radiotherapy for early stage carcinoma of the larynx. Eur Arch Otorhinolaryngol. 2011;268(10):1519–22.

19. Kaptein EM, LoPresti JS, Kaptein MJ. Is an isolated TSH elevation in chronic nonthyroidal illness "subclinical hypothyroidism"? J Clin Endocrinol Metab. 2014;99(11):4015–26.

20. Murthy V, Narang K, Ghosh-Laskar S, Gupta T, Budrukkar A, Agrawal JP. Hypothyroidism after 3-dimensional conformal radiotherapy and intensity-modulated radiotherapy for head and neck cancers: Prospective data from 2 randomized controlled trials. Head Neck. 2014;36(11):1573–80.

# "Clinicopathological features and treatment outcomes of differentiated thyroid cancer in Saudi children and adults"

Khalid Hussain AL-Qahtani[1], Mutahir A. Tunio[2*], Mushabbab Al Asiri[3], Naji J. Aljohani[4], Yasser Bayoumi[5], Khalid Riaz[2] and Wafa AlShakweer[6]

## Abstract

**Introduction:** Age is an important prognostic factor in differentiated thyroid cancer (DTC). Our aim was to evaluate differences in clinicopathological features and treatment outcomes among children and adult patients with DTC.

**Materials and methods:** We studied 27 children (below 18 years) with DTC treated during the period 2000–2012 and were compared with (a) 78 adults aged 19–25 years and (b) 52 adults aged 26–30 years treated during the same period in terms of their clinicopathological features and long term treatment outcomes. Locoregional recurrence (LRR), locoregional control (LRC), distant metastasis (DM), distant metastasis control (DMC), disease free survival (DFS) and overall survival (OS) rates were evaluated.

**Results:** Mean age of children was 13.5 years (range: 5–18), while mean age of adults was 24.6 years (range: 19–30). In children, female: male ratio was 2.85:1, and in adults female: male ratio was 7.1:1 ($P = 0.041$). No significant difference in tumor size was seen between the two groups ($P = 0.653$). According to American Thyroid Association (ATA) risk stratification classification, the children (85.2 %) were found to have at high risk as compared to adults $P = 0.001$. Post-thyroidectomy complications and RAI induced toxicities were observed more in children than adults ($P = 0.043$ and $P = 0.041$ respectively). LRR occurred in 6 (22.2 %), 9 (11.5 %) and 3 (5.8 %) in age groups of <18 years, 19–25 years and 26–30 years respectively ($P = 0.032$); while DM was seen in 10 (37.0 %), 9 (10.3 %) and 5 (9.6 %) in age groups of <18 years, 19–25 years and 26–30 years respectively ($P = 0.002$). Ten year DFS rates were 67.3 % in age group below 18 years, 82.4 % in age group of 19–25 years and 90.1 % in age group of 26–30 years ($P = 0.021$).

**Conclusion:** At the time of diagnosis, children with DTC were found to have more aggressive clinicopathological characteristics. Comparatively lower LRC, DMC and DFS rates in children warrants further multi-institutional studies.

**Keywords:** Differentiated thyroid cancers, Children, Adults, Clinicopathological characteristics, Treatment outcomes

## Background

The incidence of differentiated thyroid cancers (DTC), including papillary (PTC) and follicular (FTC) variants, is increasing exponentially over the past years throughout the world with a wide geographic variation [1]. In Kingdom of Saudi Arabia, DTC is the second most common malignancy among middle aged women [2]. DTC is relatively uncommon in children (age 18 years or below), adolescents (under 25 years old), and young adults (above 25 and below 30 years) accounting for 3–10 %.

Recent data has suggested that the frequency of DTC in children varies according to pre-puberty, puberty and adolescence growth phases [3, 4]. In contrast to adults, DTC in pre-pubertal children has some distinctive differences; such as (a) larger primary tumor at the time of diagnosis; (b) high prevalence of neck lymph nodes and distant metastases at the time of diagnosis; and (c) the high risk of recurrences [5].

DTC in children and adolescents is treated in similar fashion as that in adults, primarily because of rarity of disease in pediatric population and lack of availability of pediatric DTC treatment guidelines [6]. Fortunately, even with aggressive behavior, DTC in children has

* Correspondence: drmutahirtonio@hotmail.com
[2]Radiation Oncology, King Fahad Medical City, Riyadh, Saudi Arabia
Full list of author information is available at the end of the article

excellent prospects with use of thyroidectomy, neck dissection, radioactive iodine-131 (RAI) ablation and suppression of thyroid-stimulating hormone (TSH) secretion with levothyroxine [5, 6].

In the current study, we designed our approach towards the comparative analysis of different clinicopathological features and treatment outcomes among children, adolescents and young adults with DTC in Kingdom of Saudi Arabia.

## Methods

After formal approval from the institutional ethical committee, medical records of 157 DTC patients of age less than 30 years, who were treated at our hospital during the period of July 2000 and December 2012 were reviewed using computer based database system.

For the purpose of present study, the study population was divided in three groups; (a) children (patients below or equal to the age of 18 years), (b) young adults (aged 19 to 25 years) and (c) adults (aged 26 to < 30 years) [7].

### Demographic, clinicopathological and radiological data

Demographic and clinical data including age at the time of diagnosis, gender and symptomatology were reviewed. A detailed second review of all histopathological specimens was done by experienced histopathologist. Different histopathological characteristics, including tumor size, histopathologic variants, multifocality, tumor, lymph node and metastasis (TNM) staging were recorded. Data was collected from different imaging modalities including neck ultrasonography (USG), whole body I-131 scintigraphy (WBS), computed tomography (CT) scan of neck and chest and flourodeoxyglucose positron emission tomography (FDG-PET). Data regarding different treatment modalities including thyroidectomy, +/− neck dissection, adjuvant radioactive iodine-131 (RAI) ablation and its doses in millicurie (mCi) were also recorded.

### Statistical analysis

The primary endpoint was the disease free survival (DFS). Secondary points were; the comparative analysis of different clinicopathological features of DTC in children and adults, locoregional control (LRC), distant metastasis control (DMC) and overall survival (OS) rates.

Local recurrence (LR) was defined as the duration between surgery date and date of clinically or radiologically detectable disease in the thyroid bed and/or in cervical lymph nodes on imaging (USG, WBS, CT and FDG-PET) after evaluation of elevated thyroglobulin (TG) levels. Distant metastasis (DM) was defined as the duration between surgery date and date of documented disease outside the neck on imaging after evaluating for elevated TG. DFS was defined as the duration between surgery date and date of documented

disease reappearance/relapse, death from cancer and/or last follow-up. OS was defined as the duration between surgery date and date of patient death or last follow-up.

Chi-square or Student's t-tests were used to determine the differences in various clinical variables. Probabilities of LRC, DMC, DFS and OS rates were shown with the Kaplan-Meier method and the comparison for various survival curves was performed using log rank. All statistical analyses were performed using the computer program SPSS version 16.0.

## Results

### Demographic and clinicopathological features of cohort

The mean age at the time diagnosis of whole cohort was 22.7 years (range: 5–30). The whole cohort ($n$ = 157) was consisted of 134 (85.4 %) females and 23 (14.6 %) males. Male gender was predominant in children (25.9 %) than that in groups 19–25 years (10.3 %) and 26–30 years (15.4 %) respectively $P = 0.038$. The predominant histopathology was PTC (95.5 %) whereas FTC was seen only in 4.5 % of patients. Mean tumor size was 2.9 cm (range: 0.4–6.5) without any statistically significant difference between the children and adults ($P = 0.653$). In contrast to adults, positive lymph nodes were more evident in the children (74.1 %), $P = 0.012$. According to ATA risk stratification classification, the children (85.2 %) were found to be at higher risk as compared to other age groups $P = 0.003$. The clinicopathological and treatment characteristics are described in Table 1.

All patients underwent total or near total thyroidectomy without any difference between children and adults. However, because of palpable or radiological visible lymph nodes, the neck dissection was attempted more in children than those in other age groups (88.9 % vs. 67.9 % vs. 71.2 %) $P = 0.047$. Among 157 patients, 147 (93.6 %) patients were given adjuvant RAI ablation. Median time to RAI ablation was 8.2 weeks (6.8–16.6) from thyroidectomy and no significant differences in the frequency of adjuvant RAI ablation were observed between the children and adults ($P = 0.460$).

### Complications and Toxicities

Post-thyroidectomy complication rates were minimal; however, permanent hypocalcemia was statistically and significantly high in children and young adults ($P = 0.043$). Overall, RAI ablation was tolerated well without any grade 3 or 4 side effects; however, acute and late (any grade) complications were seen significantly higher in children and young adults ($P = 0.041$) Table 2.

### Treatment outcomes

Median follow-up period was 6.2 years (range: 2.0–10). For whole cohort, the 10-year LRC and DMC rates were

**Table 1** Comaprison of clinicopathological and treatment characteristics of children and adult patients with differentiated thyroid carcinoma at presentation

| Variables | Children with DTC (<18 years) (n =27) | Young adults with DTC (19–25 years) (n =78) | Adults with DTC (26–30 years) (n =52) | P value |
|---|---|---|---|---|
| Age (years) | | | | |
|   Mean/range/SD | 13.5 (5–18) ± 4.3 | 22.41 ± 3.3 | 27.5 ± 2.8 | 0.0001 |
|     <10 years | 8 (29.6) | 0 | 0 | |
|     11–18 years | 19 (70.4) | 0 | 0 | |
| Gender, n (%) | | | | |
|   M | 7 (25.9) | 8 (10.3) | 8 (15.4) | 0.038 |
|   F | 20 (74.1) | 70 (89.7) | 44 (84.6) | 0.160 |
| Tumor size (cm) | | | | |
|   Mean/range/SD | 2.8 (0.8–6.5) ± 1.36 | 2.8 (0.8–6.4) ±1.36 | 2.9 (0.4–6.5) ±1.62 | 0.653 |
| Histology n (%) | | | | |
|   Papillary | 27 (100) | 72 (92.3) | 51 (98.1) | 0.605 |
|   Follicular | 0 | 6 (7.7) | 1 (1.9) | |
| T stage, n (%) | | | | |
|   T1 | 12 (44.4) | 27 (34.6) | 26 (50.0) | 0.860 |
|   T2 | 11 (40.8) | 34 (43.6) | 15 (28.9) | |
|   T3 | 4 (14.8) | 15 (19.2) | 10 (19.2) | |
|   T4 | 0 | 2 (2.6) | 1 (1.9) | |
| N stage, n (%) | | | | |
|   N0 | 7 (25.9) | 42 (53.8) | 32 (61.5) | 0.012 |
|   N1 | 20 (74.1) | 36 (46.2) | 20 (38.5) | |
|   N1a | 9 (45.0) | 22 (61.1) | 11 (55.0) | |
|   N1b | 11 (55.0) | 14 (38.9) | 9 (45.0) | |
| M stage, n (%) | | | | |
|   M0 | 26 (96.3) | 77 (98.7) | 52 (100) | 0.379 |
|   M1 | 1 (3.7) | 1 (1.3) | 0 | |
| LVSI, n (%) | | | | |
|   Yes | 12 (44.4) | 27 (34.6) | 16 (30.7) | 0.031 |
|   No | 15 (55.6) | 51 (65.4) | 36 (69.3) | |
| Multifocality, n (%) | | | | |
|   Yes | 9 (33.3) | 43 (55.2) | 32 (61.5) | 0.012 |
|   No | 18 (66.6) | 35 (44.8) | 20 (38.5) | |
| Risk stratification, n (%) | | | | |
|   Low | 2 (7.4) | 17 (21.8) | 11 (21.1) | 0.003 |
|   Intermediate | 2 (7.4) | 23 (29.5) | 21 (40.4) | |
|   High | 23 (85.2) | 38 (48.7) | 20 (38.5) | |
| Surgery, n (%) | | | | |
|   Total thyroidectomy | 23 (85.2) | 68 (87.2) | 44 (84.6) | 0.065 |
|   Near total thyroidectomy | 4 (14.8) | 10 (12.8) | 8 (15.4) | |
| Neck dissection, n (%) | | | | |
|   No | 3 (11.1) | 25 (32.1) | 15 (28.8) | 0.047 |
|   Yes | 24 (88.9) | 53 (67.9) | 37 (71.2) | |
|   Central | 13 (54.2) | 30 (56.6) | 18 (48.6) | |

**Table 1** Comaprison of clinicopathological and treatment characteristics of children and adult patients with differentiated thyroid carcinoma at presentation *(Continued)*

| | | | | |
|---|---|---|---|---|
| Lateral | 11 (45.8) | 23 (43.4) | 19 (51.4) | |
| Adjuvant RAI therapy, n (%) | | | | |
| No | 1 (3.7) | 7 (9.0) | 2 (3.8) | 0.460 |
| Yes | 26 (96.3) | 71 (91.0) | 50 (96.2) | |
| 30 mCi | 0 | 4 (5.6) | 1 (2.0) | |
| 100 mCi | 7 (27.0) | 20 (28.2) | 19 (38.0) | |
| 150 mCi | 14 (53.8) | 36 (50.7) | 20 (40.0) | |
| 200 mCi | 5 (19.2) | 11 (15.5) | 10 (20.0) | |

*N* number, *DTC* differentiated thyroid cancers, *SD* standrad deviation, *M* male, *F* female, *T* tumor, *N* node, *M* metastasis, *LVSI* lymphovascular space invasion, *RAI* radioactive iodine, *mCi* millicurie

87.2 and 84.2 % respectively. The 10-year LRC and DMC rates were significantly lower in children (75.3 and 64.7 % respectively) than those young adults and adults. Total 18 LRs (11.5 %) were observed; 6/27 in children, 9/78 in young adults and 3/52 in adults (*P* = *0.032*) Table 3. The LRs were salvaged by surgery; lateral neck dissection (13 patients); completion thyroidectomy (4 patients) and excision (2 patients) followed by RAI ablation (16 patients). Similarly, total 24 DM (15.3 %) were observed; 10/27 in children, 9/78 in young adults and 5/52 in adults (*P* = *0.002*). DMs were salvaged by RAI ablation and palliative irradiation for bony lesion (one patient).

The 10-year DFS rates were 67.3 % in children, 82.4 % in young adults and 90.1 % in adults (*p* = *0.021*) Fig. 1.

There was no statistically significant difference in 10-year OS rates among all age groups (*P* = *0.075*).

## Discussion

Due to rarity of DTC in children and young adults, few major controversies regarding aggressiveness of clinical behavior and optimal treatment still persist [8]. In present study, some unusual observations related to histopathological features were observed, which are in contradiction to reported literature.

Firstly, no statistically significant difference in primary tumor volumes or presence of extrathyroidal extension (ETE) was observed between the children and adults. Previous studies have hypothesized that the tumor volumes

**Table 2** Comparative analysis of complications of surgery and toxicities of radioactive iodine ablation in our cohort

| Toxicity | Children Age below 18 years (n = 27) | Young adults Age 19–25 years (n =78) | Adults Age26-30 years (n =52) | P value |
|---|---|---|---|---|
| Thyroidectomy, n (%) | | | | |
| Hypocalcemia | 5 (18.5) | 11 (14.1) | 8 (15.4) | 0.064 |
| Transient | 4 (80.0) | 9 (81.8) | 7 (87.5) | |
| Permanent | 1 (20.0) | 2 (18.2) | 1 (12.5) | 0.043 |
| Recurrent laryngeal nerve damage | 1 (3.7) | 1 (1.3) | 1 (1.9) | 0.072 |
| RAI ablation, n (%) | | | | |
| Acute: | 16 (59.3) | 36 (46.1) | 18 (34.6) | 0.041 |
| Sialadenitis | 5 (31.3) | 12 (33.3) | 6 (33.3) | 0.071 |
| Acute sickness (nausea, vomiting) | 4 (25.0) | 17 (47.2) | 10 (55.5) | 0.042 |
| Neck pain | 7 (43.7) | 7 (19.5) | 2 (11.1) | 0.001 |
| RAI ablation, n (%) | | | | |
| Late: | 2 (7.4) | 3 (3.8) | 1 (1.9) | 0.034 |
| Sicca syndrome | 1 (50.0) | 3 (100) | 0 | |
| Nasolacrimal duct obstruction | 1 (50.0) | 0 | 1 (100) | |
| Second malignancy | 0 | 0 | 0 | |
| Infertility | 0 | 0 | 0 | |
| Lung fibrosis | 0 | 0 | 0 | |

*RAI* Radioactive iodine, *n* number

**Table 3** Pattern of failure after thyroidectomy and radioactive iodine therapy in children and adults with differentiated thyroid cancer

| Failures | Children Age below 18 years (n = 27) | Young adults Age 19–25 years (n = 78) | Adults Age 26–30 years (n =52) | P value |
|---|---|---|---|---|
| Locoregional, n (%) | 6 (22.2) | 9 (11.5) | 3 (5.8) | 0.032 |
| Thyroid bed | 1 (16.7) | 2 (22.2) | 0 | |
| Lymph nodes | 5 (83.3) | 7 (77.8) | 3 (100) | |
| Distant, n (%) | 10 (37.0) | 9 (10.3) | 5 (9.6) | 0.002 |
| Lungs | 10 (100) | 9 (100) | 4 (80.0) | |
| Bones | - | - | 1 (20.0) | |
| Locoregional + distant | 4 (14.8) | 4 (5.1) | 2 (3.8) | 0.035 |
| 10 year LRC rate | 75.3% | 87.3 % | 93.2 % | 0.001 |
| 10 year DMC rate | 64.7 % | 84.8 % | 94.2 % | 0.0001 |
| 10 year OS rate | 92.3 % | 96.2 % | 100 % | 0.079 |

n number, LRC locoregional control, DMC distant metastasis control, OS overall survival

tend to be relatively larger in children when compared to adults, probably attributed to smaller thyroid volume in children, thus higher chances of ETE and capsular invasion [3–5, 9, 10]. Similar to our results, few studies have also reported no correlation between tumor volumes and pediatric population [11–13]. However, no difference in tumor volumes or ETE among children and adults can be criticized for relatively few pre-pubertal children in our cohort. Secondly, in contrast to children, multifocality was found more prevalent in our adult cohort, which is a reasonable argument against wide practice of total thyroidectomy as primary surgical approach in children [14, 15] Thirdly, male gender was predominant in our pediatric cohort, which is likely attributed to hormonal changes during pre-puberty and puberty [16].

Further, it was also clear that larger percentage of children underwent elective neck dissections mainly because

of increased frequency of clinical or radiological cervical lymphadenopathy at the time of diagnosis. Similarly, treatment related complications were observed more in children. Large percentage of permanent hypocalcemia supports the notion of less aggressive surgery (lobectomy or hemi-thyroidectomy) for primary tumor in children, to decrease the risk of surgical complications [17, 18]. Similarly, the children experienced relatively more acute and late (any grade) RAI induced complications in our cohort. However, no RAI ablation induced second primary malignancy (SPM), lung fibrosis or infertility was observed. Possible explanation could be the short follow-up, and given lower cumulative doses of RAI in our cohort [5, 19].

In contrast to previously published data, children in our cohort experienced relatively higher all-sites recurrence rates, thus lower 10-year DFS rate (67.3 %) after extensive treatment [4, 5, 7, 9, 20, 21] which is attributed to our ATA high risk (85.2 %) pediatric cohort.

There were few limitations of our study. Firstly, since more children were rendered to neck dissections, there was a possible selection bias when it came to the number of lymph nodes found to harbor metastasis. Secondly, TSH suppression therapy complications including effects on child growth, osteoporosis and cardiovascular diseases were not studied, as children are still in growing phase, and TSH suppression therapy theoretically may affect their final height [22]. Thirdly, we did not look into molecular patterns in childhood DTC. Bongarzone I et al. initially reported that the frequency of 'Rearranged during Transcription' (RET) and 'neurotrophic tyrosine kinase receptor-1' (NTRK1) oncogenic activation is significantly higher in childhood DTC, thus contributing to childhood DTC carcinogenesis [23]. Besides RET/NTRK1, overexpression of proto-oncogenes 'MET', and 'vascular endothelial growth factor' (VEGF) have been found to cause high recurrence rate in children [24].

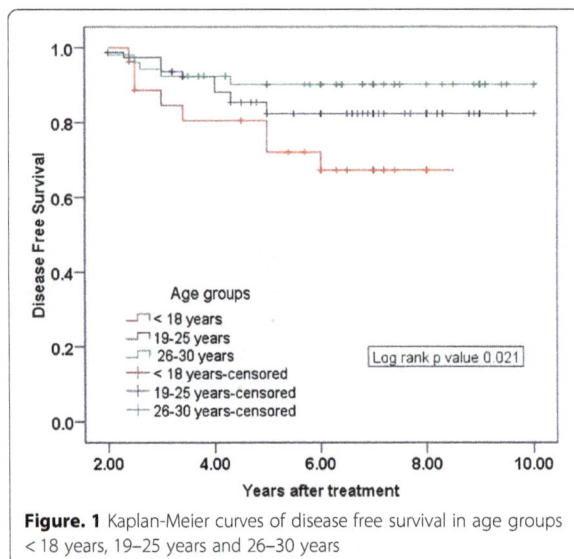

**Figure. 1** Kaplan-Meier curves of disease free survival in age groups < 18 years, 19–25 years and 26–30 years

## Conclusions

In conclusion, DTC in Saudi children is far more aggressive entity in nature as compared to adults. Children are at higher risk of treatment (thyroidectomy and RAI) related complications as compared to adults. Lower LRC, DMC and DFS rates in children after extensive therapy of thyroidectomy, neck dissection followed by RAI, TSH suppression warrants further multi-institutional studies.

### Competing interests

The authors declare that they have no competing interests.

### Authors' contributions

KQ and MT participated in the design of the study and performed the statistical analysis. MA, YB, NJ and KR collected the data and drafted the manuscript. WS carried out the histopathology data collection and edited the manuscript. MT conceived of the study, and participated in its design and coordination and helped to draft the manuscript. All authors read and approved the final manuscript.

### Acknowledgement

We are thankful to Laura Stanciu Gabriella for her efforts in the revision of manuscript and drafting.

### Interest of conflict

All authors declare no potential conflict of interest. No grant or funds have been received for this study.

### Author details

[1]Department of Otolaryngology-Head & Neck Surgery, College of Medicine, King Saud University, Riyadh, Saudi Arabia. [2]Radiation Oncology, King Fahad Medical City, Riyadh, Saudi Arabia. [3]Radiation Oncology, Comprehensive Cancer Center, King Fahad Medical City, Riyadh 59046, Saudi Arabia. [4]Endocrinology and Thyroid Oncology, King Fahad Medical City, Riyadh 59046, Saudi Arabia. [5]Radiation Oncology, NCI, Cairo University, Cairo, Egypt. [6]Histopathology, Comprehensive Cancer Center, King Fahad Medical City, Riyadh 59046, Saudi Arabia.

### References

1. Jemal A, Siegel R, Ward E, Hao Y, Xu J, Thun MJ. Cancer statistics, 2009. CA Cancer J Clin. 2009;59:225–49.
2. Hussain F, Iqbal S, Mehmood A, Bazarbashi S, ElHassan T, Chaudhri N. Incidence of thyroid cancer in the Kingdom of Saudi Arabia, 2000–2010. Hematol Oncol Stem Cell Ther. 2013;6:58–64.
3. Jarzab B, Handkiewicz-Junak D. Differentiated thyroid cancer in children and adults: same or distinct disease? Hormones (Athens). 2007;6:200–9.
4. Kim SS, Kim SJ, Kim IJ, Kim BH, Jeon YK, Kim YK. Comparison of clinical outcomes in differentiated thyroid carcinoma between children and young adult patients. Clin Nucl Med. 2012;37:850–3.
5. Jarzab B, Handkiewicz-Junak D, Wloch J. Juvenile differentiated thyroid carcinoma and the role of radioiodine in its treatment: a qualitative review. Endocr Relat Cancer. 2005;12:773–803.
6. Mihailovic J, Nikoletic K, Srbovan D. Recurrent disease in juvenile differentiated thyroid carcinoma: prognostic factors, treatments, and outcomes. J Nucl Med. 2014;55:710–7.
7. Vergamini LB, Frazier AL, Abrantes FL, Ribeiro KB, Rodriguez-Galindo C. Increase in the incidence of differentiated thyroid carcinoma in children, adolescents, and young adults: a population-based study. J Pediatr. 2014;164:1481–5.
8. Vaisman F, Corbo R, Vaisman M. Thyroid carcinoma in children and adolescents-systematic review of the literature. J Thyroid Res. 2011;2011:845362. doi:10.4061/2011/845362.
9. Dzodic R, Buta M, Markovic I, Gavrilovic D, Matovic M, Djurisic I, et al. Surgical management of well-differentiated thyroid carcinoma in children and adolescents: 33 years of experience of a single institution in Serbia. Endocr J. 2014;61:1079–86.
10. Vander Poorten V, Hens G, Delaere P. Thyroid cancer in children and adolescents. Curr Opin Otolaryngol Head Neck Surg. 2013;21:135–42.
11. Dottorini ME, Vignati A, Mazzucchelli L, Lomuscio G, Colombo L. Differentiated thyroid carcinoma in children and adolescents: a 37-year experience in 85 patients. J Nucl Med. 1997;38:669–75.
12. Spinelli C, Bertocchini A, Antonelli A, Miccoli P. Surgical therapy of the thyroid papillary carcinoma in children: experience with 56 patients < or =16 years old. J Pediatr Surg. 2004;39:1500–5.
13. Saraiva J, Ribeiro C, Melo M, Gomes L, Costa G, Carrilho F. Thyroid carcinoma in children and young adults: retrospective review of 19 cases. Acta Med Port. 2013;26:578–82.
14. Raval MV, Bentrem DJ, Stewart AK, Ko CY, Reynolds M. Utilization of total thyroidectomy for differentiated thyroid cancer in children. Ann Surg Oncol. 2010;17:2545–53.
15. Akkari M, Makeieff M, Jeandel C, Raingeard I, Cartier C, Garrel R, et al. Thyroid surgery in children and adolescents: a series of 65 cases. Eur Ann Otorhinolaryngol Head Neck Dis. 2014;131:293–7.
16. Lazar L, Lebenthal Y, Steinmetz A, Yackobovitch-Gavan M, Phillip M. Differentiated thyroid carcinoma in pediatric patients: comparison of presentation and course between pre-pubertal children and adolescents. J Pediatr. 2009;154:708–14.
17. Zimmerman D, Hay ID, Gough IR, Goellner JR, Ryan JJ, Grant CS, et al. Papillary thyroid carcinoma in children and adults: long term follow-up of 1039 patients conservatively treated at one institution during three decades. Surgery. 1988;104:1157–66.
18. Park S, Jeong JS, Ryu HR, Lee CR, Park JH, Kang SW, et al. Differentiated thyroid carcinoma of children and adolescents: 27-year experience in the yonsei university health system. J Korean Med Sci. 2013;28:693–9.
19. Van Santen HM, Aronson DC, Vulsma T, Tummers RF, Geenen MM, de Vijlder JJ, et al. Frequent adverse events after treatment for childhood-onset differentiated thyroid carcinoma: a single institute experience. Eur J Cancer. 2004;40:1743–51.
20. Hogan AR, Zhuge Y, Perez EA, Koniaris LG, Lew JI, Sola JE. Pediatric thyroid carcinoma: incidence and outcomes in 1753 patients. J Surg Res. 2009;156:167–72.
21. Giuffrida D, Scollo C, Pellegriti G, Lavenia G, Iurato MP, Pezzin V, et al. Differentiated thyroid cancer in children and adolescents. J Endocrinol Invest. 2002;25:18–24.
22. Hay ID, Gonzalez-Losada T, Reinalda MS, Honetschlager JA, Richards ML, Thompson GB. Long-term outcome in 215 children and adolescents with papillary thyroid cancer treated during 1940 through 2008. World J Surg. 2010;34:1192–202.
23. Bongarzone I, Fugazzola L, Vigneri P, Mariani L, Mondellini P, Pacini F, et al. Age-related activation of the tyrosine kinase receptor protooncogenes RET and NTRK1 in papillary thyroid carcinoma. J Clin Endocrinol Metab. 1996;81:2006–9.
24. Ramirez R, Hsu D, Patel A, Fenton C, Dinauer C, Tuttle RM, et al. Over-expression of hepatocyte growth factor/scatter factor (HGF/SF) and the HGF/SF receptor (cMET) are associated with a high risk of metastasis and recurrence for children and young adults with papillary thyroid carcinoma. Clin Endocrinol (Oxf). 2000;53:635–44.

# 16

# The relationship between upper airway collapse and the severity of obstructive sleep apnea syndrome

Russell N. Schwartz[1], Richard J. Payne[2,3*], Véronique-Isabelle Forest[2], Michael P. Hier[2], Amanda Fanous[4] and Camille Vallée-Gravel[5]

**Abstract**

**Background:** We sought to determine the ability of the endoscopic Mueller maneuver (MM) to predict the severity of OSAS based on upper airway (UA) collapse.

**Methods:** This chart review retrospectively analyzed the results of endoscopic Mueller maneuvers examining the UA on 506 patients suspected of having OSAS. There were 3 areas of UA collapse that were evaluated: velopharynx (VP), base of tongue (BOT), and lateral pharyngeal walls (LPW). A sleep study was done after the examination to assess the severity of OSAS based on the apnea-hypopnea index (AHI).

**Results:** A total of 506 patients met criteria for OSAS, with 194 mild cases ($5 \leq AHI < 15$), 163 moderate cases ($15 \leq AHI < 30$) and 149 severe cases ($30 \leq AHI$). At the VP, 30 patients had minimal collapse (mean AHI = 17); 41 patients had moderate VP collapse (mean AHI = 25); 392 patients had severe VP collapse (mean AHI = 27). At the BOT, 144 patients had minimal collapse (mean AHI = 19); 187 patients had moderate BOT collapse (mean AHI = 24); 175 patients had severe BOT collapse (mean AHI = 33). At the LPW, 158 patients had minimal collapse (mean AHI = 20); 109 patients had moderate LPW collapse (mean AHI = 25); 120 patients had severe LPW collapse (mean AHI = 33). The correlations found between VP collapse, BOT collapse, and LPW collapse and OSAS severity were: $r = 0.069$ (95 % CI; −0.022, 0.16), $r = 0.26$ (95 % CI; 0.18, 0.34) and $r = 0.22$ (95 % CI; 0.12, 0.31), respectively.

**Conclusions:** In this study, the degree of collapse of the UA at all levels, especially at the BOT and LPW levels, correlate significantly with the severity of OSAS. The Mueller maneuver helped identify patients with severe sleep apnea based on UA collapse. The MM cannot be used to diagnose OSAS, but can be a valuable tool to help the physician estimate the severity of sleep apnea and the urgency to obtain a sleep study.

**Keywords:** Obstructive sleep apnea syndrome, Mueller maneuver, Upper airway, Sleep study, Apnea-hypopnea index

## Introduction

Obstructive Sleep Apnea Syndrome (OSAS) is a condition affecting 14 % of males and 5 % of females in adults 30–70 years of age [1]. OSAS is characterized by recurrent partial or complete obstruction of the upper airway (UA) during sleep, leading to cessation of airflow, intermittent and recurrent hypoxemia and sleep fragmentation. The sites of obstruction are generally divided in three anatomical areas, which are the velopharynx (VP), the base of the tongue (BOT) and the lateral pharyngeal walls (LPW).

A sleep study is required to diagnose obstructive sleep apnea syndrome and determine its severity. Unfortunately, sleep studies are labor-intensive and waiting times to get a sleep study in a hospital can be very long, even up to a few years. Therefore, diagnosis and treatment of the condition can be delayed significantly. This

* Correspondence: rkpayne@sympatico.ca
[2]Department of Otolaryngology-Head and Neck Surgery, Sir Mortimer B. Davis-Jewish General Hospital, McGill University, 3755 Côte Ste-Catherine Road, Montreal, QC, Canada
[3]Department of Otorhinolaryngology Adult (Otl) (Ent) (Surgery), Royal Victoria Hospital, McGill University Health Center, 687 Pine Avenue West, Montreal, QC, Canada
Full list of author information is available at the end of the article

can be a real concern, especially if a patient has moderate to severe OSAS and is left untreated while waiting for the test. It is still a challenge for physicians to identify which patients would need a more urgent sleep study based on history or questionnaires alone. This study looked at the ability of the endoscopic Mueller maneuver (MM) to help predict the severity of OSAS based on UA collapse at its different levels.

The MM is a minimally invasive examination tool which has significant value due to its ease of use in clinical settings. The maneuver is done on an awake patient and can be conducted in less than a two-minute time span. The MM has mixed evidence regarding its effectiveness of predicting OSAS. Studies such as Woodson and Haganuma [2], as well as Friedman et al. [3] found no positive correlation between MM performance and OSAS. In contrast to these findings, Dreher et al. [4] found the Mueller maneuver to be predictive of OSAS based on the degree of obstruction at base of tongue and velum. The authors rationalized the divergent findings to be due to possible differences in patient cooperation as a result of the MM performed on awake patients. In the present study, the goal is to determine how well the MM maneuver can predict OSAS by observing how airway obstruction at the levels of the VP, BOT and LPW during the procedure relates to the severity of OSAS, as measured by AHI.

## Methods

This study is a retrospective chart review of 506 consecutive patients referred to a McGill University Affiliated Teaching Site otolaryngology office in Montreal, Canada for snoring, and/or suspected obstructive sleep apnea syndrome. The review (CR14-62) has been approved by the Research Ethics Committee at the Sir Mortimer B. Davis-Jewish General Hospital.

All patients completed an Epworth Sleepiness Scale (ESS) [5] and had a full head and neck examination by one of three experienced physicians, including flexible nasopharyngolaryngoscopy and MM. Patients then underwent a level 3 cardiorespiratory polygraphy that was scored using American Academy of Sleep Medicine (AASM) criteria [6]. These studies were done using a Philips Stardust II Sleep Recorder. The recordings included monitoring of respiratory effort, oro-nasal pressure, oximetry, body position, snoring sound and pulse rate channels. The number of central apneas, obstructive apneas, mixed apneas and hypopneas were measured and added to form the apnea-hypopnea index. For hypopnea, the definition used was a reduction in nasal airflow $\geq 30$ % with an associated desaturation $\geq 3$ %. The severity of OSAS was graded following a scale based on the AHI: $5 \leq \text{AHI} < 15$ (mild), $15 \leq \text{AHI} < 30$ (moderate) and $30 \leq \text{AHI}$ (severe).

The measures investigated were the relations between the three sites of obstruction based on the Mueller maneuver and BMI, and OSAS severity (AHI). The relation of OSAS severity with ESS was also investigated.

Data analysis was done using SAS, version 9.3 (Cary, NC). Continuous variables were presented as means with a standard deviation (SD). The correlation between the sites of obstruction with BMI, ESS, and AHI was done using a Spearman's correlation test using a 95 % confidence interval (CI). A multivariate multiple logistic regression analysis was done to determine if the degree of collapse using the MM predicted OSA severity and the effects of BMI, ESS and age on these associations were analyzed.

Patients who underwent a Mueller maneuver and a sleep study were included in the study. No patients were excluded on the basis of gender, age, or BMI. Patients who did not meet criteria for OSAS diagnosis (AHI <5) were excluded from the study. Patients' charts lacking data from the MM examination of airway obstruction were excluded.

There were no differences in demographic (age, BMI), ESS, or sleep characteristics (AHI) between the patients who lacked data on airway obstruction and those who were included in the study. There was also no bias towards taking measurements only in patients that had some degree of baseline airway narrowing at the UA levels.

### Endoscopic Mueller maneuver

The Mueller maneuver attempts to emulate the collapse of the UA during sleep [7]. A flexible laryngoscope is inserted through the nose of the patient into his UA and the patient is asked to perform a series of reverse Valsalvas. The examination is of short duration (less than 2 min) and is recorded. All recordings of the examinations for each patient was saved and backed up on a hard drive for later use by the scorers. The scorers were able to go back to the recordings after the consultation with the patient to insure the accuracy of their scores on the Mueller maneuver. Assessors estimated a precise percentage score for the degree of obstruction of the VP, BOT, and LPW. The scores were then sorted semi-quantitatively following a scale based on the percentage of obstruction: $\leq 50$ % (minimal), 51–75 % (moderate) and 76–100 % (severe).

### Data analysis

The data from the sleep studies and MMs were collated along with the age, gender, height, weight, and BMI. A Spearman's correlation coefficient was calculated to evaluate the association between the areas of collapse and the severity of OSAS. If a correlation were to be found, it would then be concluded that the area of obstruction that correlated would be considered as contributing to the severity of OSAS.

## Results

There were 399 male (79 %) and 107 female (21 %) subjects. The mean age was 49 years old (SD = 12) and ages ranged from 16 to 90 years. The mean BMI was 29 kg/m² (SD = 5) and ranged from 19 to 55 kg/m². The mean ESS was 9 (SD = 5) and ranged from 0 to 24.

BMI and VP collapse correlate, $r = 0.15$ (95 % CI; 0.063, 0.24). BMI and BOT collapse correlate, $r = 0.31$ (95 % CI; 0.22, 0.38). BMI and LPW collapse correlate, $r = 0.25$ (95 % CI; 0.15, 0.34). Overall, BMI and AHI correlate, $r = 0.42$ (95 % CI; 0.35, 0.49).

At the VP, females had a mean collapse of 86 % (SD = 15), while males had a mean of 85 % (SD = 16). At the base of tongue, females had a mean collapse of 60 % (SD = 20), while males had a mean of 65 % (SD = 20). At the lateral pharyngeal wall, females had a mean collapse of 55 % (SD = 22), while males had a mean of 60 % (SD = 22). Overall, females had a mean AHI of 20 (SD = 18), while males had a mean AHI of 27 (SD = 20).

### Sleep study screening findings

AHI values ranged from 5 to 122 events per hour with a mean of 26 (SD = 20) events per hour. Of the 506 total patients, 194 (38 %) had mild OSAS, 163 (32 %) had moderate OSAS, and 149 (30 %) had severe OSAS (Table 1).

### Endoscopic Mueller maneuver findings

Of the 506 patient charts, 463 had data for VP collapse, 506 had data for BOT collapse, and 387 had data for LPW collapse. Of the 463 patients with data on VP level, 30 had a minimal airway collapse at that level, 41 had a moderate airway collapse and 392 had a severe airway collapse. Among the 506 patients with BOT collapse, 144 had a minimal collapse, 187 had a moderate collapse and 175 had a severe collapse. Of 387 patients with data for obstruction at the LPW, 158 had a minimal collapse, 109 had a moderate collapse and 120 had a severe collapse (Table 2).

### Correlation between areas of collapse and OSAS severity

At the VP, patients with minimal collapse had a mean AHI of 17 (SD = 10) events per hour; patients with

moderate collapse had a mean AHI of 25 (SD = 15) events per hour; and patients with severe collapse had a mean AHI of 27 (SD = 21) events per hour. This correlation was $r = 0.069$ (95 % CI; −0.022, 0.16) (Table 2).

A positive correlation was observed under a comparative analysis between BOT percentages of collapse and AHI values, $r = 0.26$ (95 % CI; 0.18, 0.34). There was a significant rise in the mean AHI for every collapse degree. Patients with a minimal collapse at the BOT had a mean AHI of 19 (SD = 12) events per hour; patients with moderate collapse had a mean AHI of 24 (SD = 19) events per hour; patients with severe collapse had a mean AHI of 33 (SD = 24) events per hour (Table 2).

At the LPW, there was a correlation between degree of collapse and OSAS severity, $r = 0.22$ (95 % CI; 0.12, 0.31). Patients with minimal collapse had a mean AHI of 20 (SD = 16) events per hour; patients with moderate collapse had a mean AHI of 25 (SD = 19) events per hour; patients with severe collapse had a mean AHI of 33 (SD = 25) events per hour (Table 2).

### Relation between OSAS measures and Epworth sleepiness scale score

The mean ESS score for all 604 patients was 9 (SD = 5). A positive correlation was found between BOT collapse and ESS scores, $r = 0.18$ (95 % CI; 0.096, 0.26), and between LPW collapse and ESS scores, $r = 0.10$ (95 % CI; 0.0022, 0.20). The association between VP collapse and ESS scores was $r = 0.0091$ (95 % CI; −0.082, 0.10). ESS scores and AHI were positively correlated, $r = 0.19$ (95 % CI; 0.11, 0.27).

### Multiple logistic regression analysis of VP, BOT and LPW on AHI outcomes

Patients with severe compared to those with minimal VP collapse have an odds ratio (OR) of 2.75 (95 % CI; 0.99, 7.67) of being in the severe AHI category and OR = 1.64 (95 % CI; 0.68, 3.92) of being in the moderate AHI category. Patients with moderate compared to those with minimal VP collapse have OR = 2.35 (95 % CI; 0.64, 8.73) of being in the severe AHI category and OR = 3.10 (95 % CI; 1.04, 9.30) of being in the moderate AHI category (Table 3).

Patients with severe compared to those with minimal BOT collapse have OR = 5.39 (95 % CI; 2.98, 9.73) of being in the severe AHI category and OR = 1.77 (95 % CI; 1.03,

**Table 1** Distribution of the severity of OSAS at each UA level

| OSAS severity; AHI | n (%) | Mean VP collapse (%; ± SD) | Mean BOT collapse (%; ± SD) | Mean LPW collapse (%; ± SD) |
|---|---|---|---|---|
| Mild; 5 to 15 events per hour | 194(38) | 85(±18) | 59(±20) | 54(±21) |
| Moderate; 15 to 30 events per hour | 163(32) | 84(±17) | 63(±20) | 59(±22) |
| Severe; 30+ events per hour | 149(30) | 87(±12) | 72(±18) | 67(±23) |

This table shows the association between each AHI category (mild = 5 ≤ AHI < 15; moderate = 15 ≤ AHI < 30; severe = 30 ≤ AHI). n (%) = sub-sample size (percentage of overall sample). The mean collapse at each UA is shown at each level of AHI

**Table 2** Mean AHI according to the level and degree of collapse

| Velopharynx collapse | n (%) | Mean AHI (events per hour) | Standard deviation (events per hour) |
|---|---|---|---|
| Minimal | 30 (6) | 17 | 11 |
| Moderate | 41 (9) | 25 | 15 |
| Significant | 392 (85) | 27 | 21 |
| $r = 0.069$ (95 % CI; −0.022, 0.16) | | | |
| Base of Tongue Collapse | | | |
| Minimal | 144 (28) | 19 | 12 |
| Moderate | 187 (37) | 24 | 19 |
| Significant | 175 (35) | 33 | 23 |
| $r = 0.26$ (95 % CI; 0.18, 0.34) | | | |
| Lateral Pharyngeal Wall Collapse | | | |
| Minimal | 158 (41) | 20 | 16 |
| Moderate | 109 (28) | 25 | 19 |
| Significant | 120 (31) | 33 | 25 |
| $r = 0.22$ (95 % CI; 0.12, 0.31) | | | |

This table shows the mean AHI value at each degree of UA collapse (minimal = airway collapse of 0-50 %; moderate = airway collapse of 51–75 %; severe = airway collapse of 76–100 %). r and CI values are marked after each analysis

3.05) of being in the moderate AHI category. Patients with moderate compared to those with minimal BOT collapse have OR = 1.77 (95 % CI; 0.98, 3.19) of being in the severe AHI category and OR = 1.21 (95 % CI; 0.74, 1.99) of being in the moderate AHI category (Table 4).

Patients with severe compared to those with minimal LPW collapse have OR = 3.91 (95 % CI; 2.12, 7.19) of being in the severe AHI category and OR = 1.57 (95 % CI; 0.87, 2.82) of being in the moderate AHI category. Patients with moderate compared to those with minimal LPW collapse have OR = 1.96 (95 % CI; 1.04, 3.68) of being in the severe AHI category and OR = 1.27 (95 % CI; 0.72, 2.24) of being in the moderate AHI category (Table 5).

**Multiple logistic regression analysis of VP, BOT and LPW on AHI outcomes and the effects of BMI, age, and ESS**
Accounting for BMI, age and ESS, patients with severe compared to those with minimal VP collapse

**Table 3** VP odds ratio estimates

| Effect | AHI | Point estimate | 95 % confidence limits | |
|---|---|---|---|---|
| VP severe vs mild | severe | 2.751 | 0.987 | 7.669 |
| VP severe vs mild | moderate | 1.636 | 0.682 | 3.921 |
| VP moderate vs mild | severe | 2.354 | 0.635 | 8.725 |
| VP moderate vs mild | moderate | 3.106 | 1.037 | 9.304 |

This table shows the odds ratio estimates of OSAS severity (based on AHI) for different severities of VP collapse

**Table 4** BOT odds ratio estimates

| Effect | AHI | Point estimate | 95 % confidence limits | |
|---|---|---|---|---|
| BOT severe vs mild | severe | 5.386 | 2.983 | 9.727 |
| BOT severe vs mild | moderate | 1.773 | 1.030 | 3.050 |
| BOT moderate vs mild | severe | 1.769 | 0.982 | 3.186 |
| BOT moderate vs mild | moderate | 1.212 | 0.740 | 1.985 |

This table shows the odds ratio estimates of OSAS severity (based on AHI) for different severities of BOT collapse

have OR = 1.77 (95 % CI; 0.60, 5.20) of being in the severe AHI category and OR = 1.44 (95 % CI; 0.59, 3.49) of being in the moderate AHI category. Patients with moderate compared to those with minimal VP collapse have OR = 1.66 (95 % CI; 0.42, 6.63) of being in the severe AHI category and OR = 2.83 (95 % CI; 0.93, 8.57) of being in the moderate AHI category (Table 6).

Accounting for BMI, age and ESS, patients with severe compared to those with minimal BOT collapse have OR = 3.18 (95 % CI; 1.69, 5.99) of being in the severe AHI category and OR = 1.54 (95 % CI; 0.87, 2.72) of being in the moderate AHI category. Patients with moderate compared to those with minimal BOT collapse have OR = 1.40 (95 % CI; 0.75, 2.60) of being in the severe AHI category and OR = 1.15 (95 % CI; 0.70, 1.90) of being in the moderate AHI category (Table 7).

Accounting for BMI, age and ESS, patients with severe compared to those with minimal LPW collapse have OR = 2.53 (95 % CI; 1.32, 4.87) of being in the severe AHI category and OR = 1.40 (95 % CI; 0.77, 2.57) of being in the moderate AHI category. Patients with moderate compared to those with minimal LPW collapse have OR = 1.72 (95 % CI; 0.88, 3.33) of being in the severe AHI category and OR = 1.21 (95 % CI; 0.68, 2.16) of being in the moderate AHI category (Table 8).

**Discussion**
The Wisconsin Cohort Study found that the prevalence of OSAS in people aged 30–60 years was 9–24 % for males and 4–9 % for females. It is also widely recognized that BMI is a serious risk factor for OSAS. It was mentioned in the Wisconsin Cohort study that a one

**Table 5** LPW odds ratio estimates

| Effect | AHI | Point estimate | 95 % confidence limits | |
|---|---|---|---|---|
| LPW severe vs mild | severe | 3.905 | 2.121 | 7.187 |
| LPW severe vs mild | moderate | 1.568 | 0.873 | 2.817 |
| LPW moderate vs mild | severe | 1.960 | 1.043 | 3.682 |
| LPW moderate vs mild | moderate | 1.269 | 0.720 | 2.238 |

This table shows the odds ratio estimates of OSAS severity (based on AHI) for different severities of LPW collapse

**Table 6** VP odds ratio estimates accounting for BMI, age and ESS

| Effect | AHI | Point estimate | 95 % confidence limits | |
|--------|-----|----------------|--------|--------|
| VP severe vs mild | severe | 1.773 | 0.604 | 5.204 |
| VP severe vs mild | moderate | 1.439 | 0.593 | 3.491 |
| VP moderate vs mild | severe | 1.662 | 0.417 | 6.631 |
| VP moderate vs mild | moderate | 2.827 | 0.932 | 8.574 |
| BMI | severe | 1.165 | 1.108 | 1.224 |
| BMI | moderate | 1.052 | 1.002 | 1.104 |
| Age | severe | 1.024 | 1.002 | 1.046 |
| Age | moderate | 1.017 | 0.998 | 1.037 |
| ESS | severe | 1.070 | 1.022 | 1.120 |
| ESS | moderate | 1.024 | 0.980 | 1.070 |

This table shows the odds ratio estimates of OSAS severity (based on AHI) for different severities of VP collapse after accounting for BMI, age and ESS. It also indicates the odds ratio estimates of OSAS severity (based on AHI) of BMI, age and ESS individually

**Table 8** LPW odds ratio estimates accounting for BMI, age and ESS

| Effect | AHI | Point estimate | 95 % confidence limits | |
|--------|-----|----------------|--------|--------|
| LPW severe vs mild | severe | 2.532 | 1.318 | 4.866 |
| LPW severe vs mild | moderate | 1.404 | 0.765 | 2.573 |
| LPW moderate vs mild | severe | 1.715 | 0.884 | 3.325 |
| LPW moderate vs mild | moderate | 1.214 | 0.682 | 2.161 |
| BMI | severe | 1.152 | 1.087 | 1.220 |
| BMI | moderate | 1.034 | 0.979 | 1.092 |
| Age | severe | 1.027 | 1.003 | 1.050 |
| Age | moderate | 1.020 | 0.999 | 1.041 |
| ESS | severe | 1.065 | 1.010 | 1.123 |
| ESS | moderate | 1.047 | 0.997 | 1.100 |

This table shows the odds ratio estimates of OSAS severity (based on AHI) for different severities of LPW collapse after accounting for BMI, age and ESS. It also indicates the odds ratio estimates of OSAS severity (based on AHI) of BMI, age and ESS individually

standard deviation difference in BMI was associated with a 4-fold increase in OSAS prevalence [8]. In our study, BMI was significantly associated with VP, BOT and LPW collapse as well as with AHI. With a predominance of males, the mean age of 49 years, and patients with high BMIs, our cohort is representative of patients with OSAS [9].

Various studies have been conducted in an attempt to find a correlation between the degree and area of UA collapse and the severity of OSAS using different modalities [7, 10]. These modalities include tri-dimensional magnetic resonance imaging (MRI) [11], cine and sleep-MRI [12], computed tomography (CT) [13], critical pressure measurement (Pcrit) [14], negative expiratory pressure

**Table 7** BOT odds ratio estimates accounting for BMI, age and ESS

| Effect | AHI | Point estimate | 95 % confidence limits | |
|--------|-----|----------------|--------|--------|
| BOT severe vs mild | severe | 3.177 | 1.686 | 5.987 |
| BOT severe vs mild | moderate | 1.536 | 0.869 | 2.716 |
| BOT moderate vs mild | severe | 1.400 | 0.754 | 2.596 |
| BOT moderate vs mild | moderate | 1.147 | 0.692 | 1.899 |
| BMI | severe | 1.151 | 1.095 | 1.210 |
| BMI | moderate | 1.046 | 0.997 | 1.097 |
| Age | severe | 1.032 | 1.010 | 1.053 |
| Age | moderate | 1.022 | 1.003 | 1.042 |
| ESS | severe | 1.055 | 1.008 | 1.105 |
| ESS | moderate | 1.031 | 0.988 | 1.076 |

This table shows the odds ratio estimates of OSAS severity (based on AHI) for different severities of BOT collapse after accounting for BMI, age and ESS. It also indicates the odds ratio estimates of OSAS severity (based on AHI) of BMI, age and ESS individually

technique (NEP) [15], drug induced sleep endoscopy (DISE) [16] and Mueller maneuver [2–4, 7, 10, 17, 18, 21]. Our study aimed at finding such a relationship using the Mueller maneuver.

In this study, the Mueller maneuver was investigated for its predictive value of the severity of OSAS diagnosis. This maneuver is simple, safe, low cost, and can be part of a routine flexible laryngoscopy done during the head and neck examination. Studies have divergent opinions concerning MM statistical reliability. A 1994 study by Petri et al. found no predictive value in the Mueller maneuver for uvulopalatopharyngoplasty (UPPP) success rate [17]. Patients who primarily had retropalatal obstruction as judged by MM had only a 40 % response to UPPP. On the other hand, Li et al. later found clinical value for MM in improving outcomes from UPPP [18]. This study is not looking at the correlation between the MM and surgical outcomes. We were evaluating if the degree of obstruction seen with the MM could correlate with the severity of OSAS to guide the physician and the patients on the urgency to test for OSAS. We believe the MM is an effective procedure to observe upper airway collapse and its degree and we showed that the greater the collapse in the UA, the greater the chance of having more severe OSAS.

It must be noted that because our study involves the subjective evaluations of three different physicians on the degree of upper airway obstruction, there may be inherent inter-observer variation. A recent study by Ramji et al. [19] tested inter- and intra-rater agreement on sixty-one recorded videos of children undergoing a sleep nasopharyngoscopy. The authors concluded that there was validation for this procedure with good inter- and intra-rater agreement. The study was done using non-expert raters who did not perform the sleep nasopharyngoscopy routinely and were at various stages in their otolaryngology career. In the present study, the three physicians who scored the degree of collapse during the Mueller maneuver would be considered expert raters. All three are trained to perform the endoscopy and have routinely performed the procedure over many years. This cannot ensure that inter-rater variation is reliable in the present study; however it gives more confidence that the results were not biased in this manner.

In our study, a scale similar to the one used to grade the degree of obstruction of the UAs in studies on drug-induced sleep endoscopy was used (≤50 % obstruction = minimal collapse, 51–75 % obstruction = moderate collapse, 76–100 % obstruction = significant collapse). The degree of UA obstruction correlated with AHI at each level studied, mainly at the BOT and LPW. The VP level discriminates weakly compared to the other two levels and this may be explained by the fact that the velum collapses in the majority of patients with OSAS.

From the multivariate multiple logistic regression analysis, it is clear that the strongest effects are seen at the BOT and LPW levels. More specifically, there is a higher likelihood that a patient with severe BOT collapse compared to one with minimal BOT collapse would have severe OSAS. The analysis shows that, while other variables such as BMI, age and ESS scores accentuate this effect, the conclusions still hold true above and beyond these variables. In addition, there is a higher likelihood that a patient with severe LPW collapse compared to one with minimal LPW collapse would have severe OSAS. The analysis also shows that this holds true when accounting for variables such as BMI, age, and ESS scores.

The regression analysis results show significant odds ratios for predicting severe OSAS based on BOT and LPW observations of collapse. These results are important to the purpose of the study, as it shows that the Mueller maneuver may be used as a clinical screening device for predicting the probability of having severe OSAS, and therefore be prioritized for a sleep study.

Other studies have shown correlations between upper airway and OSAS. Santiago-Recuerda et al. [20] conducted a study on 40 morbidly obese women to determine the relationship of upper airway changes and OSAS. They found that the oropharyngeal area at maximal inspiration was negatively correlated with AHI ($r = -0.423$, $p = 0.044$). This study used computed tomography assessments of the upper airway. More recently, Kum et al. [21] used the Mueller maneuver to measure collapse at the retrolingual level and found the LPW obstruction site to be correlated with AHI in OSAS patients. A similar obstruction grading scale was used in the present study; however, our results indicate an important relationship between the BOT and OSAS in addition to the relationship between the LPW

and OSAS. To our knowledge, the present study is the first showing a relationship between BOT collapse, LPW collapse and OSAS severity using our graded obstruction scale based on the ease of the MM technique.

## Conclusions

In this study, the Mueller maneuver helped identify patients with severe sleep apnea based on UA collapse. MM cannot be used to diagnose OSAS, but can be a valuable tool to help the physician estimate the severity of sleep apnea and the urgency to obtain a sleep study. This examination can be performed in the physician's office as a part of the routine head and neck examination. It allows for physicians to identify patients with significant collapse at the BOT and LPW, and as a result prioritize them for a formal sleep study.

### Abbreviations
OSAS: Obstructive sleep apnea syndrome; UA: Upper airway; VP: Velopharynx; BOT: Base of Tongue; LPW: Lateral pharyngeal walls; MM: Mueller maneuver; ESS: Epworth Sleepiness Scale; AASM: American Academy of Sleep Medicine; SD: Standard deviation; CI: Confidence interval; r: Correlation Statistic; OR: Odd ratio; MRI: Magnetic Resonance Imaging; CT: Computed Tomography; Pcrit: Critical pressure measurement; NEP: Negative expiratory pressure technique; DISE: Drug-induced sleep endoscopy; UPPP: Uvulopalatopharyngoplasty.

### Competing interests
The authors declare that they have no competing interests.

### Authors' contributions
The original idea was conceived and the study was designed by RP. RS and AF were responsible for creating and completing the database. The original manuscript was created by RS and was reviewed and approved by all authors. RS, RP, VF, MH, and AF all made valuable contributions and changes to the manuscript leading to its completion.

### Acknowledgements
We would like to acknowledge The ENT Specialty Group for providing the space to perform Mueller maneuvers and the collection of data.

### Financial Support/Disclosures
Funding from the BioMed Central Membership of Canadian Society of Otolaryngology – Head and Neck Surgery.

### Author details
[1]Faculty of Science, McGill University, 845 Rue Sherbrooke West, Montréal, QC, Canada. [2]Department of Otolaryngology-Head and Neck Surgery, Sir Mortimer B. Davis-Jewish General Hospital, McGill University, 3755 Côte Ste-Catherine Road, Montreal, QC, Canada. [3]Department of Otorhinolaryngology Adult (Otl) (Ent) (Surgery), Royal Victoria Hospital, McGill University Health Center, 687 Pine Avenue West, Montreal, QC, Canada. [4]Department of Otolaryngology-Head and Neck Surgery, McGill Executive Institute, McGill University, 1001 Rue Sherbrooke West, Montreal, QC,. Canada. [5]Faculty of Medicine, McGill University, 845 Rue Sherbrooke West, Montréal, QC, Canada.

### References
1.  Peppard PE, Young T, Barnet JH, Palta M, Hagen EW, Hla KM. Increased prevalence of sleep-disordered breathing in adults. Am J Epidemiol. 2013;177(9):1006–14. PubMed Abstract | Publisher Full Text.

2.  Woodson BT, Haganuma H. Comparison of methods of airway evaluation in bstructive sleep apnea syndrome. Otolaryngol Head Neck Surg. 1999;120(4):460. PubMed Abstract.

3.  Friedman M, Tanyeri H, La Rosa M, Landsberg R, Vaidyanathan K, Pieri S, et al. Clinical predictors of obstructive sleep apnea. Laryngoscope. 1999;109(12):1901–7. PubMed Abstract | Publisher Full Text.

4.  Dreher A, de la Chaux R, Klemens C, Werner R, Baker F, Barthlen G, et al. Correlation between otorhinolaryngologic evaluation and severity of obstructive sleep apnea syndrome in snorers. Arch Otolaryngol Head Neck Surg. 2005;131(2):95–8. PubMed Abstract | Publisher Full Text.

5.  Johns MW. Daytime sleepiness, snoring, and obstructive sleep apnea. The Epworth Sleepiness Scale. Chest. 1993;103(1):30–6. PubMed Abstract | Publisher Full Text.

6.  Berry RB, Budhiraja R, Gottlieb DJ, Gozal D, Iber C, Kapur VK, et al. Rules for scoring respiratory events in sleep: update of the 2007 AASM Manual for the Scoring of Sleep and Associated Events. Deliberations of the Sleep Apnea Definitions Task Force of the American Academy of Sleep Medicine. J Clin Sleep Med. 2012;8(5):597–619. PubMed Abstract.

7.  Tunçel U, Inançli HM, Kürkçüoğlu SS, Enöz M. Can the Müller maneuver detect multilevel obstruction of the upper airway in patients with obstructive sleep apnea syndrome? Kulak Burun Bogaz Ihtis Derg. 2010;20(2):84–8. PubMed Abstract | Publisher Full Text.

8.  Finn L, Young T, Palta M, Fryback DG. Sleep-disordered breathing and self-reported general health status in the Wisconsin Sleep Cohort Study. SLEEP. 1998;21(7):701–6. PubMed Abstract | Publisher Full Text.

9.  Deng X, Gu W, Li Y, Liu M, Li Y, Gao X. Age-Group-Specific Associations between the Severity of Obstructive Sleep Apnea and Relevant Risk Factors in Male and Female Patients. PLoS One. 2014;9(9):e107380. PubMed Abstract | Publisher Full Text.

10. Herzog M, Metz T, Schmidt A, Bremert T, Venohr B, Hosemann W, et al. The prognostic value of simulated snoring in awake patients with suspected sleep-disordered breathing: introduction of a new technique of examination. SLEEP. 2006;29(11):1456–62. PubMed Abstract | Publisher Full Text.

11. Togeiro SM, Chaves Jr CM, Palombini L, Tufik S, Hora F, Nery LE. Evaluation of the upper airway in obstructive sleep apnoea. Indian J Med Res. 2010;131:230–5. PubMed Abstract | Publisher Full Text.

12. Moon IJ, Han DH, Kim JW, Rhee CS, Sung MW, Park JW, et al. Sleep magnetic resonance imaging as a new diagnostic method in obstructive sleep apnea syndrome. Laryngoscope. 2010;120(12):2546–54. PubMed Abstract | Publisher Full Text.

13. Ryan CF, Lowe AA, Li D, Fleetham JA. Three-dimensional upper airway computed tomography in obstructive sleep apnea. A prospective study in patients treated by uvulopalatopharyngoplasty. Am Rev Respir Dis. 1991;144(2):428–32. PubMed Abstract | Publisher Full Text.

14. Kirkness JP, Peterson LA, Squier SB, McGinley BM, Schneider H, Meyer A, et al. Performance characteristics of upper airway critical collapsing pressure measurements during sleep. Sleep. 2011;34(4):459–67. PubMed Abstract | Publisher Full Text.

15. Romano S, Salvaggio A, Lo Bue A, Marrone O, Insalaco G. A negative expiratory pressure test during wakefulness for evaluating the risk of obstructive sleep apnea in patients referred for sleep studies. Clinics (Sao Paulo). 2011;66(11):1887–94. PubMed Abstract | Publisher Full Text.

16. Borek RC, Thaler ER, Kim C, Jackson N, Mandel JE, Schwab RJ. Quantitative airway analysis during drug-induced sleep endoscopy for evaluation of sleep apnea. Laryngoscope. 2012;122(11):2592–9. PubMed Abstract | Publisher Full Text.

17. Petri N, Suadicani P, Wildschiødtz G, Bjørn-Jørgensen J. Predictive value of Müller maneuver, cephalometry and clinical features for the outcome of uvulopalatopharyngoplasty. Evaluation of predictive factors using discriminant analysis in 30 sleep apnea patients. Acta Otolaryngol. 1994;114(5):565–71. PubMed Abstract | Publisher Full Text.

18. Li W, Ni D, Jiang H, Zhang L. Predictive value of sleep nasendoscopy and the Müller maneuver in uvulopalatopharyngoplasty for the obstructive sleep apnea syndrome. Lin Chuang Er Bi Yan Hou Ke Za Zhi. 2003;17(3):145–6. PubMed Abstract | Publisher Full Text.

19. Ramji M, Biron VL, Jeffery CC, Côté DW, El-Hakim H. Validation of pharyngeal findings on sleep nasopharyngoscopy in children with snoring/sleep disordered breathing. J Otolaryngol Head Neck Surg. 2014;43:13. PubMed Abstract | Publisher Full Text.

20. Santiago-Recuerda A, Gómez-Terreros FJ, Caballero P, Martin-Duce A, Soleto MJ, Vesperinas G, et al. Relationship between the upper airway and obstructive sleep apnea-hypopnea syndrome in morbidly obese women. Obes Surg. 2007;17(7):996. PubMed Abstract | Publisher Full Text.

21. Kum RO, Ozcan M, Yilmaz YF, Gungor V, Yurtsever Kum N, Unal A. The Relation of the Obstruction Site on Muller's Maneuver with BMI, Neck Circumference and PSG Findings in OSAS. Indian J Otolaryngol Head Neck Surg. 2014;66(2):167–72. PubMed Abstract | Publisher Full Text.

# 17

# Ototoxicity of acetic acid on the guinea pig cochlea

Takafumi Yamano[1,2*], Hitomi Higuchi[2], Takashi Nakagawa[2] and Tetsuo Morizono[3]

## Abstract

**Background:** To evaluate the ototoxicity of acetic acid solutions.

**Methods:** Compound action potentials (CAPs) of the eighth nerve were measured in guinea pigs before and after the application of acetic acid in the middle ear cavity. The pH values of the acetic acid solutions were pH 3.0, 4.0, and 5.0, and the application times were 30 min, 24 h, and 1 week.

**Results:** Acetic acid solution (pH 3.0, $N = 3$) for 30 min caused no significant elevation in CAP threshold at 4 kHz, but a significant elevation in the threshold was noted for 8 kHz and clicks. Acetic acid solutions (pH 4.0 $N = 6$, 5.0 $N = 5$) for 30 min caused no significant elevation in CAP. Acetic acid solution (pH 4.0) for 24 h ($N = 5$) caused significant elevations of the CAP threshold for 8 kHz, 4 kHz, and for clicks. Acetic acid (pH 5.0) for 24 h ($N = 3$) caused a significant elevation of the CAP threshold for 4 kHz, but not for 8 kHz or clicks. Acetic acid (pH 5.0) for 1 week ($N = 3$) caused a small but significant elevation CAP the threshold for 8 kHz and 4 kHz tone bursts, but no significant change was noted for clicks.

**Conclusions:** We found a significant toxic effect of acetic acid in guinea pigs on eighth-nerve compound action potentials when the pH was 5.0 or lower. Clearly, the stronger the acidity, and longer the exposure time, the more the CAP threshold was elevated.

## Background

The purpose of this study is to elucidate the effect of various acidity of acetic acid on the guinea pig cochlea. Ototoxicity of Burow's solution on the guinea pig cochlea was reported by us (1). Main ingredient of Burow's solution is 13 % aluminum acetate. Original Burow's solution has a pH 3.5 which caused a significant reduction of compound action potential (CAP) when applied in the middle ear cavity for 30 min, while a two fold diluted Burow's solution (pH 4.4) caused no reduction in CAP threshold. No study has been performed to determine ototoxicity of acetic acid with various pH.

## Methods

This protocol was approved by Fukuoka University Animal Ethics Committee.

* Correspondence: yamano@college.fdcnet.ac.jp
[1]Section of Otorhinolaryngology, Department of Medicine, Fukuoka Dental College, 2-15-1 Tamura,Sawara-ku, Fukuoka 814-0193, Japan
[2]Department of Otorhinolaryngology, Fukuoka University School of Medicine, Jounan-ku Nanakuma 7-45-1, Fukuoka 814-0180, Japan
Full list of author information is available at the end of the article

### Animals

To evaluate the ototoxicity of various acidity (pH) of acetic acid, alubino Hartley guinea pigs of both genders (in total $N = 30$) were used. Animals selected had an average body weight between 300 and 400 g and had a positive Prayer reflex.

### Acetic acid

The test solution was freshly prepared by the Pharmacy Department of our University Hospital, and the pH was measured and adjusted to 3.0, 4.0, and 5.0, before each experiment. Osmotic pressure of acetic acid studied was 300 mOsm, the molecular weight was 60.

### Surgical procedure

The animals were anesthetized with sodium pentobarbital (30 mg/kg), and were secured in a custom-made head holder. Xylocaine (Astra Zeneca PLC, Osaka, Japan) 0.5 % was infiltrated into the surgical area before making the skin incision for access to the middle ear cavity. The tympanic bulla was exposed using a retro-auricular incision. A small hole, about 2 mm in diameter, was made using a dental drill, and the round window membrane was visualized with a 40× operating microscope.

## Sound system

Asynchronous tone bursts of 4 kHz, 8 kHz (1-ms rise and fall time, 10- ms plateau time), and click sounds were given as stimuli at a pulse rate of 20 per second, from 80 dB (re 20μPa) to thresholds with 10 dB decrements. The speaker used was a Telephonics TDH-39P, and the sound source was placed 10 cm away from the auricle. The free field sound pressure was monitored and calibrated with a Brüel & Kjær half-inch condenser microphone.

## Recording system and CAP measurement

An 0.08-mm-diameter Teflon-insulated silver wire with an exposed ball tip was carefully placed with a micromanipulator on the peripheral round window membrane. An Ag-AgCl reference electrode was placed in the neck muscles. The obtained CAP responses were averaged 200 times with a Traveler Express ER-22 (Biologic Systems Corp. USA.)

## Application of acetic acid

After the initial CAP was measured, the middle ear cavity was filled with acetic acid of various acidity. The amount of fluid necessary to fill the middle ear cavity was about 0.2 mls. Prior to CAP measurement, middle ear cavity of each animal was thoroughly dried using a tissue paper wick. We evaluated the following: (1–3) the effect on the action potential threshold of acetic acid (pH 3.0, 4.0, and 5.0) at 30 min after topical application, (4-5) the effect of 24 h application of acetic acid (pH 4.0, 5.0), (6) the effect of 1 week application of acetic acid (pH5.0).

## Analysis of the data

A threshold response was defined as an N1-P1 signal with amplitude of 10 μV. The change in the sound pressure level in decibels before and after drug application was defined as a change in hearing. The threshold change before and after drug application was compared, and a paired t-test was used to define statistical significance.

## Bacteriology

The bacteriostatic activity of acetic acid was studied using a disk diffusion assay. Bacteria obtained from patients of our clinic was two stocks of MRSA, which were diluted to $10^6$ FCU/ml, and cultured on an agar plate for 24 h. Acetic acid with pH 3.0, 4.0, 5.0, either 50 μl or 75 μl, was dropped on an 8 mm diameter disk, and placed on the agar plate. At another 24 h, the diameter

of zones of inhibition of bacterial growth on the agar plate was measured.

## Results

Figure 1 shows changes in CAP threshold in decibel loss before and 30 min after saline control. No significant reduction in CAP was observed brfore and after saline application.

Figure 2 shows changes in CAP threshold in decibel loss from control at 30 min. For 4 kHz, no significant elevation in CAP threshold was noted. For click stimulation and for 8 kHz, a significant elevation of the threshold was noted.

Figure 3 shows changes in CAP with acetic acid pH 4.0 at 30 min. No significant elevation in CAP threshold was noted at 30 min. Significant difference exists between pH 3.0 and pH 4.0 solution at 30 min. Figure 4 shows the results from acetic acid pH 5.0 at 30 min. No change in CAP threshold was noted at 30 min.

At 24 h, acetic acid (pH 4.0) caused significant elevation of CAP threshold for 8 kHz, 4 kHz, and for click sounds (Fig. 5). Compared with the results at 30 min, ototoxicity became evident at 24 h.

At 24 h, acetic acid (pH 5.0) caused a significant elevation of CAP threshold with tone burst of 4 kHz, but no significant elevation for 8 kHz or for click sounds (Fig. 6).

At 1 week, acetic acid (pH 5.0) caused small but a significant elevation in CAP threshold for 8 kHz and 4 kHz tone burst. No significant change was noted for click sound (Fig. 7).

## Bacteriology

The diameter of the zone of inhibition for two stocks of MRSA is shown in Table 1. The zone of inhibition in mm is shown. The larger zones of inhibition indicate better antimicrobial effect. Either 50 μl or 75 μl, was used. The diameter of the disk was 8 mm. At 24 h, Bacteriostatic activity was noted for pH 3.0, 4.0, and 5.0.

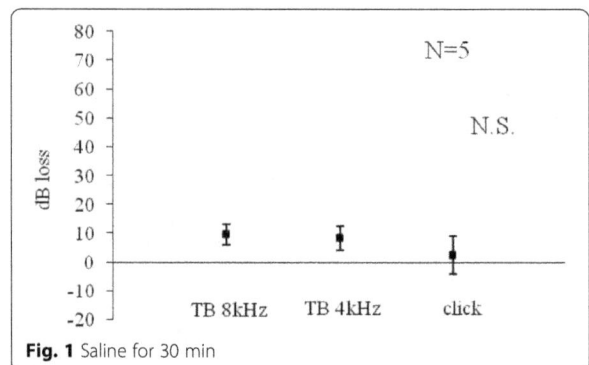

**Fig. 1** Saline for 30 min

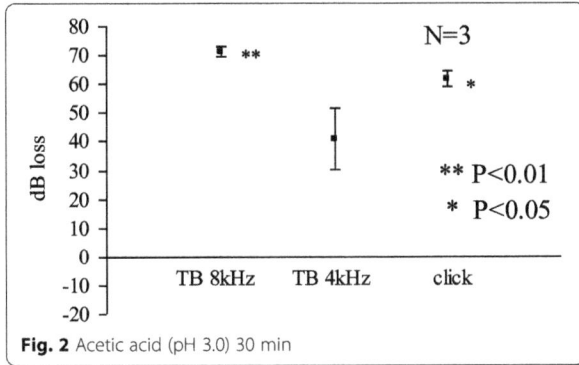

**Fig. 2** Acetic acid (pH 3.0) 30 min

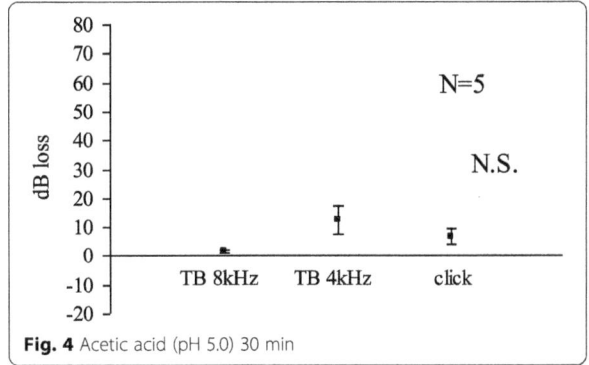

**Fig. 4** Acetic acid (pH 5.0) 30 min

The bacteriostatic activity was concentration dependent. A larger amount of acetic acid caused more bacteriostatic activity.

## Discussion

The bactericidal effect of acetic acid has been well known empirically. Recently, Burrow's solution has gained popularity as effective solution in treating intractable ear discharge with fungi and with methicillin-resistant *staphylococcus aureus* (MRSA). The primary ingredient of this solution is acetic acid and 13 % aluminum acetate. In our previous study [1], use of original Burrow's solution (pH3.5) for 30 min caused a significant elevation of CAP threshold, a two-fold diluted Burrow's solution (pH 4.4) for 30 min caused no change in CAP threshold [1].

VoSol otic solution (ECR Pharmaceuticals Co. Inc) is a commonly available ear drops in the USA, which contains 2 % acetic acid in a propylene glycol vehicle containing propylene glycol diacetate (3 %), benzentonoum chloride (0.02 %), and sodium acetate (0.015 %). This otic solution is buffered at pH3.0 for use in the external canal. Adverse effect of VoSol solution has been reported previously [2–4]. Application of 2 % acetic acid or VoSol on the round window membrane caused a reduction of pH in the perilymph, in the endolymph, and a reduction of endocochlear DC potentials (EP). The reduction started only a few minutes after the application. They concluded that otic preparation containing acetic acid penetrates the round window membrane within a few minutes, and causes an inhibition of Na+, K-ATPase activity of the stria vascularis. The effect was much stronger for the VoSol solution than for acetic acid, probably due to synergistic effects of acetic acid and propylene glycol. Propylene glycol causes damage of the round window membrane, thus the diffusion of acetic acid becomes greater.

Thorp et al [5–7] reported antibacterial activity of acetic acid and Burow's solution in vitro and also in vivo. However, otototoxic effect of this solution was not addressed. No systemic study has been performed to determine the ototoxicity of acetic acid alone.

We varied the pH of acetic acid to 3.0, 4.0, and 5.0. Also we varied the duration of acetic acid in the middle ear cavity for 30 min, 24 h, and 1 week.

We found a significant toxic effect of acetic acid in guinea pigs on eighth nerve compound action potentials (CAP).

Clearly, stronger the acidity, more the elevation of CAP threshold, and longer the exposure time, more the elevation of CAP threshold.

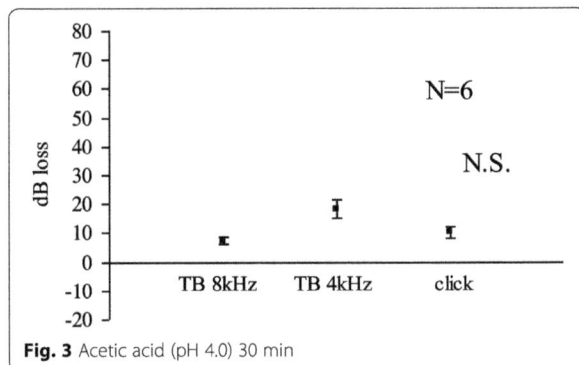

**Fig. 3** Acetic acid (pH 4.0) 30 min

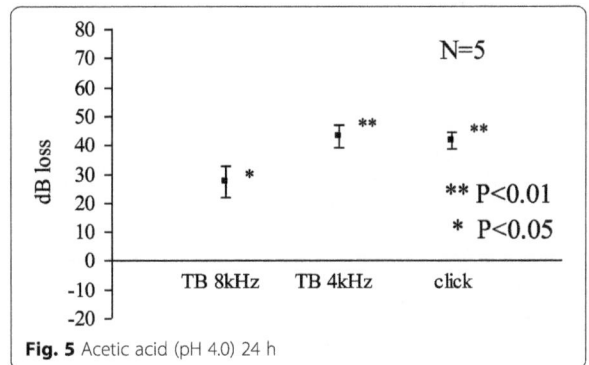

**Fig. 5** Acetic acid (pH 4.0) 24 h

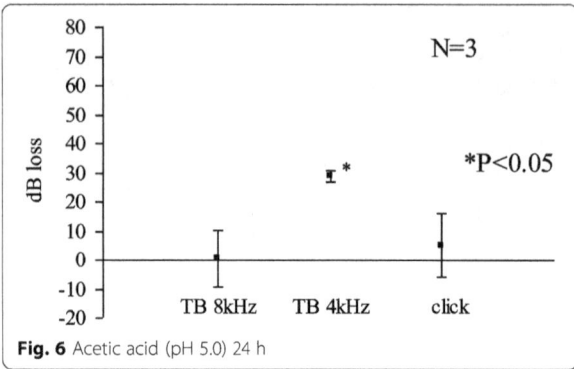

**Fig. 6** Acetic acid (pH 5.0) 24 h

We limited the use of animals as small as possible yet to obtain significant results. In the Figs. 1, 2, 3 and 4, standard errors shown as a vertical line indicated that the variability of the change among animals in each groups is small.

In the group of Acetic acid (pH5.0) for 1 week, probably most of the acetic acid leaked out from Eustachian tube at the time we took the measurement. Also, tissue fluids from the middle ear mucosa would dilute the acetic acid. Comparison of the group of acetic acid (pH 5.0) for 30 min, 24 h and 1 week revealed that longer exposure time is more harmful to the cochlea, suggesting the toxic effect of the acetic acid is not reversible.

It is impossible to completely exclude the possibility of a conductive hearing loss caused by the fluid in the tympanic bulla. However, we believe conductive component of the hearing loss is minimum after drying the middle ear cavity with wicks of tissue paper.

Although acidic solutions have been used in the middle ear cavity as ear drops or irrigation, ototoxicity of the acidic solution has not been addressed adequately. Our previous study [1] showed Burrow's solution with pH 3.5 for 30 min caused a significant reduction in CAP, yet a two-fold dilute Burrow's solution (pH 4.4) for 30 min caused no reduction in CAP. Our current

**Table 1** Bacteriostatic activity for either 50 or 75 μl of acetic acid

|        |        | pH3.0 | pH4.0 | pH5.0 |
|--------|--------|-------|-------|-------|
| MRSA1  | 50 μL  | 35    | 32    | 21    |
|        | 75 μL  | 39    | 33    | 26    |
| MRSA2  | 50 μL  | 37    | 30    | 23    |
|        | 75 μL  | 40    | 35    | 26    |
|        |        |       |       | (mm)  |

experiment suggests ototoxicity becomes evident at pH 3.0 at 30 min, which is in good agreement with the previous study.

In the clinical settings, it is advisable to avoid allowing the solution to contact the round window membrane for extended times.

## Conclusions

No systemic study has been performed to determine the ototoxicity of acetic acid alone. We varied the pH of acetic acid to 3.0, 4.0, and 5.0. Also we varied the duration of acetic acid in the middle ear cavity for 30 min, 24 h, and 1 week.

We found a significant toxic effect of acetic acid in guinea pigs on eighth nerve compound action potentials (CAP) when the pH is 5.0 or less. Clearly, stronger the acidity, more the elevation of CAP threshold, and longer the exposure time, more the elevation of CAP threshold.

**Competing interests**
The authors declare that they have no competing interests.

**Authors' contributions**
TY: data collection and review, conception of the study design, surgery and writing of the manuscript; HH: surgery and revision of the initial manuscript; TN: analysis and interpretation of data; TM: proposal of the study, surgery, and revision of the final manuscript. All authors read and approved the final manuscript.

**Author details**
[1]Section of Otorhinolaryngology, Department of Medicine, Fukuoka Dental College, 2-15-1 Tamura,Sawara-ku, Fukuoka 814-0193, Japan. [2]Department of Otorhinolaryngology, Fukuoka University School of Medicine, Jounan-ku Nanakuma 7-45-1, Fukuoka 814-0180, Japan. [3]Nishi Fukuoka Hospital, Nishi-ku Ikino-matsubara 3-18-8, Fukuoka 819-8555, Japan.

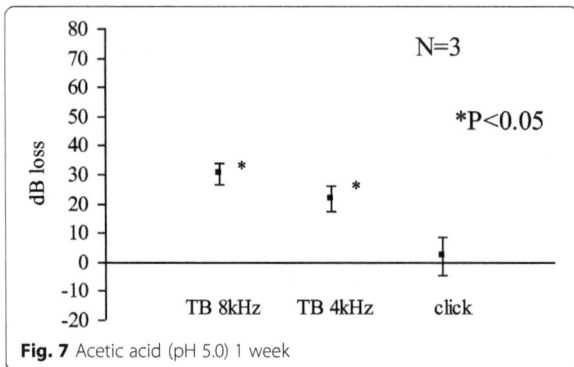

**Fig. 7** Acetic acid (pH 5.0) 1 week

**References**
1.  Sugamura M, Yamano T, Higuchi H, Takase H, Yoshimura H, Nakagawa T, et al. Ototoxicity of Burow solution on the guinea pig cochlea. Am J Otolaryngol. 2012;33:595–9.
2.  Ikeda K, Morizono T. The preparation of acetic acid for use in otic drops and its effect on endocochlear potential and pH in inner ear fluid. Am J Otolaryngol. 1989;10:382–5.
3.  Morizono T. Toxicity of ototopical drugs: Animal modeling. Ann Otol Rhinol Laryngol. 1990;99:42–5.
4.  Jinn TH, Kim PD, Russell PT, Church CA, John EO, Jung TT, et al. Determination of ototoxicity of common otic drops using isolated cochlear outer hair cells. Laryngoscope. 2001;111:2105–8.

5.  Thorp MA, Kruger J, Oliver S, Nilssen EL, Prescott CA. Antibacterial activity of acetic acid and Burow's solution as topical otologic preparations. J Laryng Otol. 1998;112:925–8.
6.  Thorp MA, Oliver SP, Kruger J, Prescott CA. Determination of the lowest dilution of aluminum acetate solution able to inhibit in vitro growth of organisms commomly found in chronic suppurative otitis media. J Laryng Otol. 2000;114:830–1.
7.  Thorp MA, Gardiner IB, Prescot CA. Burow's solution in the treatment of active mucosal chronic suppurative otitis media determining an effective dilution. J Laryngol Otol. 2000;114:432–6.

# 18

# Clinicopathological features and treatment outcomes of the rare, salivary duct carcinoma of parotid gland

Khalid Hussain AL-Qahtani[1], Mutahir A. Tunio[3]*, Yasser Bayoumi[2], Venkada Manickam Gurusamy[3], Fahad Ahmed A. Bahamdain[4] and Hanadi Fatani[5]

## Abstract

**Background:** Salivary ductal carcinoma (SDC) of parotid gland is a rare and aggressive entity; accounting for 1–3 % of all malignant salivary gland tumors, 0.2 % of epithelial salivary gland neoplasms, 0.5 % of salivary gland carcinomas, and 1.1 % of parotid gland carcinomas. Here in we aimed to evaluate the clinico-pathological features and treatment outcomes of parotid gland SDC in Saudi population.

**Methods:** Among 38 patients with parotid malignancies, who were treated in two major tertiary care referral cancer centers between December 2007 and December 2014, seven cases (18.4 %) were found to have SDC, which were investigated for clinicopathological features, locoregional recurrences (LRRs), distant metastasis (DM) and survival rates.

**Results:** Mean age of cohort was 62.3 years (range: 41–83) and female predominant (71.4 %). All patients underwent total parotidectomy and ipsilateral neck dissection. Mean tumor size was 3.4 cm (range: 2.1–5.3); perineural invasion (85.8 %); lymph node involvement (42.9 %); and HER-2 neu overexpression (28.6 %). Postoperative radiation therapy (PORT) was given to six patients (dose: 50–66 Gy). Median follow-up was 20.2 months (range: 11–48). LRRs were seen in five (71.4 %) patients (base of skull, 3 patients; cervical nodes, one patient; parotid bed, one patient). LRRs were salvaged with resection (two patients) and re-irradiation (one patient with base of skull). DM in lungs was seen in three patients (42.8 %); one treated with carboplatin/paclitaxel based chemotherapy. The 4-year disease free and overall survival rates were 16.7 % and 40 % respectively.

**Conclusion:** SDC of parotid gland is a rare and aggressive entity, and most of LRRs were seen in the base of skull, which warrants inclusion of base of skull in clinical target volume in PORT planning. Role of anti HER-2 targeted therapy in SDC with HER-2 neu overexpression needs further investigations.

**Keywords:** Salivary ductal carcinoma, Parotid gland, Saudi population

## Background

Salivary ductal carcinoma (SDC) of parotid gland is a rare and aggressive entity; accounting for 1–3 % of all malignant salivary gland tumors, 0.2 % of epithelial salivary gland neoplasms, 0.5 % of salivary gland carcinomas, and 1.1 % of parotid gland carcinomas [1, 2]. SDC of parotid gland has been classified as high grade tumors along with high-grade mucoepidermoid carcinoma and carcinoma ex pleomorphic adenoma in the updated World Health Organisation (WHO) classification of salivary gland tumors [3]. The histopathological features of SDC of parotid gland are similar to those of breast ductal carcinoma requiring a differential diagnosis with possible metastasis through immunohistochemistry (IHC) analysis among patients with a previous history of breast carcinoma [4].

The standard treatment for SDC of parotid gland is total parotidectomy, ipsilateral neck dissection followed by postoperative radiation therapy with or without concurrent chemotherapy; however, SDC of parotid gland has grave dismal prognosis [5].

* Correspondence: drmutahirtonio@hotmail.com
[3]Radiation Oncology, King Fahad Medical City, Riyadh 59046, Saudi Arabia
Full list of author information is available at the end of the article

Here in, we describe and discuss the clinicopathological characteristics and treatment outcomes SDC of parotid gland in our population.

## Methods

After formal approval from the institutional review committee, medical records of 38 patients with confirmed parotid gland malignancies, who were treated in two cancer centers of Riyadh, Saudi Arabia during the period of December 2007 and December 2014, were reviewed using digital database system. Patients with SDC of parotid gland were retrieved in following manner;

### Demographic, clinicopathological and radiological variables

Demographic and clinical data including age at the diagnosis, gender, and signs and symptoms at the time of presentation were reviewed. A detailed second review of all histopathological specimens was performed by experienced histopathologist. Different histopathological parameters, including the tumor size, lymphovascular space invasion (LVSI), perineural invasion (PNI), margin status, lymph node involvement and tumor, lymph node and metastasis (TNM) staging were recorded. Data from different imaging modalities, including computed tomography (CT) scan of neck and chest, magnetic resonance imaging (MRI) and flourodeoxyglucose positron emission tomography (FDG-PET) was collected. Data regarding different treatment modalities, including the type of parotidectomy and neck dissection, postoperative radiation therapy (PORT), and its doses were also recorded.

### Statistical analysis

The primary endpoint was locoregional control (LRC). Secondary points were the distant metastasis control (DMC), disease free survival (DFS) and overall survival (OS) rates. Locoregional recurrence (LRR) was defined as, the duration between the parotidectomy and the date of clinically or radiologically detectable disease in the parotid bed or in cervical lymph nodes on imaging. Distant metastasis (DM) was defined as, the duration between the parotidectomy and the date of documented disease outside the neck on imaging. Similarly, DFS was defined as, the duration between the parotidectomy and the date of documented disease reappearance/relapse, death from cancer and/or last follow-up (censored). The OS was defined as, the duration between the surgery and the date of patient death or last follow-up (censored). Probabilities of LRC, DMC, DFS and OS rates were shown with the Kaplan-Meier method, and the comparisons for various survival curves were performed using log rank. All statistical analyses were performed using the computer program SPSS version 16.0. Relevant literature was searched through PubMed/MED-LINE, CANCERLIT, EMBASE, Cochrane Library database, Web of Science, Academic Search Premier, and CINAHL using the terms "(salivary duct carcinoma, ductal carcinoma parotid, Stensen duct carcinoma of parotid. These terms were then combined for search for prospective, retrospective, randomized, controlled, review articles.

## Results

Among thirty eight patients with parotid malignant tumors who were treated in our centers between December 2007 and December 2014, seven cases (18.4 %) were found to have SDC. Mean age of cohort was 62.3 years (range: 41–83), with female preponderance (71.4 %). The common presentation at the diagnosis was the parotid swelling. In two patients (28.6 %), facial nerve palsy was seen at the time of diagnosis. Patient characteristics are shown in Table 1.

All patients underwent total parotidectomy and modified ipsilateral neck dissection. Mean tumor size was 3.4 cm (range: 2.1–5.3). Predominant histopathological pattern was the neoplasm was comprised of cribriform growth pattern with central comedo necrosis, and tumor cells were polygonal with distinct cell borders, with pleomorphic nuclei and increased mitotic activity (Fig. 1a and b). PNI was observed in 6/7 cases (85.8 %), while LVSI was seen in 3/7 patients (42.9 %). Lymph node involvement was observed in 3/7 cases (42.9 %). HER-2 neu was overexpressed in 2/7 cases (28.6 %).

PORT via IMRT was given to 6/7 cases (85.8 %). Indications were positive margins (66.7 %), and lymph node metastasis (50 %). Median delay between surgery and PORT was 6 weeks (range: 5.5–8). The treatment fields encompassed the tumor bed and upper neck (4 patients), and tumor bed and entire neck (2 patients). Cranial border of PORT fields were kept at base of skull in 2 patients. Mean dose for PORT was 61.3 Gy (range: 50–66 Gy), given as daily 2 Gy/fraction, 5 days/week over 6–6.5 weeks (30–33 fractions).

Median follow-up was 20.2 months (range: 11–48). LRRs were seen in five (71.4 %) patients. One LRR was in patient without PORT, Two LRRs were marginal near PORT fields (mastoid air cells/base of skull; 3 patients) Fig. 2a and b; two LRRs were seen in-field PORT (cervical nodes; one patient, parotid bed; one patient) Fig. 3. LRRs were salvaged with resection (two patients) and re-irradiation via IMRT (one patient with base of skull recurrence) and systemic chemotherapy (one patient). DM in lungs was seen in three patients (42.8 %); one treated with carboplatin/paclitaxel based chemotherapy. At the time of analysis, four patients (57.2 %) were alive and were disease free. The median time to survival was 15.8 months. The 4-year LRC, DMC, DFS and OS rates were 20.8 %, 40 %, 16.7 % and 40 % respectively Fig. 4a and b.

**Table 1** Patient characteristics

| Patient | Age /gender | Symptoms | Treatment | Pathology | Recurrence | Metastasis | Died | Follow-up period |
|---|---|---|---|---|---|---|---|---|
| 1. | 52/F | Left parotid swelling, facial nerve palsy | Total parotidectomy and ipsilateral MND | Tumor size: 2 × 3 cm; LVSI -; PNI-; 0/20 LN; HER-2 neu +++; Margins-; | Base of skull with ICE (VI,VIII,IX,X,XI CN palsy) Treated with Palliative RT 25 /10 | Bilateral Lungs | Yes | 14 months |
| 2. | 41/M | Right parotid swelling | Total parotidectomy + ipsilateral MND → RT 60 Gy/30 fractions | Tumor size: 3 × 3 cm,; LVSI-, PNI+; 0/30LN; HER-2 neu +++; margins- | No | No | No | 11 months |
| 3. | 83/M | Right parotid swelling | Total Parotidectomy + ipsilateral MND → RT 50 Gy/25 fractions | Tumor size: 2 × 2 cm,; LVSI-;PNI+; 0/10 LN; HER-2 neu -; margins+, | No | Bilateral Lungs | Yes | 13 months |
| 4. | 43/F | Right parotid swelling | Total parotidectomy + ipsilateral MND → 66 GY/33 fractions | Tumor size: 4 × 3 cm,; LVSI+; PNI+; HER-2 neu -; skin +; 2/30LN+; margins+ | Mastoid air cells and base of skull Treated with Reirradiation 60 Gy/30 fractions | No | No | 27 months |
| 5. | 65/F | Right parotid swelling | Total parotidectomy + ipsilateral MND → RT 66 Gy/33 fractions | Tumor size: 4 × 4 cm; LVSI-; PNI+; HER-2 neu -; 5/14 LN+; margins+, | Ipsilateral Neck nodes level III, IV Treated with salvage LND | No | No | 12 months |
| 6. | 81/F | Right parotid swelling, facial nerve palsy | Total parotidectomy + ipsilateral MND → RT 66 Gy/33 fractions | Tumor size: 5 × 5 cm; LVSI+; PNI+; HER-2 neu -; 3/21LN+; margins + | Mastoid air cells and base of skull treated with chemotherapy | Bilateral Lung treated with Carboplatin/Paclitaxel chemotherapy | Yes | 16 months |
| 7. | 71/F | Left parotid swelling | Total parotidectomy + ipsilateral MND → RT 60 Gy/30 fractions | Tumor size: 3 × 3 cm; LVSI +; 0/22LN; PNI+; HER-2 neu -; margins- | Tumor bed Treated with resection Pathology 1.2 cm SDC | No | No | 48 months |

*F* female, *M* male, *MLND* modified neck dissection, *RT* radiation therapy, *LVSI* lymphovascular space invasion, *PNI* perineural invasion, *LN* lymph nodes, *ICE* intracranial extension, *SDC* salivary duct carcinoma

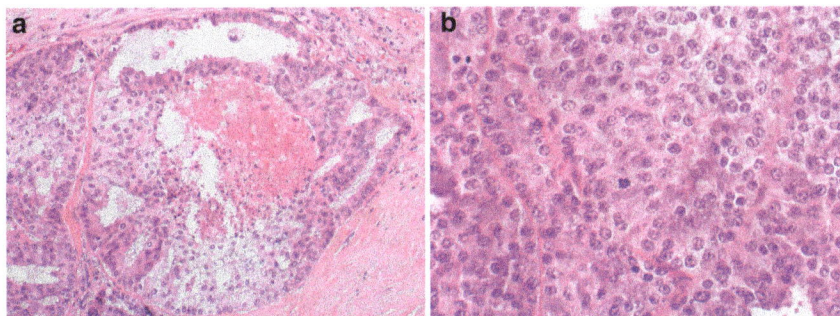

**Fig. 1 a** Neoplasm is comprised of cribriform growth pattern with central comedo necrosis (H & E stain, 200 X magnifications); **b** neoplastic cells have polygonal morphology, distinct cell borders, moderately pleomorphic nuclei and increased mitotic activity (H & E stain, 400 X magnifications)

## Discussion

SDC is an extremely rare and aggressive malignancy of the salivary glands. Owing to its rare nature, clinical data is scanty and only a few clinical studies comprise more than 50 SDC patients [4, 6–8]. To date, largest SDC study has been reported from the Surveillance, Epidemiology, and End Results (SEER) database, based on 228 patients [9]. This review reported that poor prognostic factors for OS and DFS in SDC patients were age 50 years or above, tumor size, and lymph node involvement. However, this study was criticized for the diagnostic bias. Similar other studies have been mentioned in Table 2 [3, 4, 6–8, 10–21]. However, none of these studies has evaluated clinico-pathological features, DFS and OS in SDC of the parotid gland separately, which was the aim of present study. Reason for lower incidence of facial nerve involvement at the time of diagnosis (28.6 %) in our series as compared to reported data can be explained by the fact that the preoperative facial nerve function was not available for many patients, so facial nerve sacrifice at the time of parotidectomy was used as a surrogate for preoperative facial nerve palsy.

Our series was predominantly female gender (71.4 %), which is in agreement with one study by Hosal AS et al. [15], while other studies have shown a male preponderance ranging from 53.8 % to 94.7 % [11, 19]. In present study, relatively high incidence of pathological positive cervical lymph nodes (42.9 %) was found in agreement with reported literature, and it warrants routine use of prophylactic ipsilateral neck dissection in SDC of the parotid gland. Similarly, the percentage of pathologically positive PNI (85.8 %) was significantly high in our series, which supports the notion that CTV should include the cranial nerves involved and the corresponding parts of the base of skull in cases of pathologically positive PNI [22]. Interestingly, in our series, no contralateral neck recurrence was seen, therefore the role of prophylactic contralateral neck irradiation needs further investigation.

HER-2 neu overexpression (28.6 %) was much lower than those reported in literature [3, 6, 13]. Recent data has shown that HER-2 neu overexpression and targeted therapy with Trastuzumab therapy is associated with improved DFS and OS rates [23]. Given the limited published data on use of adjuvant or maintenance Trastuzumab in SDC of parotid

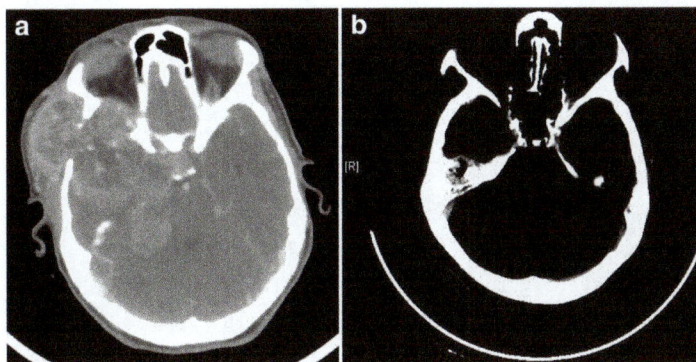

**Fig. 2 a** CT head axial image (patient # 1) showing a destructive recurrent mass in the right sphenoid wing, extending into middle and posterior cranial fossae with destruction of a large portion of the skull base; **b** CT head (patient # 4) demonstrating heterogeneous soft tissue recurrent mass involving the right mastoid air cells, mastoid bone and occipital bone associated with bone destruction

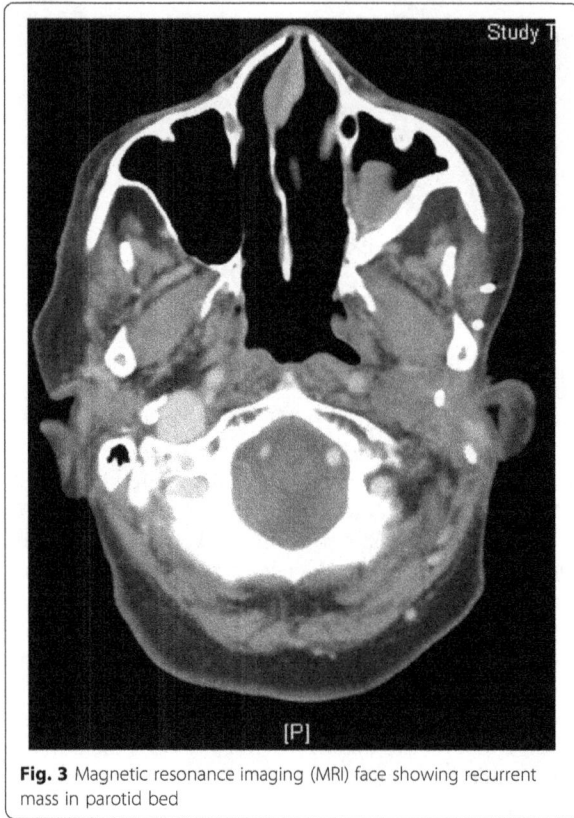

**Fig. 3** Magnetic resonance imaging (MRI) face showing recurrent mass in parotid bed

gland, it might also be useful to develop future Trastuzumab trials in SDC from HER-2 neu positive breast cancer [24]. As SDC of parotid gland has morphologic and molecular similarity to breast cancer, it is recommended that apart from regular histopathological examination, additional immunohistochemical staining including HER-2 neu, Ki-67, p16, p53, estrogen receptors (ER), progesterone receptors (PR), epithelial membrane antigen (EMA), and carcinoembryonic antigen (CEA) should be performed, as proposed by many studies [25, 26].

In contrast to other studies, about 60 % of LRRs were seen in base of skull (PORT was given in 2 patients) in our series, which further supports the hypothesis of inclusion of base of skull in CTV during PORT for these patients as in patients with parotid gland adenoid cystic carcinoma [27]. One LRR in base of skull was salvaged by re-irradiation using IMRT with acceptable toxicity. However, data from re-irradiation in adenoid cystic carcinoma has shown that most of LRRs following re-irradiation occur within the re-irradiated high-dose region, therefore more data regarding dose escalation and delayed toxicity is required [28].

Our study has few limitations. A relatively small number of patients were studied, due to the rarity of SDC in our population. Further, PORT fields, techniques and doses varied somewhat in our study.

## Conclusions

SDC of parotid gland is rare and aggressive entity. Despite extensive treatment by parotidectomy, neck dissection and PORT; a large proportion of patients developed all-sites recurrences. Base of skull should be included

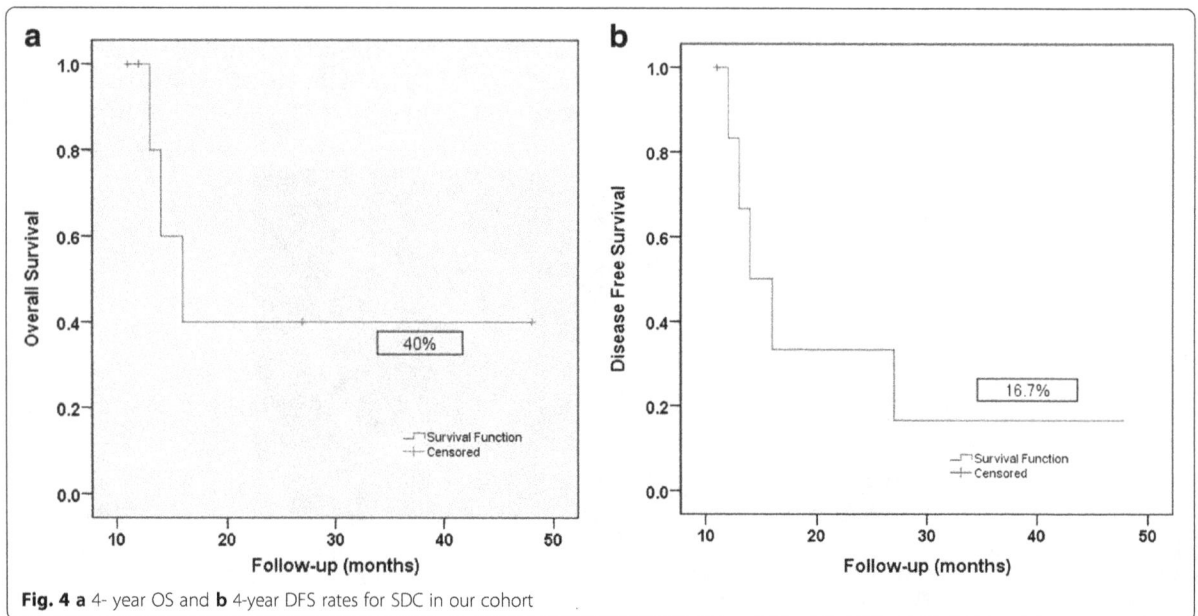

**Fig. 4 a** 4- year OS and **b** 4-year DFS rates for SDC in our cohort

Clinicopathological features and treatment outcomes of the rare, salivary duct carcinoma...

137

**Table 2** Previously published studies on salivary duct carcinoma of Parotid gland

| Study | Patients | Parotid SDC | LN + | PNI | HER-2 neu expression | PORT | Follow-up Mean | LRR | DM | OS |
|---|---|---|---|---|---|---|---|---|---|---|
| Huang X, et al. [3] | 117 M (63.6 %) | 7 (63.6 %) | 6 (54.5 %) | 5 (45.5 %) | 9 (81.8) | 8 (72.7 %) Dose: 50–60 | 30 months | 2 (18.2 %) | 2 (18.2 %) | 2-year 75 % |
| Jaehne M, et al. [4] | 50 30 M (60 %) | 39 (78 %) | 28 (56 %) | - | - | 36 (72 %) | 24 months | 24 (48 %) | 24 (48 %) | 66 % |
| Gilbert MR, et al. [6] | 75 53 M (71 %) | 62 (83 %) | 54 (72 %) | 52 (69 %) | 23 (31 %) | 31 (41 %) | 55 months | 0 | 0 | 3 year 50 % |
| Johnston ML, et al. [7] | 54- | 49 (90.7 %) | 38 (67 %) | - | - | 48 (89 %) Dose: 60 Gy | 68.4 months | 16 (29.6 %) | 28 (51.8 %) | 43 % |
| Roh JL, et al [8] | 56 | 34 (62 %) | 38 (67 %) | - | - | 21 (37.5) | 60 months | | 71 % | 44 % |
| Kim TH, et al. [10] | 15 12 M (80 %) | 12 (80 %) | 9 (60 %) | 8 (53.3 %) | - | 15 (100 %) | 38 months | 2 (13.3 %) | 7 (47 %) | 93 % |
| Shi S, et al. [11] | 38 36 M (94.7 %) | 38 (100) | - | - | - | - | 48 months | - | - | 45 % |
| Kim JY, et al. [12] | 35 30 M (85.7 %) | 22 (62.9 %) | 26 (74.3 %) | 12 (34.3 %) | - | 31 (88.6 %) | 36 months | 9 (25.7 %) | 6 (17.2 %) | 55.1 % |
| Brandwein-Gensler M, et al. [13] | 19 | - | - | - | 10 (52.6 %) | - | 30 months | - | - | 68.4 % |
| Luna MA, et al. [14] | 30 19 M (63.3 %) | 24 (80 %) | 16 (66.7 %) | - | - | - | 24 months | 16 (66.7 %) | 16 (66.7 %) | 30 % |
| Colmenero Ruiz C, et al. [15] | 9 7 M (77.8 %) | 8 (88.9 %) | 3 (37.5 %) | - | - | 7 (87.5 %) | 30 months | 5 (55.6 %) | 3 (33.5 %) | 33 % |
| Delgado R, et al. [16] | 15 12 M (80 %) | 13 (86.7 %) | 2 (13.3 %) | - | - | 9 (60 %) | - | 5 (33 %) | 6 (40 %) | 47 % |
| Guzzo M, et al. [17] | 26 14 M (53.8 %) | 21 (80.7 %) | 15 (57.7 %) | - | - | 17 (65.4 %) | 60 months | 11 (42.3 %) | 12 (46.2 %) | 46 % |
| Hosal AS, et al. [18] | 15 7 M (46.7 %) | 12 (80 %) | 11 (73.3 %) | - | - | 14 (93.3 %) | 48 months | 8 (53.3 %) | 7 (46.7 %) | 43 % |
| Ko YH, et al. [19] | 27 16 M (56.3 %) | 21 (77.8 %) | 10 (37.1 %) | - | - | 19 (70.4 %) | 30 months | 9 (33.3 %) | 15 (55.6 %) | 44 % |
| Afzelius LE, et al. [20] | 12 7 M (58.3 %) | 12 (100 %) | 5 (41.7 %) | - | - | 12 (100 %) | 60 months | 3 (25 %) | 6 (50 %) | 42 % |
| Lewis JE, et al. [21] | 26 17 M (65.4 %) | 23 (88.5 %) | 19 (73.1 %) | - | - | 13 (50 %) | 60 months | 15 (57.7 %) | 11 (43 %) | 43 % |
| Our study | 7 2 M (28.6 %) | 7 (100 %) | 3 (42.9 %) | 6 (85.8 %) | 2 (28.6 %) | 6 (85.8 %) | 20.2 months | 5 (71.4 %) | 3 (42.8 %) | 40 % |

SDC salivary duct carcinoma, M male, LN lymph nodes, PNI Perineural invasion, PORT postoperative radiotherapy, LRR locoregional recurrence, DM distant metastasis, OS overall survival

routinely in CTV during PORT, and HER-2 neu status should also be examined routinely in all these patients. Further, large multi-institutional studies regarding the role of re-irradiation, systemic chemotherapy, trastuzumab are warranted to suggest optimal treatment approaches for SDC of parotid gland.

## Competing interests
The authors declare that they have no competing interests.

## Authors' contributions
KQ, YB and MT participated in the design of the study and performed the statistical analysis. VMG, YB and FAB collected the data and drafted the manuscript. HF carried out the histopathology data collection and edited the manuscript. All authors read and approved the final manuscript.

## Acknowledgement
We are thankful to Laura Stanciu Gabriella for her efforts in the revision of manuscript and drafting.

## Author details
[1]Department of Otolaryngology-Head & Neck Surgery, College of Medicine, King Saud University, Riyadh, Saudi Arabia. [2]Radiation Oncology, NCI, Cairo University, Cairo, Egypt. [3]Radiation Oncology, King Fahad Medical City, Riyadh 59046, Saudi Arabia. [4]Faculty of Medicine, King AbdulAziz University, Riyadh 59046, Saudi Arabia. [5]Histopathology, Comprehensive Cancer Center, King Fahad Medical City, Riyadh 59046, Saudi Arabia.

## References
1. Pont E, Pla A, Cruz Mojarrieta J, Ferrandis E, Brotons S, Vendrell JB. Salivary duct carcinoma: diagnostic clues, histology and treatment. Acta Otorrinolaringol Esp. 2013;64:150–3.
2. Xie S, Yang H, Bredell M, Shen S, Yang H, Jin L, Zhang S. Salivary duct carcinoma of the parotid gland: A case report and review of the literature. Oncol Lett. 2015;9:371–4.
3. Huang X, Hao J, Chen S, Deng R. Salivary duct carcinoma: A clinopathological report of 11 cases. Oncol Lett. 2015;10:337–41.
4. Jaehne M, Roeser K, Jaekel T, Schepers JD, Albert N, Loning T. Clinical and immunohistologic typing of salivary duct carcinoma: a report of 50 cases. Cancer. 2005;103:2526–33.
5. Nabili V, Tan JW, Bhuta S, Sercarz JA, Head CS. Salivary duct carcinoma: a clinical and histologic review with implications for trastuzumab therapy. Head Neck. 2007;29:907–12.
6. Gilbert MR, Sharma A, Schmitt NC, Johnson JT, Ferris RL, Duvvuri U, Kim S. A 20-Year Review of 75 Cases of Salivary Duct Carcinoma. JAMA Otolaryngol Head Neck Surg. 2016. doi:10.1001/jamaoto.2015.3930.
7. Johnston ML, Huang SH, Waldron JN, Atenafu EG, Chan K, Cummings BJ, Gilbert RW, Goldstein D, Gullane PJ, Irish JC, Perez-Ordonez B, Weinreb I, Bayley A, Cho J, Dawson LA, Hope A, Ringash J, Witterick IJ, O'Sullivan B, Kim J. Salivary duct carcinoma: Treatment, outcomes, and patterns of failure. Head Neck. 2015. doi:10.1002/hed.24107.
8. Roh JL, Lee JI, Choi SH, Nam SY, Kim SO, Cho KJ, Kim SB, Kim SY. Prognostic factors and oncologic outcomes of 56 salivary duct carcinoma patients in a single institution: high rate of systemic failure warrants targeted therapy. Oral Oncol. 2014;50:e64–6.
9. Jayaprakash V, Merzianu M, Warren GW, Arshad H, Hicks Jr WL, Rigual NR, Sullivan MA, Seshadri M, Marshall JR, Cohan DM, Zhao Y, Singh AK. Survival rates and prognostic factors for infiltrating salivary duct carcinoma: Analysis of 228 cases from the Surveillance, Epidemiology, and End Results database. Head Neck. 2014;36:694–70.
10. Kim TH, Kim MS, Choi SH, Suh YG, Koh YW, Kim SH, Choi EC, Keum KC. Postoperative radiotherapy in salivary ductal carcinoma: a single institution experience. Radiat Oncol J. 2014;32:125–31.
11. Shi S, Fang Q, Liu F, Zhong M, Sun C. Prognostic factors and survival rates for parotid duct carcinoma patients. J Craniomaxillofac Surg. 2014;42:1929–31.
12. Kim JY, Lee S, Cho KJ, Kim SY, Nam SY, Choi SH, Roh JL, Choi EK, Kim JH, Song SY, Shin HS, Chang SK, Ahn SD. Treatment results of post-operative

radiotherapy in patients with salivary duct carcinoma of the major salivary glands. Br J Radiol. 2012;85:e947–52.
13. Brandwein-Gensler M, Hille J, Wang BY, Urken M, Gordon R, Wang LJ, Simpson JR, Simpson RH, Gnepp DR. Low-grade salivary duct carcinoma: description of 16 cases. Am J Surg Pathol. 2004;28:1040–44.
14. Luna MA, Batsakis JG, Ordonez NG, Mackay B, Tortoledo ME. Salivary gland adenocarcinomas: a clinicopathologic analysis of three distinctive types. Semin Diagn Pathol. 1987;4:117–35.
15. Colmenero Ruiz C, Patron Romero M, Martin PM. Salivary duct carcinoma: a report of nine cases. J Oral Maxillofac Surg. 1993;51:641–6.
16. Delgado R, Vuitch F, Albores-Saavedra J. Salivary duct carcinoma. Cancer. 1993;72:1503–12.
17. Guzzo M, Di Palma S, Grandi C, Molinari R. Salivary duct carcinoma: clinical characteristics and treatment strategies. Head Neck. 1997;19:126–33.
18. Hosal AS, Fan C, Barnes L, Myers EN. Salivary duct carcinoma. Otolaryngol Head Neck Surg. 2003;129:720–5.
19. Ko YH, Roh JH, Son YI, Chung MK, Jang JY, Byun H, Baek CH, Jeong HS. Expression of mitotic checkpoint proteins BUB1B and MAD2L1 in salivary duct carcinomas. J Oral Pathol Med. 2010;39:349–55.
20. Afzelius LE, Cameron WR, Svensson C. Salivary duct carcinoma-a clinicopathologic study of 12 cases. Head Neck Surg. 1987;9:151–6.
21. Lewis JE, McKinney BC, Weiland LH, Ferreiro JA, Olsen KD. Salivary duct carcinoma. Clinicopathologic and immunohistochemical review of 26 cases. Cancer. 1996;77:223–30.
22. Shinoto M, Shioyama Y, Nakamura K, Nakashima T, Kunitake N, Higaki Y, Sasaki T, Ohga S, Yoshitake T, Ohnishi K, Asai K, Hirata H, Honda H. Postoperative radiotherapy in patients with salivary duct carcinoma: clinical outcomes and prognostic factors. J Radiat Res. 2013;54:925–30.
23. Limaye SA, Posner MR, Krane JF, Fonfria M, Lorch JH, Dillon DA, Shreenivas AV, Tishler RB, Haddad RI. Trastuzumab for the treatment of salivary duct carcinoma. Oncologist. 2013;18:294–300.
24. McKeage K, Perry CM. Trastuzumab: a review of its use in the treatment of metastatic breast cancer overexpressing HER2. Drugs. 2002;62:209–43.
25. Masubuchi T, Tada Y, Maruya S, Osamura Y, Kamata SE, Miura K, Fushimi C, Takahashi H, Kawakita D, Kishimoto S, Nagao T. Clinicopathological significance of androgen receptor, HER2, Ki-67 and EGFR expressions in salivary duct carcinoma. Int J Clin Oncol. 2015;20:35–44.
26. Simpson RH, Skalova A, Di Palma S, Leivo I. Recent advances in the diagnostic pathology of salivary carcinomas. Virchows Arch. 2014;465:371–84.
27. Garden AS, Weber RS, Morrison WH, Ang KK, Peters LJ. The influence of positive margins and nerve invasion in adenoid cystic carcinoma of the head and neck treated with surgery and radiation. Int J Radiat Oncol Biol Phys. 1995;32:619–26.
28. Jensen AD, Poulakis M, Nikoghosyan AV, Chaudhri N, Uhl M, Munter MW, Herfarth KK, Debus J. Re-irradiation of adenoid cystic carcinoma: analysis and evaluation of outcome in 52 consecutive patients treated with raster-scanned carbon ion therapy. Radiother Oncol. 2015;114:182-8.

# 19

# Reconsidering first-line treatment for obstructive sleep apnea

Brian W. Rotenberg[1,4*], Claudio Vicini[2], Edward B. Pang[3] and Kenny P. Pang[3]

## Abstract

**Background:** Continuous positive airway pressure (CPAP) is typically recommended as first line therapy for obstructive sleep apnea, but the adherence rate of CPAP is problematic. This study's objective was to systematically review the literature relating to CPAP as first line therapy for OSA and compare it to surgical literature on the same topic.

**Methods:** A systematic review was conducted according to PRISMA guidelines, examining Medline-Ovid, Embase, and Pubmed databases. The primary search objective was to identify all papers reporting the results of (1) randomized clinical trials (RCT) of CPAP for the treatment of adults with OSA; and (2) both randomized and non-randomized clinical trials and case series on the surgical treatment of OSA in adults. A PhD-level biostatistician first screened papers, and then those that met study criteria were retrieved and analyzed using standardized forms for each author. The primary outcomes were adherence rates of CPAP.

**Results:** A total of 82 controlled clinical trials for CPAP and 69 controlled and non-controlled surgery trials were identified for analysis. Variation in CPAP use within reported RCT trials were identified, and the majority of patients in the studies would eventually be considered non-adherent to CPAP.

**Conclusions:** When considering the numerous patient-related factors that come into play when CPAP is prescribed, the concept of CPAP as gold-standard therapy for OSA should be reconsidered. In many cases surgery can provide a better overall outcome. This study's results suggest that certain patients with OSA may be managed more effectively with surgery than CPAP, without confounding issues of treatment adherence.

**Keywords:** Obstructive sleep apnea, Uvulopalatoplasty, CPAP

## Background

Obstructive sleep apnea (OSA) is considered part of a group of disorders that cover a continuum ranging from habitual snoring (simple snoring) to moderate or severe OSAS. OSA is characterized by repetitive apnea and/or hypopnea during sleep. Due to relaxation of the upper airway pharyngeal and tongue muscles during sleep the airway narrows and collapses resulting in hypoxaemia, increased sympathetic overdrive, increased blood pressure, and hypercapnia. These add hypoxic stress to the

brain and heart. Apneic and hypopneic events may occur numerous times per night, resulting in arousals from sleep and sleep disruptions causing sleep fragmentation leading to excessive daytime sleepiness. These repeated cyclic oxygen desaturations and a fragmented sleep architecture lead to sympathetic overdrive, interrupted sleep, and reduced percentage of slow wave sleep, translating into symptoms of daytime somnolence, morning headaches, poor concentration, memory loss, a higher risk of car accidents, depression and marital discord.

OSA has a strong association with hypertension, atherosclerosis, and cerebrovascular accidents (strokes) [1]. Studies have also shown a higher mortality rate among patients with cardiovascular disease who also have OSA [1]. It has been long purported that nasal continuous

* Correspondence: brian.rotenberg@sjhc.london.on.ca
[1]Department of Otolaryngology–Head and Neck Surgery, Western University, London, Ontario, Canada
[4]St. Joseph's Hospital, Room B2-501, 268 Grosvenor Street, London, ON N6A 4V2, Canada
Full list of author information is available at the end of the article

positive airway pressure (CPAP) is the "gold" standard in the treatment of OSA, and there is no doubt that CPAP is effective when used properly and according to AASM standards. However, it is also well known that due to problematic patient adherence, the real world effectiveness of CPAP is low, with a large proportion of users abandoning the machine within one year of prescription. Such patients cannot be said to be effectively treated. Surgery for OSA on the other hand does not rely on any form of long-term patient adherence, and when the right patient is matched with the right pharyngeal procedure in order to maximize success, long-term strong results have been shown. When considering all OSA patients it is recognized that overall treatment success rates with surgery are lower than via CPAP, but this does not hold true for the subset of patients with appropriate apnea-specific surgical anatomy wherein rates of successful surgical OSA treatment are very high. Moreover the issue of CPAP adherence has generally not been examined during these debates; to make an effective comparison adherence must be taken into account when studying the impact on OSA of CPAP versus surgery. CPAP, an efficacious therapy with inconsistent adherence, can potentially be equivalent to surgery, that being a "partial" therapy with complete adherence. It is the issue of treatment effectiveness versus adherence (the relationship of the two defining success) that is at the crux of the matter.

This study's objective was to systematically review the literature relating to CPAP as first line therapy for OSA and then compare it to surgical literature on the same topic.

## Methods

Our review was carried out in accordance with the preferred reporting items for systematic review and meta-analysis protocols (PRISMA-P) 2015 statement. A comprehensive systematic literature review was conducted using the Medline-Ovid, Embase, and Pubmed databases.

The primary search objective was to identify all papers reporting the results of (1) randomized clinical trials (RCT) of CPAP for the treatment of adults with OSA; and (2) both randomized and non-randomized clinical trials and case series on the surgical treatment of OSA in adults. The first step was a locate and review all of the studies listed for analysis in three major literature reviews, a Cochrane Collaboration review [1] and a second systematic literature review published by the National Institutes of Health Research (NIHR) [2] on the use of CPAP for the treatment of OSA, and a second Cochrane Collaboration review on its surgical management [3]. The second step was an extensive search of the PubMed/MedLine database, initiated using the following

combined search terms: "randomized clinical trial and obstructive sleep apnea" ($n = 1083$); "CPAP and randomized clinical trial and obstructive sleep apnea" ($n = 357$); and "surgery and obstructive sleep apnea and clinical trial" ($n = 603$). From these lists, studies were identified that (a) did not replicate studies already found and (b) were otherwise eligible for inclusion. The third and final step was a review of all reference lists and tables of other studies found within papers identified in the second step. A PhD level biostatistician performed all three of the search steps.

Articles were considered for inclusion into the study by reviewing the titles and abstracts of all retrieved studies. The senior study authors BWR and KPP did this and results were compiled to ensure no studies were missed. The full text of selected studies were then analyzed to ensure that the following inclusion criteria were met: diagnosis of obstructive sleep apnea, no confounding data for central sleep apnea, and the paper referred to either CPAP or surgical treatment of OSA.

## Results

A total of 82 controlled clinical trials for CPAP and 69 controlled and non-controlled surgery trials were identified for analysis (note that non-controlled trials were accepted for surgery because of the relatively few controlled trials). The CPAP studies included trials comparing CPAP versus sub-therapeutic (sham) CPAP [4–34], CPAP versus an oral placebo [33, 35–43], CPAP versus conservative or no therapy [10, 22, 44–54], CPAP versus an oral appliance [4, 5, 36, 51, 55–63], CPAP versus postural therapy [64–67], and CPAP alone assessing different means to modify adherence (e.g., with vs. without a humidifying element) [8, 21, 30, 68–79]. The surgical trials assessed a variety of single- and multi-stage procedures incorporating uvuloplasty [22, 80–117], mandibular advancement [118, 119], laser treatments [120–125], radiofrequency tissue reduction and other lingual procedures [117, 125–134], and palate implants [135–141], in addition to five trials specifically evaluating the safety versus risks of OSA surgery, including its safety as an outpatient/same-day procedure [142–146]. The PRISMA charts seen in Figs. 1 and 2 summarize the study flow, and Additional files 1, 2, and Table 1 summarize the results of the search strategy.

## Discussion of findings

Currently, continuous positive airway pressure (CPAP) is considered the gold standard treatment for patients with obstructive sleep apnea, be it mild, moderate or severe. This is the conclusion expressed in both a recently-published Cochrane Collaboration review [1] and a second systematic literature review published by the National Institutes of Health Research (NIHR) [2]. Surgical approaches are hardly discussed at all in either of these two

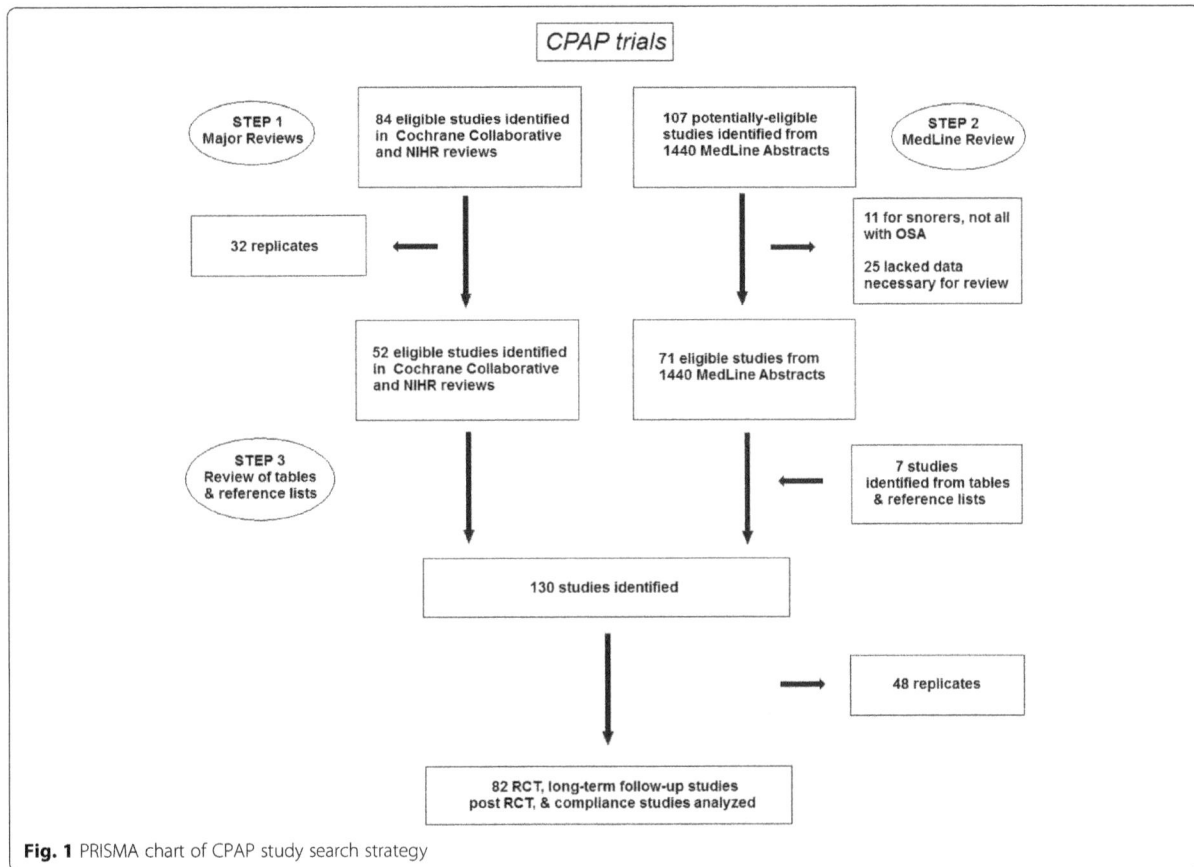

**Fig. 1** PRISMA chart of CPAP study search strategy

reviews, largely on the basis of the lack of randomized controlled trials (RCTs). A closer look at the evidence however reveals that surgery may indeed play a primary role in many patients with OSA.

First, although a large number of RCTs have been published documenting the benefits of CPAP relative to sub-therapeutic (sham) CPAP [3–33], an oral placebo [32, 34–43], conservative or no therapy [9, 21, 42, 44–53], various oral appliances [3, 4, 35, 50, 54–62], and postural therapy [63–66], numerous limitations of these RCTs must be considered. First among these is the short duration of follow-up that has been almost ubiquitous amongst CPAP trials, the vast majority having final assessments within weeks of the initial treatment, and only a small handful extending beyond 3 to 4 months [46, 56], 6 months [3, 52], 1 year [9, 21], or beyond [44]. A couple of additional long-term cohort studies emerged from RCT, following patients, open label, to and beyond 1 year [3, 62]. This contrasts, however, with the much more long-term follow-up generally performed for surgical trials, where follow-up to and beyond 6 months is the norm, with several investigative groups reporting on outcomes beyond 1 year.

A second issue pertains to adherence with CPAP, a well-documented problem that warrants concern. In our review of 83 CPAP trials (Additional file 1), the average patient in bed for 7 h across these 83 closely supervised clinical trials was not using it an average of 32.9 % of the time. When the nights per week of CPAP non-use have been examined, the percentages range from 10 to 40 % [5, 35, 50, 55, 67–70] These are problematic percentages given that several published RCT have documented that at least a minimum level of CPAP use of 5–6 h per night is required to reap benefits from it [9, 37, 40, 68, 71]. There is therefore a sizeable subset of patients on CPAP who either cease to use it altogether, or fail to use it enough hours per night and/or nights per week to achieve clinically-significant benefits.

The issue of adherence is generally a non-issue with surgery, especially beyond the initial recovery period. Once a patient's anatomy is changed, it should remain so. How effective is surgery? Admittedly, there are far fewer EBM (evidence-based medicine) level 1 RCT and many more EBM level 4 case series for OSA surgery, as should be expected given the ethical and methodological obstacles associated with performing double-blinded or

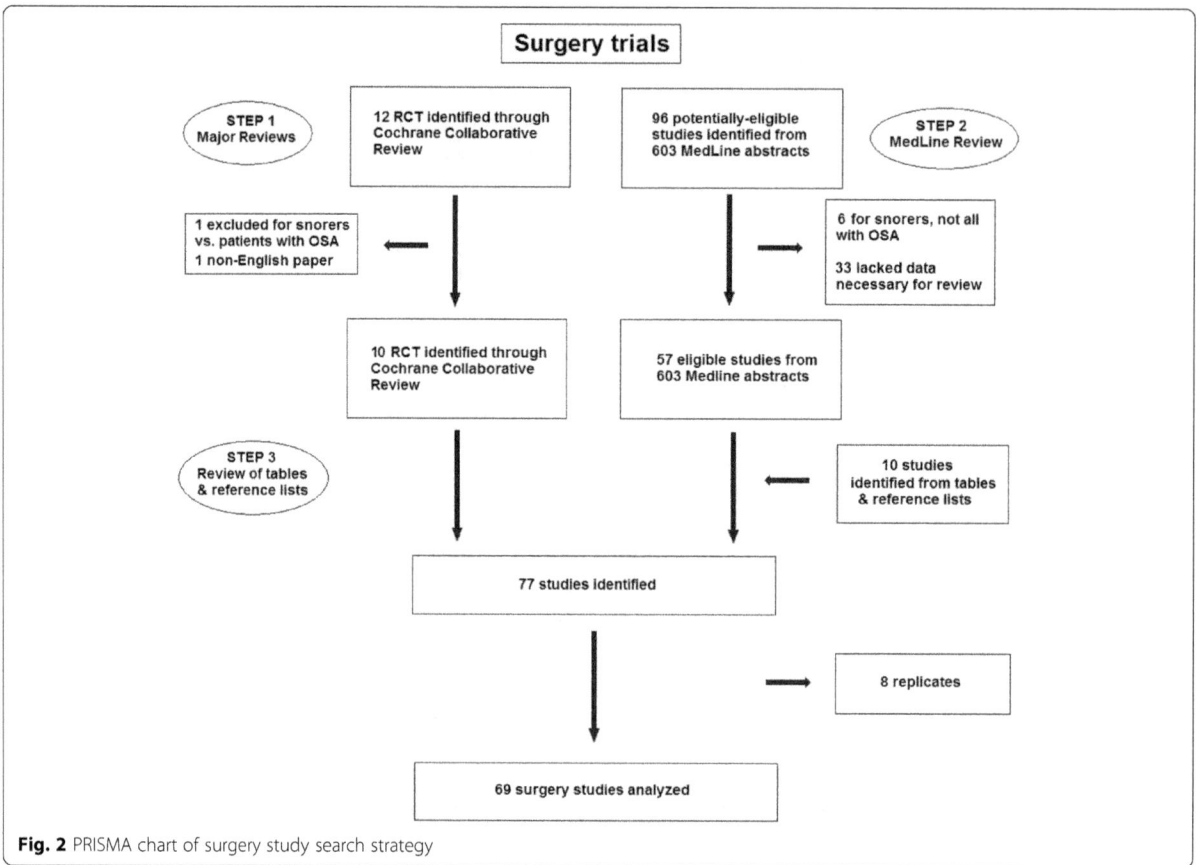

**Fig. 2** PRISMA chart of surgery study search strategy

**Table 1** CPAP versus surgery comparisons

| First author - year | EBM rating | Study design | Treatment groups | Study findings | Study limitations/issues |
|---|---|---|---|---|---|
| Woodson 2003 | 1 | RCT | nCPAP vs. RFTR vs. sham RFTR | Relative to sham Rx, rxn time & fastest rxn time both improved post-RFTR ($p = 0.03$ & $0.02$) but not on CPAP. | Very poor CPAP compliance (~16 h/week); |
| | | | | ESS ↓ similarly with RFTR & CPAP ($-2.1$ vs. $-2.3$, $p = 0.005$ & $0.02$). SNORE25 score ↓ w/both ($p < 0.001$ vs. $0.005$) | Different # of Rx sessions in RFTR (4.5) vs. sham RFTR (2.9) groups |
| Ceylan 2009 | 3 | nonRCT | TC-RFTR vs. nCPAP | Both RFTR & CPAP → ↓AHI ($28.5 \rightarrow 15.7$ vs $29.6 \rightarrow 16.1$, both $p < 0.001$; NS); ↓ESS ($11.1 \rightarrow 8.4$, $p = 0.003$ vs $10.8 \rightarrow 8.2$, $p = 0.003$; NS); | Non-random allocation to Rx/potential selection bias; |
| | | | | ↓CT90 ($15.2 \rightarrow 11.1$ % vs $14.3 \rightarrow 10.7$ %, both $p < 0.001$; NS); & ↑LSAT ($88.4 \rightarrow 93.5$, $p = 0.03$ vs $86.8 \rightarrow 94.6$ %, $p < 0.001$, NS). 53.8 vs. 52.4 % responders | Compliance with CPAP not reported |
| Weaver 2004 | 1 | pop. survey | UPPP ± TE ± SP ± other vs. CPAP | 1339/18,754 (7.1 %) died w/ CPAP vs. 71/2072 (3.4 %) post-op. Adjusting for age, gender, race, year of Rx & co-morbidities, | Retrospective analysis; potential confounders missing |
| | | | | MR ↑ 31 % (95 % CI 3–67 %) w/CPAP ($p = 0.03$) | (e.g., severity of OSA, overall health status) |

even controlled surgical trials. This being said, only 24 of the CPAP RCT described above were truly blinded, pitting therapeutic CPAP against sub-therapeutic (and thereby, sham) CPAP, rendering all comparisons, especially of subjective measures like the patient's level of sleepiness and quality of life, at least somewhat suspect. Clearly, all subjects in these studies knew that they were using an oral appliance, an oral placebo or nothing versus nasal CPAP. Interestingly, and harkening back to the issue of adherence, though CPAP tended to improve objective measures of OSA to a greater degree than oral appliances, patients consistently and decidedly preferred the latter [35, 55, 57, 60].

The limitations of EBM level 4 evidence set aside, among the 1802 patients who underwent OSA surgery across the 53 studies we analyzed, more than half (957, 53.1 %) were deemed to have experienced a 'good response'. This is despite the consistent use of strict criteria for a 'response' that ranged from Sher's criteria of no less than a 50 % reduction in AHI to a level of 20 events/hour or less [79], criteria that were used in 20 of the studies [80–99]; to being as stringent as no less than a 50 % reduction in RDI (which is similar to the AHI but also incorporates near-hyponeic events) to a level of 20 events/hour or less [100–106]; no less than a 50 % reduction in either AHI or RDI (the latter also incorporating near-hyponeic events) to a level of 15 or even 10 events/hour or less [91, 107–110]; and reducing AHI or RDI to ≤10 or even 5 events/hour [111–114] (Additional file 2). Mandibular/maxillo-mandibular advancement procedures had an especially high success (good response) rate of 87.0 % [84, 107, 115]. Moreover, there appeared to be a dose–response effect, with more aggressive procedures incorporating UPPP more effective than less aggressive procedures like tongue tissue ablation (Additional file 2), and more repetitions of treatments like laser- or radiofrequency- aided tissue reduction more effective than fewer repetitions [116].

Only three studies directly have compared CPAP and OSA surgery: one a randomized clinical trial comparing therapeutic radiofrequency-aided tissue reduction (RFTR), sham RFTR and nasal CPAP [117]; one a non-randomized clinical trial comparing RFTR and nasal CPAP [83]; and the third a population survey assessing long-term mortality among over 20,000 U.S. veterans who underwent either UPPP or CPAP therapy between October 1997 and September 2001 within the Veterans Affairs hospital system [118]. These results are summarized in Table 1. With the first study [117], subjective sleepiness, as measured with the Epworth Sleepiness scale (ESS), decreased to the same extent with RFTR & CPAP (−2.1 vs. −2.3, $p = 0.005$ & 0.02), as did the patients' level of snoring, as measured with the SNORE25 ($p < 0.001$ vs. 0.005), both effects superior to sham RFTR ($p < 0.001$).

However, objective sleepiness, measured as each patient's average and shortest reaction time, only improved with RFTR ($p = 0.03$ and $p = 0.02$ versus sham therapy, respectively). In the non-randomized trial [83], RFTR and CPAP significantly reduced AHI versus baseline ($28.5 \rightarrow 15.7$ vs. $29.6 \rightarrow 16.1$, both $p < 0.001$; no significant inter-treatment difference), with similar significant reductions noted for the ESS score ($11.1 \rightarrow 8.4$, $p = 0.003$ vs. $10.8 \rightarrow 8.2$, $p = 0.003$; NS) and the percentage of time with oxygen saturation below 90 % ($15.2 \rightarrow 11.1$ % vs. $14.3 \rightarrow 10.7$ %, both $p < 0.001$; NS). The two treatments also produced a similar increase in the patient's lowest recorded nocturnal oxygen saturation level ($88.4 \rightarrow 93.5$, $p = 0.03$ vs. $86.8 \rightarrow 94.6$ %, $p < 0.001$; NS). Overall, 53.8 and 52.4 % of patients were deemed to be treatment 'responders' (NS).

Perhaps most alarming of these results are those of the survival study [118], in which 1339 out of 18,754 patients on CPAP died over the course of observation (7.1 %) versus just 71 of 2072 (3.4 %) post-operatively. Adjusting for patient age, gender, race, year of treatment and co-morbid illnesses, there still was a 31 % (95 % CI: 3–67 %) increase in mortality among CPAP patients ($p = 0.03$) versus their post-UPPP counterparts. It may be that some patients receiving CPAP were considered too ill to be surgical candidates, a confounder that would falsely elevate the CPAP mortality rate. It is also important to acknowledge that the study authors were not able to adjust for OSA severity or account for CPAP adherence. Nonetheless, it is clear that all prior assumptions that CPAP is both more effective and safer than surgery as first-line treatment for OSA warrant re-evaluation.

In summary, though it is true that the evidence supporting CPAP over surgery as first-line therapy for OSA is more strongly supported by EBM level 1 evidence, closer inspection reveals major limitations of that evidence and reasons to suspect that this long-held assumption should now be questioned. Among these limitations are the very short-term follow-up of almost all CPAP trials (versus the longer follow-up of surgical trials); the very high degree of CPAP non-adherence that, in the vast majority of trials, was not accounted for by intent-to-treat analysis; failure to identify any significant advantage of CPAP over surgery in the two trials in which these two approaches were compared directly; and the apparent 30 % increased mortality observed in veterans who received CPAP versus surgical treatment in the U.S. between 1997 and 2001. Surgery appears to be clinically successful long-term in at least half of OSA patients, in terms of reducing their AHI to normal or near-normal levels. Given all of this, the time has come to rethink our CPAP-first approach to the OSA patient, especially in those patients in whom adherence, for whatever reason, might be considered an issue. Within that context however it is also imperative that surgeons understand that changing the current care ladder means also stressing the importance of correct patient selection and an appropriate consent process.

As a systematic review, this study is limited to the quality of the included studies. Because it is a collection of findings from various other studies, it provides an overview of the direction of literature but is unable to show new findings. This study is also limited in the fact that only English language articles are considered, which may introduce a language bias. However, studies are published from a variety of centers internationally. Because this study is not a meta-analysis, study results have not been statistically combined for more powerful results. One additional caveat is that studies were only graded by a traditional EBM approach as opposed to the more sophisticated Cochrane GRADE tool. This may introduce some level of bias to the priorities given to the various studies. However the large volume of literature reviewed for this paper should adequately compensate for that.

## Conclusion

This review illustrates the need for an in-depth, thorough and critical analysis of the available treatment options for the OSA patient. Although CPAP is often documented as the gold standard or mandatory first line therapy for patients with OSA, a careful assessment of the outcomes provided by the literature does not support this assertion, especially when the concept of CPAP adherence is taken into account. Clinicians should consider a patient-centered approach to care wherein the patient's individual anatomical characteristics are evaluated in context of their OSA severity and treatment goals, and then tailor intervention to individual needs. In many patients beneficial surgical results may supplant the role of the CPAP machine when considering first line therapy.

## Additional files

**Additional file 1: Table S1.** CPAP comparisons. (DOCX 60 kb)
**Additional file 2: Table S2.** Surgery findings. (DOCX 43 kb)

#### Competing interests
The authors declare that they have no competing interests.

#### Authors' contributions
BR conducted the study design, and the majority of the writing. KP and EP assisted with writing, as well as compiling the data tables. CV assisted with intellectual contributions and editing of the paper. All authors read and approved the final manuscript.

#### Acknowledgments
The authors would like to acknowledge Dr. Kevin White for his invaluable help with statistical analysis.

**Author details**
[1]Department of Otolaryngology–Head and Neck Surgery, Western University, London, Ontario, Canada. [2]Head & Neck Department, ASL of Romagna, ENT and Oral Surgery Unit, Morgagni-Pierantoni Hospital (Forlì), Ospedale degli Infermi (Faenza), Forlì, Italy. [3]Asia Sleep Centre, Paragon, Singapore. [4]St. Joseph's Hospital, Room B2-501, 268 Grosvenor Street, London, ON N6A 4V2, Canada.

**References**
1. Giles TL, Lasserson TJ, Smith B, White J, Wright JJ, Cates CJ. Continuous positive airways pressure for obstructive sleep apnoea in adults: a Cochrane Collaboration Review. Etobicoke, Canada: John Wiley & Sons, Ltd; 2008. Issue 4, 1–103.
2. McDaid C, Griffin S, Weatherly H, et al. Continuous positive airway pressure devices for the treatment of obstructive sleep apnoea-hypopnoea syndrome: a systematic review and economic analysis. Southampton, UK: National Institutes of Health Research Health Technology Assessment Program; 2009.1–162.
3. Sundaram S, Lim J, Lasserson TJ. Surgery for obstructive sleep apnoea in adults: A Cochrane Collaboration Review. Etobicoke, Canada: John Wiley & Sons, Ltd; 2009. 1, 1–72.
4. Aarab G, Lobbezoo F, Heymans MW, Hamburger HL, Naeije M. Long-term follow-up of a randomized controlled trial of oral appliance therapy in obstructive sleep apnea. Respiration. 2011;82(2):162–8.
5. Aarab G, Lobbezoo F, Hamburger HL, Naeije M. Oral appliance therapy versus nasal continuous positive airway pressure in obstructive sleep apnea: a randomized, placebo-controlled trial. Respiration. 2011;81(5):411–9.
6. Ancoli-Israel S, Palmer BW, Cooke JR, et al. Cognitive effects of treating obstructive sleep apnea in Alzheimer's disease: a randomized controlled study. J Am Geriatr Soc. 2008;56(11):2076–81.
7. Arias MA, Garcia-Rio F, Alonso-Fernandez A, Martinez I, Villamor J. Pulmonary hypertension in obstructive sleep apnea: effects of continuous positive airway pressure: a randomized, controlled cross-over study. Eur Heart J. 2006;27(9):1106–13.
8. Bakker J, Campbell A, Neill A. Randomized controlled trial comparing flexible and continuous positive airway pressure delivery: effects on adherence, objective and subjective sleepiness and vigilance. Sleep. 2010;33(4):523–9.
9. Barbe F, Mayoralas LR, Duran J, et al. Treatment with continuous positive airway pressure is not effective in patients with sleep apnea but no daytime sleepiness. a randomized, controlled trial. Ann Intern Med. 2001;134(11):1015–23.
10. Barbe F, Duran-Cantolla J, Capote F, et al. Long-term effect of continuous positive airway pressure in hypertensive patients with sleep apnea. Am J Respir Crit Care Med. 2010;181(7):718–26.
11. Becker HF, Jerrentrup A, Ploch T, et al. Effect of nasal continuous positive airway pressure treatment on blood pressure in patients with obstructive sleep apnea. Circulation. 2003;107(1):68–73.
12. Campos-Rodriguez F, Grilo-Reina A, Perez-Ronchel J, et al. Effect of continuous positive airway pressure on ambulatory BP in patients with sleep apnea and hypertension: a placebo-controlled trial. Chest. 2006;129(6):1459–67.
13. Coughlin SR, Mawdsley L, Mugarza JA, Wilding P, Calverley PM. Cardiovascular and metabolic effects of CPAP in obese males with OSA. Eur Respir J. 2007;29(4):720–7.
14. Cross MD, Mills NL, Al-Abri M, et al. Continuous positive airway pressure improves vascular function in obstructive sleep apnoea/hypopnoea syndrome: a randomised controlled trial. Thorax. 2008;63(7):578–83.
15. Dimsdale JE, Loredo JS, Profant J. Effect of continuous positive airway pressure on blood pressure : a placebo trial. Hypertension. 2000;35(1 Pt 1):144–7.
16. Duran-Cantolla J, Aizpuru F, Montserrat JM, et al. Continuous positive airway pressure as treatment for systemic hypertension in people with obstructive sleep apnoea: randomised controlled trial. BMJ. 2010;341:c5991. doi:10.1136/bmj.c5991.
17. Egea CJ, Aizpuru F, Pinto JA, et al. Cardiac function after CPAP therapy in patients with chronic heart failure and sleep apnea: a multicenter study. Sleep. 2008;9(6):660–6.
18. Henke KG, Grady JJ, Kuna ST. Effect of nasal continuous positive airway pressure on neuropsychological function in sleep apnea-hypopnea

syndrome. A randomized, placebo-controlled trial. Am J Respir Crit Care Med. 2001;163(4):911–7.

19. Hui DS, To KW, Ko FW, et al. Nasal CPAP reduces systemic blood pressure in patients with obstructive sleep apnoea and mild sleepiness. Thorax. 2006;61(12):1083–90.

20. Jenkinson C, Davies RJ, Mullins R, Stradling JR. Comparison of therapeutic and subtherapeutic nasal continuous positive airway pressure for obstructive sleep apnoea: a randomised prospective parallel trial. Lancet. 1999;353(9170):2100–5.

21. Jenkinson C, Davies RJ, Mullins R, Stradling JR. Long-term benefits in self-reported health status of nasal continuous positive airway pressure therapy for obstructive sleep apnoea. QJM. 2001;94(2):95–9.

22. Lojander J, Maasilta P, Partinen M, Brander PE, Salmi T, Lehtonen H. Nasal-CPAP, surgery, and conservative management for treatment of obstructive sleep apnea syndrome. Chest. 1996;110:114–9.

23. Loredo JS, Ancoli-Israel S, Kim EJ, Lim WJ, Dimsdale JE. Effect of continuous positive airway pressure versus supplemental oxygen on sleep quality in obstructive sleep apnea: a placebo-CPAP-controlled study. Sleep. 2006;29(4):564–71.

24. Marshall NS, Neill AM, Campbell AJ, Sheppard DS. Randomised controlled crossover trial of humidified continuous positive airway pressure in mild obstructive sleep apnoea. Thorax. 2005;60(5):427–32.

25. Marshall NS, Neill AM, Campbell AJ. Randomised trial of adherence with flexible (C-Flex) and standard continuous positive airway pressure for severe obstructive sleep apnea. Sleep Breath. 2008;12(4):393–6.

26. Montserrat JM, Ferrer M, Hernandez L, et al. Effectiveness of CPAP treatment in daytime function in sleep apnea syndrome: a randomized controlled study with an optimized placebo. Am J Respir Crit Care Med. 2001;164(4):608–13.

27. Norman D, Loredo JS, Nelesen RA, et al. Effects of continuous positive airway pressure versus supplemental oxygen on 24-hour ambulatory blood pressure. Hypertension. 2006;47(5):840–5.

28. Pepperell JC, Ramdassingh-Dow S, Crosthwaite N, et al. Ambulatory blood pressure after therapeutic and subtherapeutic nasal continuous positive airway pressure for obstructive sleep apnea: a randomised parallel trial. Lancet. 2002;359(9302):204–10.

29. Robinson GV, Smith DM, Langford BA, Davies RJ, Stradling JR. Continuous positive airway pressure does not reduce blood pressure in nonsleepy hypertensive OSA patients. Eur Respir J. 2006;27(6):1229–35.

30. Sharma SK, Agrawal S, Damodaran D, et al. CPAP for the metabolic syndrome in patients with obstructive sleep apnea. N Engl J Med. 2011;365(24):2277–86.

31. Siccoli MM, Pepperell JC, Kohler M, Craig SE, Davies RJ, Stradling JR. Effects of continuous positive airway pressure on quality of life in patients with moderate to severe obstructive sleep apnea: data from a randomized controlled trial. Sleep. 2008;31(11):1551–8.

32. West SD, Nicoll DJ, Wallace TM, Matthews DR, Stradling JR. Effect of CPAP on insulin resistance and HbA1c in men with obstructive sleep apnoea and type 2 diabetes. Thorax. 2007;62(11):969–74.

33. Engleman HM, Martin SE, Deary IJ, Douglas NJ. Effect of continuous positive airway pressure treatment on daytime function in sleep apnoea/hypopnoea syndrome. Lancet. 1994;343(8897):572–5.

34. Spicuzza L, Bernardi L, Balsamo R, Ciancio N, Polosa R, Di MG. Effect of treatment with nasal continuous positive airway pressure on ventilatory response to hypoxia and hypercapnia in patients with sleep apnea syndrome. Chest. 2006;130(3):774–9.

35. Barnes M, Houston D, Worsnop CJ, et al. A randomized controlled trial of continuous positive airway pressure in mild obstructive sleep apnea. Am J Respir Crit Care Med. 2002;165(6):773–80.

36. Barnes M, McEvoy RD, Banks S, et al. Efficacy of positive airway pressure and oral appliance in mild to moderate obstructive sleep apnea. Am J Respir Crit Care Med. 2004;170(6):656–64.

37. Engleman HM, Gough K, Martin SE, Kingshott RN, Padfield PL, Douglas NJ. Ambulatory blood pressure on and off continuous positive airway pressure therapy for the sleep apnea/hypopnoea syndrome: effects in "non-dippers". Sleep. 1996;19(5):378–81.

38. Engleman HM, Martin SE, Deary IJ, Douglas NJ. Effect of CPAP therapy on daytime function in patients with mild sleep apnoea/hypopnoea syndrome. Thorax. 1997;52(2):114–9.

39. Engleman HM, Martin SE, Kingshott RN, Mackay TW, Deary IJ, Douglas NJ. Randomised placebo controlled trial of daytime function after continuous

positive airway pressure (CPAP) therapy for the sleep apnoea/hypopnoea syndrome. Thorax. 1998;53(5):341–5.

40. Engleman HM, Kingshott RN, Wraith PK, Mackay TW, Deary IJ, Douglas NJ. Randomized placebo-controlled crossover trial of continuous positive airway pressure for mild sleep Apnea/Hypopnea syndrome. Am J Respir Crit Care Med. 1999;159(2):461–7.

41. Faccenda JF, Mackay TW, Boon NA, Douglas NJ. Randomized placebo-controlled trial of continuous positive airway pressure on blood pressure in the sleep apnea-hypopnea syndrome. Am J Respir Crit Care Med. 2001;163(2):344–8.

42. McArdle N, Douglas NJ. Effect of continuous positive airway pressure on sleep architecture in the sleep apnea-hypopnea syndrome: a randomized controlled trial. Am J Respir Crit Care Med. 2001;164(8 Pt 1):1459–63.

43. McArdle N, Kingshott R, Engleman HM, Mackay TW, Douglas NJ. Partners of patients with sleep apnoea/hypopnoea syndrome: effect of CPAP treatment on sleep quality and quality of life. Thorax. 2001;56(7):513–8.

44. Ballester E, Badia JR, Hernandez L, et al. Evidence of the effectiveness of continuous positive airway pressure in the treatment of sleep apnea/hypopnea syndrome. Am J Respir Crit Care Med. 1999;159(2):495–501.

45. Barbe F, Duran-Cantolla J, Sanchez-de-la-Torre M, et al. Effect of continuous positive airway pressure on the incidence of hypertension and cardiovascular events in nonsleepy patients with obstructive sleep apnea: a randomized controlled trial. JAMA. 2012;307(20):2161–8.

46. Chakravorty I, Cayton RM, Szczepura A. Health utilities in evaluating intervention in the sleep apnoea/hypopnoea syndrome. Eur Respir J. 2002;20(5):1233–8.

47. Drager LF, Bortolotto LA, Figueiredo AC, Krieger EM, Lorenzi GF. Effects of continuous positive airway pressure on early signs of atherosclerosis in obstructive sleep apnea. Am J Respir Crit Care Med. 2007;176(7):706–12.

48. Drager LF, Pedrosa RP, Diniz PM, et al. The effects of continuous positive airway pressure on prehypertension and masked hypertension in men with severe obstructive sleep apnea. Hypertension. 2011;57(3):549–55.

49. Hsu CY, Vennelle M, Li HY, Engleman HM, Dennis MS, Douglas NJ. Sleep-disordered breathing after stroke: a randomised controlled trial of continuous positive airway pressure. J Neurol Neurosurg Psychiatry. 2006;77(10):1143–9.

50. Kaneko Y, Floras JS, Usui K, et al. Cardiovascular effects of continuous positive airway pressure in patients with heart failure and obstructive sleep apnea. N Engl J Med. 2003;348(13):1233–41.

51. Lam B, Sam K, Mok WY, et al. Randomised study of three non-surgical treatments in mild to moderate obstructive sleep apnea. Thorax. 2007;62(4):354–9.

52. Mansfield DR, Gollogly NC, Kaye DM, Richardson M, Bergin P, Naughton NT. Controlled trial of continuous positive airway pressure in obstructive sleep apnea and heart failure. Am J Respir Crit Care Med. 2004;169(3):361–6.

53. Monasterio C, Vidal S, Duran J, et al. Effectiveness of continuous positive airway pressure in mild sleep apnea-hypopnea syndrome. Am J Respir Crit Care Med. 2001;164(6):939–43.

54. Redline S, Adams N, Strauss ME, Roebuck T, Winters M, Rosenberg C. Improvement of mild sleep-disordered breathing with CPAP compared with conservative therapy. Am J Respir Crit Care Med. 1998;157:858–65.

55. Engleman HM, McDonald JP, Graham D, et al. Randomized crossover trial of two treatments for sleep apnea/hypopnea syndrome: continuous positive airway pressure and mandibular repositioning splint. Am J Respir Crit Care Med. 2002;166(6):855–9.

56. Ferguson KA, Ono T, Lowe AA, Keenan SP, Fleetham JA. A randomized crossover study of an oral appliance vs nasal-continuous positive airway pressure in the treatment of mild-moderate obstructive sleep apnea. Chest. 1996;109:1269–75.

57. Ferguson KA, Ono T, Lowe AA, al-Majed S, Love LL, Fleetham JA. A short-term controlled trial of an adjustable oral appliance for the treatment of mild to moderate obstructive sleep apnea. Thorax. 1997;52(4):362–8.

58. Gagnadoux F, Fleury B, Vielle B, et al. Titrated mandibular advancement versus positive airway pressure for sleep apnoea. Eur Respir J. 2009;34(4):914–20.

59. Hoekema A, Stegenga B, Wijkstra PJ, van der Hoeven JH, Meinesz AF, De Bont LG. Obstructive sleep apnea therapy. J Dent Res. 2008;87(9):882–7.

60. Randerath WJ, Heise M, Hinz R, Ruehle KH. An individually adjustable oral appliance vs continuous positive airway pressure in mild-to-moderate obstructive sleep apnea syndrome. Chest. 2002;122(2):569–75.

61. Tan YK, L'Estrange PR, Luo YM, et al. Mandibular advancement splints and continuous positive airway pressure in patients with obstructive sleep apnoea: a randomized cross-over trial. Eur J Orthod. 2002;24(3):239–49.

62. Trzepizur W, Gagnadoux F, Abraham P, et al. Microvascular endothelial function in obstructive sleep apnea: Impact of continuous positive airway pressure and mandibular advancement. Sleep Med. 2009;10(7):746–52.

63. Doff MH, Hoekema A, Wijkstra PJ, et al. Oral appliance versus continuous positive airway pressure in obstructive sleep apnea syndrome: a 2-year follow-up. Sleep. 2013;36(9):1289–96.

64. Jokic R, Klimaszewski A, Crossley M, Sridhar G, Fitzpatrick MF. Positional treatment vs continuous positive airway pressure in patients with positional obstructive sleep apnea syndrome. Chest. 1999;115(3):771–81.

65. Permut I, Diaz-Abad M, Chatila W, et al. Comparison of positional therapy to CPAP in patients with positional obstructive sleep apnea. J Clin Sleep Med. 2010;6(3):238–43.

66. Skinner MA, Kingshott RN, Jones DR, Homan SD, Taylor DR. Elevated posture for the management of obstructive sleep apnea. Sleep Breath. 2004;8(4):193–200.

67. Skinner MA, Kingshott RN, Jones DR, Taylor DR. Lack of efficacy for a cervicomandibular support collar in the management of obstructive sleep apnea. Chest. 2004;125(1):118–26.

68. Ballard RD, Gay PC, Strollo PJ. Interventions to improve adherence in sleep apnea patients previously non-compliant with continuous positive airway pressure. J Clin Sleep Med. 2007;3(7):706–12.

69. Engleman HM, Martin SE, Douglas NJ. Adherence with CPAP therapy in patients with the sleep apnoea/hypopnoea syndrome. Thorax. 1994;49(3):263–6.

70. Kohler M, Stoewhas AC, Ayers L, et al. Effects of continuous positive airway pressure therapy withdrawal in patients with obstructive sleep apnea: a randomized controlled trial. Am J Respir Crit Care Med. 2011;184(10):1192–9.

71. Kryger MH, Berry RB, Massie CA. Long-term use of a nasal expiratory positive airway pressure (EPAP) device as a treatment for obstructive sleep apnea (OSA). J Clin Sleep Med. 2011;7(5):449–53B.

72. Kushida CA, Berry RB, Blau A, et al. Positive airway pressure initiation: a randomized controlled trial to assess the impact of therapy mode and titration process on efficacy, adherence, and outcomes. Sleep. 2011;34(8):1083–92.

73. Roecklein KA, Schumacher JA, Gabriele JM, Fagan C, Baran AS, Richert AC. Personalized feedback to improve CPAP adherence in obstructive sleep apnea. Behav Sleep Med. 2010;8(2):105–12.

74. Ruhle KH, Franke KJ, Domanski U, Nilius G. Quality of life, adherence, sleep and nasopharyngeal side effects during CPAP therapy with and without controlled heated humidification. Sleep Breath. 2010;15(3):479–85.

75. Ryan S, Doherty LS, Nolan GM, McNicholas WT. Effects of heated humidification and topical steroids on adherence, nasal symptoms, and quality of life in patients with obstructive sleep apnea syndrome using nasal continuous positive airway pressure. J Clin Sleep Med. 2009;5(5):422–7.

76. To KW, Chan WC, Choo KL, Lam WK, Wong KK, Hui DS. A randomized cross-over study of auto-continuous positive airway pressure versus fixed-continuous positive airway pressure in patients with obstructive sleep apnoea. Respirology. 2008;13(1):79–86.

77. Vennelle M, White S, Riha RL, Mackay TW, Engleman HM, Douglas NJ. Randomized controlled trial of variable-pressure versus fixed-pressure continuous positive airway pressure (CPAP) treatment for patients with obstructive sleep apnea/hypopnea syndrome (OSAHS). Sleep. 2010;33(2):267–71.

78. Weaver TE, Maislin G, Dinges DF, et al. Relationship between hours of CPAP use and achieving normal levels of sleepiness and daily functioning. Sleep. 2007;30(6):711–9.

79. Wolkove N, Baltzan M, Kamel H, Dabrusin R, Palayew M. Long-term adherence with continuous positive airway pressure in patients with obstructive sleep apnea. Can Respir J. 2008;15(7):365–9.

80. Cahali MB. Lateral pharyngoplasty: a new treatment for obstructive sleep apnea hypopnea syndrome. Laryngoscope. 2003;113(11):1961–8.

81. Friedman M, Ibraham H, Lee G, Joseph NJ. Combined uvulopalatopharyngoplasty and radiofrequency tongue base reduction for treatment of obstructive sleep apnea/hypopnea syndrome. Otolaryngol Head Neck Surg. 2003;129(6):611–21.

82. Hendler BH, Costello BJ, Silverstein K, Yen D, Goldberg A. A protocol for uvulopalatopharyngoplasty, mortised genioplasty, and maxillomandibular advancement in patients with obstructive sleep apnea: an analysis of 40 cases. J Oral Maxillofac Surg. 2001;59(8):892–9.

83. Lee NR, Givens Jr CD, Wilson J, Robins RB. Staged surgical treatment of obstructive sleep apnea syndrome: a review of 35 patients. J Oral Maxillofac Surg. 1999;57(4):382–5.

84. Li KK. Surgical therapy for adult obstructive sleep apnea. Sleep Med Rev. 2005;9(3):201–9.

85. Miller FR, Watson D, Malis D. Role of the tongue base suspension suture with The Repose System bone screw in the multilevel surgical management of obstructive sleep apnea. Otolaryngol Head Neck Surg. 2002;126(4):392–8.

86. Nelson LM. Combined temperature-controlled radiofrequency tongue reduction and UPPP in apnea surgery. Ear Nose Throat J. 2001;80(9):640–4.

87. Neruntarat C. Hyoid myotomy with suspension under local anesthesia for obstructive sleep apnea syndrome. Eur Arch Otorhinolaryngol. 2003;260(5):286–90.

88. Neruntarat C. Genioglossus advancement and hyoid myotomy under local anesthesia. Otolaryngol Head Neck Surg. 2003;129(1):85–91.

89. Neruntarat C. Uvulopalatal flap for obstructive sleep apnea: short-term and long-term results. Laryngoscope. 2011;121(3):683–7.

90. Terris DJ, Kunda LD, Gonella MC. Minimally invasive tongue base surgery for obstructive sleep apnoea. J Laryngol Otol. 2002;116(9):716–21.

91. Vilaseca I, Morello A, Montserrat JM, Santamaria J, Iranzo A. Usefulness of uvulopalatopharyngoplasty with genioglossus and hyoid advancement in the treatment of obstructive sleep apnea. Arch Otolaryngol Head Neck Surg. 2002;128(4):435–40.

92. Walker-Engstrom ML, Wilhelmsson B, Tegelberg A, Dimenas E, Ringqvist I. Quality of life assessment of treatment with dental appliance or UPPP in patients with mild to moderate obstructive sleep apnoea. A prospective randomized 1-year follow-up study. J Sleep Res. 2000;9(3):303–8.

93. Walker-Engstrom ML, Tegelberg A, Wilhelmsson B, Ringqvist I. 4-year follow-up of treatment with dental appliance or uvulopalatopharyngoplasty in patients with obstructive sleep apnea: a randomized study. Chest. 2002;121(3):739–46.

94. Weaver EM, Woodson BT, Yueh B, et al. Studying Life Effects & Effectiveness of Palatopharyngoplasty (SLEEP) Study: subjective outcomes of isolated uvulopalatopharyngoplasty. Otolaryngol Head Neck Surg. 2011;144(4):623–31.

95. Wilhelmsson B, Tegelberg A, Walker-Engstrom ML, et al. A prospective randomized study of a dental appliance compared with uvulopalatopharyngoplasty in the treatment of obstructive sleep apnoea. Acta Otolaryngol. 1999;119(4):503–9.

96. Aneeza WH, Marina MB, Razif MY, Azimatun NA, Asma A, Sani A. Effects of uvulopalatopharyngoplasty: a seven year review. Med J Malaysia. 2011;66(2):129–32.

97. Baradaranfar MH, Edalatkhah M, Dadgarnia MH, et al. The effect of uvulopalatopharyngoplasty with tonsillectomy in patients with obstructive sleep apnea. Indian J Otolaryngol Head Neck Surg. 2015;67 Suppl 1:29–33.

98. Lee JM, Weinstein GS, O'Malley Jr BW, Thaler ER. Transoral robot-assisted lingual tonsillectomy and uvulopalatopharyngoplasty for obstructive sleep apnea. Ann Otol Rhinol Laryngol. 2012;121(10):635–9.

99. MacKay SG, Carney AS, Woods C, et al. Modified uvulopalatopharyngoplasty and coblation channeling of the tongue for obstructive sleep apnea: a multi-centre Australian trial. J Clin Sleep Med. 2013;9(2):117–24.

100. Pang KP, Tan R, Puraviappan P, Terris DJ. Anterior palatoplasty for the treatment of OSA: three-year results. Otolaryngol Head Neck Surg. 2009;141(2):253–6.

101. Verse T, Baisch A, Maurer JT, Stuck BA, Hormann K. Multilevel surgery for obstructive sleep apnea: short-term results. Otolaryngol Head Neck Surg. 2006;134(4):571–7.

102. Weaver EM, Maynard C, Yueh B. Survival of veterans with sleep apnea: continuous positive airway pressure versus surgery. Otolaryngol Head Neck Surg. 2004;130(6):659–65.

103. Yang HB, Wang Y, Dong MM. Effect of Han-uvulopalatopharyngoplasty on flow-mediated dilatation in patients with moderate or severe obstructive sleep apnea syndrome. Acta Otolaryngol. 2012;132(7):769–72.

104. Yaremchuk K, Tacia B, Peterson E, Roth T. Change in Epworth Sleepiness Scale after surgical treatment of obstructive sleep apnea. Laryngoscope. 2011;121(7):1590–3.

105. Yu S, Liu F, Wang Q, et al. Effect of revised UPPP surgery on ambulatory BP in sleep apnea patients with hypertension and oropharyngeal obstruction. Clin Exp Hypertens. 2010;32(1):49–53.

106. Djupesland G, Schrader H, Lyberg T, Refsum H, Lilleas F, Godtlibsen OB. Palatopharyngoglossoplasty in the treatment of patients with obstructive sleep apnea syndrome. Acta Otolaryngol Suppl. 1992;492:50–4.

107. Ramirez SG, Loube DI. Inferior sagittal osteotomy with hyoid bone suspension for obese patients with sleep apnea. Arch Otolaryngol Head Neck Surg. 1996;122(9):953–7.

108. Elasfour A, Miyazaki S, Itasaka Y, Yamakawa K, Ishikawa K, Togawa K. Evaluation of uvulopalatopharyngoplasty in treatment of obstructive sleep apnea syndrome. Acta Otolaryngol Suppl. 1998;537:52–6.

109. Hendler B, Silverstein K, Giannakopoulos H, Costello BJ. Mortised genioplasty in the treatment of obstructive sleep apnea: an historical perspective and modification of design. Sleep Breath. 2001;5(4):173–80.

110. Dattilo DJ, Drooger SA. Outcome assessment of patients undergoing maxillofacial procedures for the treatment of sleep apnea: comparison of subjective and objective results. J Oral Maxillofac Surg. 2004;62(2):164–8.

111. Dattilo DJ, Aynechi M. Modification of the anterior mandibular osteotomy for genioglossus advancement with hyoid suspension for obstructive sleep apnea. J Oral Maxillofac Surg. 2007;65(9):1876–9.

112. Li HY, Wang PC, Hsu CY, Chen NH, Lee LA, Fang TJ. Same-stage palatopharyngeal and hypopharyngeal surgery for severe obstructive sleep apnea. Acta Otolaryngol. 2004;124(7):820–6.

113. Hathaway B, Johnson JT. Safety of uvulopalatopharyngoplasty as outpatient surgery. Otolaryngol Head Neck Surg. 2006;134(4):542–4.

114. Baugh R, Burke B, Fink B, Garcia R, Kominsky A, Yaremchuk K. Safety of outpatient surgery for obstructive sleep apnea. Otolaryngol Head Neck Surg. 2013;148(5):867–72.

115. Rotenberg BW, Theriault J, Gottesman S. Redefining the timing of surgery for obstructive sleep apnea in anatomically favorable patients. Laryngoscope. 2014;124 Suppl 4:S1–9.

116. Cahali MB, Formigoni GG, Gebrim EM, Miziara ID. Lateral pharyngoplasty versus uvulopalatopharyngoplasty: a clinical, polysomnographic and computed tomography measurement comparison. Sleep. 2004;27(5):942–50.

117. Thomas AJ, Chavoya M, Terris DJ. Preliminary findings from a prospective, randomized trial of two tongue-base surgeries for sleep-disordered breathing. Otolaryngol Head Neck Surg. 2003;129(5):539–46.

118. Bettega G, Pepin JL, Veale D, Deschaux C, Raphael B, Levy P. Obstructive sleep apnea syndrome. fifty-one consecutive patients treated by maxillofacial surgery. Am J Respir Crit Care Med. 2000;162(2 Pt 1):641–9.

119. Li KK, Powell NB, Riley RW, Troell RJ, Guilleminault C. Long-term results of maxillomandibular advancement surgery. Sleep Breath. 2000;4(3):137–40.

120. Ferguson KA, Heighway K, Ruby RR. A randomized trial of laser-assisted uvulopalatoplasty in the treatment of mild obstructive sleep apnea. Am J Respir Crit Care Med. 2003;167(1):15–9.

121. Finkelstein Y, Stein G, Ophir D, Berger R, Berger G. Laser-assisted uvulopalatoplasty for the management of obstructive sleep apnea: myths and facts. Arch Otolaryngol Head Neck Surg. 2002;128(4):429–34.

122. Kyrmizakis DE, Chimona TS, Papadakis CE, et al. Laser-assisted uvulopalatoplasty for the treatment of snoring and mild obstructive sleep apnea syndrome. J Otolaryngol. 2003;32(3):174–9.

123. Lin CC, Lee KS, Chang KC, Wu KM, Chou CS. Effect of laser-assisted uvulopalatoplasty on oral airway resistance during wakefulness in obstructive sleep apnea syndrome. Eur Arch Otorhinolaryngol. 2006;263(3):241–7.

124. Mickelson SA. Laser-assisted uvulopalatoplasty for obstructive sleep apnea. Laryngoscope. 1996;106(1 Pt 1):10–3.

125. Atef A, Mosleh M, Hesham M, Fathi A, Hassan M, Fawzy M. Radiofrequency vs laser in the management of mild to moderate obstructive sleep apnoea: does the number of treatment sessions matter? J Laryngol Otol. 2005;119(11):888–93.

126. Ceylan K, Emir H, Kizilkaya Z, et al. First-choice treatment in mild to moderate obstructive sleep apnea: single-stage, multilevel, temperature-controlled radiofrequency tissue volume reduction or nasal continuous positive airway pressure. Arch Otolaryngol Head Neck Surg. 2009;135(9):915–9.

127. Powell NB, Riley RW, Guilleminault C. Radiofrequency tongue base reduction in sleep-disordered breathing: A pilot study. Otolaryngol Head Neck Surg. 1999;120(5):656–64.

128. Riley RW, Powell NB, Li KK, Weaver EM, Guilleminault C. An adjunctive method of radiofrequency volumetric tissue reduction of the tongue for OSAS. Otolaryngol Head Neck Surg. 2003;129(1):37–42.

129. Steward DL, Weaver EM, Woodson BT. Multilevel temperature-controlled radiofrequency for obstructive sleep apnea: extended follow-up. Otolaryngol Head Neck Surg. 2005;132(4):630–5.

130. Stuck BA, Starzak K, Hein G, Verse T, Hormann K, Maurer JT. Combined radiofrequency surgery of the tongue base and soft palate in obstructive sleep apnoea. Acta Otolaryngol. 2004;124(7):827–32.

131. Woodson BT, Nelson LM, Mickelson S, Huntley T, Sher A. A multi-institutional study of radiofrequency volumetric tissue reduction for OSAS. Otolaryngol Head Neck Surg. 2001;125(4):303–11.

132. Woodson BT. A tongue suspension suture for obstructive sleep apnea and snorers. Otolaryngol Head Neck Surg. 2001;124(3):297–303.

133. Woodson BT, Steward DL, Weaver EM, Javaheri S. A randomized trial of temperature-controlled radiofrequency, continuous positive airway pressure, and placebo for obstructive sleep apnea syndrome. Otolaryngol Head Neck Surg. 2003;128(6):848–61.

134. Bassiouny A, El Salamawy A, Abd El-Tawab M, Atef A. Bipolar radiofrequency treatment for snoring with mild to moderate sleep apnea: a comparative study between the radiofrequency assisted uvulopalatoplasty technique and the channeling technique. Eur Arch Otorhinolaryngol. 2007;264(6):659–67.

135. Friedman M, Schalch P, Lin HC, Kakodkar KA, Joseph NJ, Mazloom N. Palatal implants for the treatment of snoring and obstructive sleep apnea/hypopnea syndrome. Otolaryngol Head Neck Surg. 2008;138(2):209–16.

136. Nordgard S, Stene BK, Skjostad KW. Soft palate implants for the treatment of mild to moderate obstructive sleep apnea. Otolaryngol Head Neck Surg. 2006;134(4):565–70.

137. Pang KP, Terris DJ. Modified cautery-assisted palatal stiffening operation: new method for treating snoring and mild obstructive sleep apnea. Otolaryngol Head Neck Surg. 2007;136(5):823–6.

138. Walker RP, Levine HL, Hopp ML, Greene D, Pang K. Palatal implants: a new approach for the treatment of obstructive sleep apnea. Otolaryngol Head Neck Surg. 2006;135(4):549–54.

139. Walker RP, Levine HL, Hopp ML, Greene D. Extended follow-up of palatal implants for OSA treatment. Otolaryngol Head Neck Surg. 2007;137(5):822–7.

140. Back LJ, Liukko T, Rantanen I, et al. Radiofrequency surgery of the soft palate in the treatment of mild obstructive sleep apnea is not effective as a single-stage procedure: A randomized single-blinded placebo-controlled trial. Laryngoscope. 2009;119(8):1621–7.

141. Huang TW, Cheng PW, Fang KM. Concurrent palatal implants and uvulopalatal flap: safe and effective office-based procedure for selected patients with snoring and obstructive sleep apnea syndrome. Laryngoscope. 2011;121(9):2038–42.

142. Kezirian EJ, Weaver EM, Yueh B, et al. Incidence of serious complications after uvulopalatopharyngoplasty. Laryngoscope. 2004;114(3):450–3.

143. Strocker AM, Cohen AN, Wang MB. The safety of outpatient UPPP for obstructive sleep apnea: a retrospective review of 40 cases. Ear Nose Throat J. 2008;87(8):466–8.

144. Rotenberg B, Hu A, Fuller J, Bureau Y, Arra I, Sen M. The early postoperative course of surgical sleep apnea patients. Laryngoscope. 2010;120(5):1063–8.

145. Pang KP, Siow JK, Tseng P. Safety of multilevel surgery in obstructive sleep apnea: a review of 487 cases. Arch Otolaryngol Head Neck Surg. 2012;138(4):353–7.

146. Kandasamy T, Wright ED, Fuller J, Rotenberg BW. The incidence of early post-operative complications following uvulopalatopharyngoplasty: identification of predictive risk factors. J Otolaryngol Head Neck Surg. 2013;42(1):15.

# 20

# In vivo Wnt pathway inhibition of human squamous cell carcinoma growth and metastasis in the chick chorioallantoic model

Shannon F. Rudy[1,5], J. Chad Brenner[1,2], Jennifer L. Harris[4], Jun Liu[4], Jianwei Che[4], Megan V. Scott[2,6], John Henry Owen[1], Christine M. Komarck[1], Martin P. Graham[1], Emily L. Bellile[3], Carol R. Bradford[1,2], Mark EP Prince[1,2†] and Thomas E. Carey[1,2*†]

## Abstract

**Background:** Head and neck squamous cell carcinoma (HNSCC) is an aggressive cancer with poor overall survival. New therapeutic strategies that target specific molecular lesions driving advanced disease are needed. Herein we demonstrate the utility of the chicken chorioallantoic membrane (CAM) assay for in vivo human HNSCC tumor growth and metastasis and the tumor suppressive effects of a new chemotherapeutic agent.

**Methods:** We tested anti-metastatic effects of a WNT pathway inhibitor, WNT974 (also known as LGK974), which targets porcupine (PORCN) the palmityl-transferase that is essential for secretion of Wnt proteins. CAM assays were performed with 8 HNSCC cell lines: UM-SCC-1, UM-SCC-10A, UM-SCC-10B, UM-SCC-11A, UM-SCC-14A UM-SCC-17A, UM-SCC-17B, UM-SCC-25, and UM-SCC-34.

**Results:** UM-SCC-1 (University of Michigan Squamous Cell Carcinoma cell line) CAM xenografts contain CD44+ and ALDH+ cancer stem cell (CSC) proportions similar to UM-SCC-1 mouse xenografts supporting the applicability of the CAM assay for study of CSCs. Inhibition of WNT signaling by the PORCN inhibitor WNT974 reduced metastatic spread of UM-SCC cells, especially in UM-SCCs with Notch1 deficiency.

**Conclusions:** Our data demonstrate decreased tumor growth and metastases in tumors from cell lines that showed in vitro responses to WNT974, providing evidence that this agent may have a role in future HNSCC therapy.

**Keywords:** In vivo cancer model, WNT pathway inhibition, WNT974, Human squamous cell carcinoma, Chorioallantoic membrane, UM-SCC, Cell lines, NOTCH1 mutation

## Background

Head and neck squamous cell carcinoma (HNSCC) is the sixth most common form of cancer worldwide [1]. Despite therapeutic strides made in the field of oncology in recent years, the prognosis of HNSCC remains very poor, in large part due to the highly invasive nature of this cancer which often results in extensive local invasion, early dissemination into regional lymph nodes, and metastatic spread of the disease [2]. At the time of diagnosis, two-thirds of patients already have locoregionally advanced disease, defined as Stage 3 or 4. The overall five year overall survival rates for all stages of larynx and oral and pharynx cancer ranges from 63–66 percent respectively [3]. For patients with advanced disease the introduction of adjuvant concurrent chemoradiotherapy has improved survival by roughly 12 %, which corresponds to an improvement in overall 5 year survival from 45 % in 1973 to 53.2 % in 2005 [4]. Given these considerations, there is a clear need for therapeutic advances in this field, and those that will have the most

* Correspondence: careyte@med.umich.edu
†Equal contributors
[1]Department of Otolaryngology/Head Neck Surgery, University of Michigan School of Medicine, Ann Arbor, MI 48109-5616, USA
[2]Comprehensive Cancer Center, University of Michigan School of Medicine, Ann Arbor, MI 48109-5616, USA
Full list of author information is available at the end of the article

meaningful impact are likely to come in the form of modalities that treat the genetic drivers of advanced-staged disease [5].

The Wnt signaling pathway is an appealing target, as this developmental pathway has been implicated in a large number of human cancers, with recent evidence for an oncogenic role in HNSCC [6]. Deregulation of Wnt signaling from mutation or abnormal expression of pathway components has been implicated to play a role in invasive growth patterns in HNSCC [7]. Normally, the Wnt signal transduction pathway leads to activation of pathways regulating the cytoskeleton, cellular calcium levels and beta-catenin protein expression and transcriptional activation (reviewed in [8–13]). Briefly, the pathway is activated by either autocrine or paracrine signaling through a combination of up to nineteen different Wnt ligands acting on Frizzled receptors. In the absence of Wnt receptor activation, two scaffolding tumor suppressor proteins in the beta-catenin destruction complex called adenomatous polyposis coli (APC) and axin bind to beta-catenin enabling the kinases CK1 and glycogen synthase kinase 3 to sequentially phosphorylate the amino terminus of beta-catenin. The resulting phosphorylated footprint targets beta-catenin for proteasomal degradation. Once activated by Wnt, the Frizzled receptors inhibit the destruction complex through incompletely understood mechanisms. Together, this leads to an accumulation of β-catenin protein, which can then translocate to the nucleus to form a complex with LEF/TCF proteins to regulate transcription of proliferation associated genes.

A small molecule inhibitor of the Wnt-pathway, LGK974, was recently described [14]. The drug name LGK974 has been renamed and is now synonymous with the name WNT974. WNT974 is the name that will be used to reference this compound in this manuscript. WNT974 compound is a potent small molecule inhibitor of Porcupine (PORCN), a membrane-bound O-acyltransferase that adds a palmityol group to Wnt ligands. This modification is essential for Wnt secretion and Frizzled activation. In vitro studies showed a potent inhibitory effect of WNT974 on Wnt signaling, as evidenced by decreased expression of downstream target genes, such as *AXIN2*, as well as reduced Wnt-dependent phosphorylation of LRP6. Of the 96 HNSCC cell lines analyzed, 31 demonstrated a pharmacodymanic (PD) *AXIN2* mRNA reduction response and were thus considered as cell lines that were responsive to treatment with WNT974. Interestingly, there was an enriched rate of response to WNT974 among head and neck cancer cell lines with Notch1 loss-of-function (LOF) mutations [14].

Like Wnt, Notch is also a developmental pathway gene that has recently been implicated in HNSCC

tumorigenesis [15–17]. While Notch gain-of-function mutations have been demonstrated in T-cell leukemias and some other forms of cancer, a tumor suppressor role for the Notch pathway has also been suggested in a number of human cancers, including in HNSCC, in which *NOTCH1* LOF mutations were found in 10–15 % of tumors and abnormalities of the Notch pathway in 66 % of patients [18]. The Notch pathway has been proposed to have an inhibitory effect on Wnt signaling in some cell types [19, 20] with evidence suggesting that activated Notch1 signaling suppresses β-catenin signaling in cells that should normally undergo differentiation from the basal layer of the epidermis [17]. With these considerations in mind, we designed an experiment to test the effectiveness of Wnt pathway inhibition with WNT974 on in vivo tumor growth and distant metastasis using the chick chorioallantoic membrane (CAM) assay and human squamous cell carcinoma cell lines. The chick CAM is a multilayered epithelium that consists of ectoderm, mesoderm, and endoderm, as well as extracellular matrix proteins such as laminin and type I collagen, a composition that mimics the tumor environment in humans [21]. Consequently, CAM assays are a well-established in vivo model that has been used to study angiogenesis and tumor invasion in several types of human cancer, including prostate carcinoma, glioma, and bowel cancer [22–24]. Here, we sought to further illustrate the feasibility for study of head and neck cancer cell lines using the CAM assay, determine if HNSCC cancer stem cells (CSCs) can be identified and isolated from primary tumors grown on the CAM, and test the hypothesis that UM-SCC cell line CAM xenograft tumor growth and metastasis can be impaired by WNT974.

## Methods

The aim of this study was to determine the feasibility of the chicken chorioallantoic membrane assay for assessing in vivo tumor response to a novel WNT pathway inhibitor, WNT974, in human head and neck cancer cell lines.

### Ethics consent and permissions

The UM-SCC-1, -10A, -10B, -11A, 14A -17A, -17B, -25, and -34 cell lines were derived in our laboratory from human head and neck tumor explants taken during surgical resection from patients treated at the University of Michigan. The cell line donor-patients gave written informed consent for the use of their tissue to create cell lines in studies reviewed and approved by the University of Michigan Medical School (Ann Arbor) IRBMED institutional review board.

## Cell lines

The cell lines have been carefully characterized in our laboratory for HNSCC characteristics and each has been genotyped at a minimum of 10 microsatellite markers (Profiler Plus, Invitrogen) to confirm their unique origin [25]. Cell lines with the same number and a letter, i.e. were from the same donor and were derived from primary and recurrent (UM-SCC 10A and UM-SCC-10B) or primary and metastatic (UM-SCC-17A, UM-SCC-17B), lesions respectively. Cells were cultured in Dulbecco modified Eagle medium (Gibco, Life Technologies) containing 2 mM L-glutamine, 1 % nonessential amino acids, 1 % penicillin-streptomycin (Invitrogen), and 10 % fetal bovine serum in a humidified atmosphere of 5 % carbon dioxide at 37 °C. All cell lines were tested for mycoplasma using the MycoAlert Detection Kit (Cambrex) to ensure that they were free from contamination prior to use in these experiments.

The use of fertilized chicken eggs is exempt from vertebrate animal use approval.

## Chick Chorioallantoic Membrane (CAM) Assay

Fertilized white leghorn chicken eggs were obtained from Charles River Labs (Norwich, CT). The use of fertilized chicken eggs is exempt from vertebrate animal use approval. The eggs were kept in an incubator at 99.5 degrees Fahrenheit at a humidity range of 45–55 %. Eight days following arrival, the embryos were assessed for viability, performed by trans-illumination of the egg in a dark room to identify the presence of an embryo and surrounding blood vessels. A 1 cm$^2$ window was drawn on the egg shell overlying the most vascularized area of each viable embryo. Two small holes were then bored into the egg shell, one in the center of the window and the other at the apex of the egg, overlying a naturally occurring air pocket. A rubber pipette bulb was used to suction a small amount of air out of this apical pocket, causing the chorioallantoic membrane to drop downward, away from the vent hole in the drawn window. The window was then opened using a Dremel 1100-N/25 7.2-Volt Stylus Lithium-Ion Cordless Rota Drill (Robert Bosch Tool Company) and was covered with a piece of clear adhesive tape to protect the embryo and prevent dehydration. This window served as the site for subsequent cancer cell inoculation in our preliminary experiment, and cancer cell and drug inoculation in our WNT974 treatment experiment (See Liu, Min et al Translational Oncology 6:273-281, 2013 for illustrations of the model).

Seven days after the administration of cancer cells, the chick eggs were opened with sterile scissors, and primary tumors were dissected out and weighed. The chick embryos were then dissected, removing the lungs and livers which were immediately placed on ice in labeled 10 mL

conical containers. The samples were stored in the -80 degree C freezer until DNA extraction.

## DNA extraction and analysis

Chick embryo livers and lungs were thawed, rinsed with 5 mL PBS and homogenized with a handheld homogenizer (Omni International) using a sterile tip for each sample. DNA extraction was performed using the QIAgen DNeasy Blood & Tissue Kit (QIAGEN Group), following the manufacturer's specifications. Purified DNA was quantified using a spectrophotometer, adjusted to a concentration of 0.2ug/uL, and stored at -20 degrees C. Quantitative PCR (qPCR) was performed on the DNA samples using primers specific for a human Alu sequence. Alu sequences are primate-specific, and thus their detection in chick organs represents disseminated human cells, or cancer metastases. The copy threshold, or CT, values of the liver and lung specimens from the eight HNSCC cell lines were compared to the CT values of the negative controls of the respective organ. Student T-tests were used to compare the CT values of both organs of each cell line to the respective negative control.

## Applicability assay

The initial experiments were designed to demonstrate feasibility of the CAM assay for use with HNSCC cancer cells using eight cell lines (UM-SCC-1, -10A, -10B, -11A, -17A, -17B, -25, and -34)..The cells were grown in 150 cm$^2$ plastic flasks, trypsinized, counted, and resuspended in a mixture of 10 % matrigel (BD Biosciences) and 90 % DMEM for a total volume of 30uL per eggs such that each egg received 2.5 million cancer cells. The prepared chick eggs were removed from the incubator, and the cancer cell suspension was laid on top of the chorioallantoic membrane using a 100uL pipette tips. For each cell line, five eggs were each inoculated. An additional ten eggs received a 30uL suspension of 10 % matrigel and 90 % DMEM with no cancer cells to serve as treatment, embryo viability, and specificity controls.

## Flow cytometry

UM-SCC-1 cancer cells were administered to an additional ten eggs for cancer stem cell analysis. Seven days following cancer cell administration, primary tumors were dissected from eight viable embryos and placed on ice in 15 mL tubes filled with DMEM media. Tumor tissue was minced and digested in DMEM/ F12 (Gibco) with 1x collagenase/hyaluronidase (Stem Cell Technologies). After two hours of digestion, the mixture was strained through a 40 μm sieve and the cells were counted before being prepared for flow cytometry. CD44 expression was detected using an APC-conjugated antibody (BD Pharmingen). Aldehyde dehydrogenase (ALDH) expression was detected using the ALDEFLUOR kit (StemCell Technologies). The aldefluor substrate freely diffuses into cells and reacts with human aldehyde dehydrogenase enzyme, producing a fluorescent reaction product that is proportional to the enzymatic activity. This reaction does not occur in the chicken host cells.

Tumor cells from the primary tumors of the eight viable chick embryos were pooled together to gather sufficient cells for an adequate assessment of CSCs in the tumors grown on the CAM. Fluorescence-activated cell sorting gates were established for ALDH expression using the inhibited control (DEAB) along the fluorescein isothiocyanate (FITC) channel with excitation and emission wavelengths of approximately 495 nm/521 nm. For CD44 expression, cell sorting gates were established using the APC-conjugated isotype control along the allophycocyanin (APC) channel with excitation and emission wavelengths of approximately 650 nm/660 nm.

### WNT974 treatment assay

To test the effect of Wnt pathway inhibition on tumor growth and distant metastasis we first performed a dose-finding assay with WNT974 to assess for potential toxicity of this pathway inhibitor on chick embryos. Three drug concentrations were tested, 0.1 µM, 0.31 µM, and 1 µM. µM. For each drug concentration, five chick eggs were dosed every other day for a total of four doses. An additional five eggs were treated with 5uL DMSO (the WNT974 vehicle) to control for vehicle toxicity to the embryos. This assay showed minimal toxicity of these drug concentrations on the chick embryos, with all five embryos given 1 µM WNT974 remaining viable and phenotypically normal through harvesting. Thus 1 µM was selected as the treatment dose. Four UM-SCC cell lines were selected to test the effect of WNT974 on tumor growth on the CAM and on distant metastases to liver and lung. Two cell lines, UM-SCC-11A and -25, were shown via deep exome sequencing to have *Notch1* mutations (UM-SCC-25 contains a nonsense LOF mutation, and UM-SCC-11A contains a missense mutation), and both exhibited a pharmacodynamic (PD) change in *AXIN2* mRNA expression in response to WNT974 during the in vitro analysis performed by GNF. A third cell line, UM-SCC-1, containing wildtype *NOTCH1*, also showed a PD response to WNT974. The fourth line, UM-SCC-14A, also wildtype for *NOTCH1*, was a PD non-responder in vitro. The CAM assay was prepared as described above. For each cell line, 2.5 million cells were administered to each of 32 eggs (performed in separate assays per cell line due to limited incubator space). Of these, half served as treatment eggs and the other half were vehicle control eggs. The treatment arm received 5 µL of 1 µM WNT974 once daily, every other day starting the day of cancer cell inoculation for a total of four

doses. The control arm received 5uL DMSO every other day for a total of four doses. There were also 5 manipulation-only control eggs per cell line, which were injected with 30 µL of 10 % matrigel and 90 % DMEM but no cancer cells. Eggs were opened seven days following cancer cell administration, all identifiable primary tumors dissected and weighed, the lung and liver tissues harvested and DNA was purified as described above.

### Statistical analysis

An *a priori* power calculation was performed. Given a Type I error rate of 0.05 and power of approximately 85 %, it was determined that a sample size of at least 9 tumors in each treatment group was needed to detect a treatment effect size of 1.5 standard deviations in magnitude. For each of the four cell lines, tumor weights for the treatment and non-treatment groups were recorded and compared using two-tailed T-tests. Given the need to run the assay twice for each cell line due to space limitations, an ANOVA model for each cell line was used to evaluate treatment effect controlling for assay batch as a main effect and as potential effect modifier in the model parameterization. These analyses revealed no significant batch effect in any of the four cell lines, thus allowing pooling of the data from both batches. The qPCR cycle threshold (CT) values for both the liver and lung specimens in the treatment group for each cell line were compared to the CT values of the corresponding organ and cell line using a two-tailed T-test, generating a P-value for both the liver and lungs in each cell line. P-values $<0.05$ were considered statistically significant.

### Results
#### UM-SCC cell lines grow and metastasize in CAM assays

Five chick embryos were implanted with cancer cells for each of the eight UMSCC cell lines tested in this study. For each cell line, the number of viable embryos examined for tumor growth is given following the cell line: UM-SCC-1: 5, UM-SCC-10A: 3, UM-SCC-10B: 4, UM-SCC-11A: 5, UM-SCC-17A: 3, UM-SCC-17B: 5, UM-SCC-25: 5, and UM-SCC-34: 4 embryos. Of the viable embryos, a subset was randomly chosen for primary tumor dissection and weighing. Tumor weights ranged from 27.4 to 82.4 mg with consistency within cell lines (all weights within two fold of one another) and less consistency between cell lines (up to a fourfold difference in tumor weights). To assess the metastatic ability of these cell lines in this assay, quantitative PCR performed on DNA isolated from the livers of xenograft bearing animals and negative control specimens are shown in Fig. 1. This demonstrated that all eight of the cell lines metastasized to the livers of the developing chicks. qPCR was also performed on DNA isolated from the chick lungs. However, only one negative

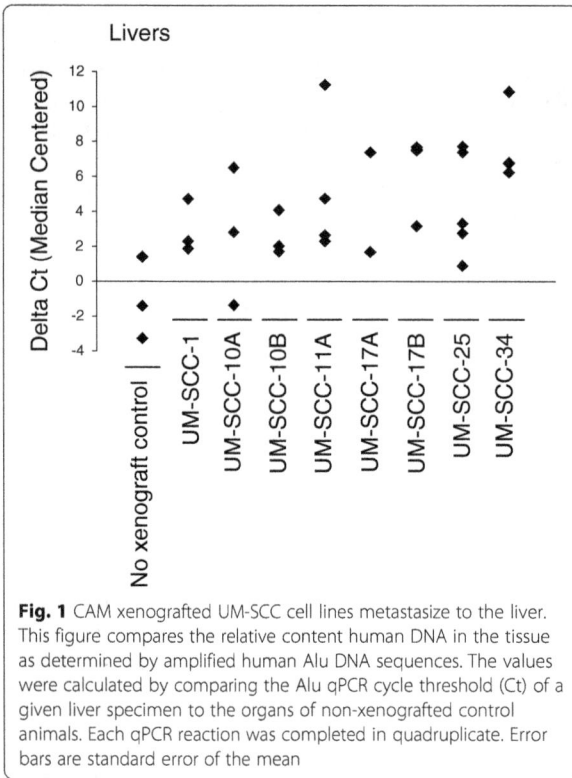

**Fig. 1** CAM xenografted UM-SCC cell lines metastasize to the liver. This figure compares the relative content human DNA in the tissue as determined by amplified human Alu DNA sequences. The values were calculated by comparing the Alu qPCR cycle threshold (Ct) of a given liver specimen to the organs of non-xenografted control animals. Each qPCR reaction was completed in quadruplicate. Error bars are standard error of the mean

control was included in the qPRC analysis due to the initial poor egg viability, and therefore these data have not been included in Fig. 1.

### CAM assays as a cancer stem cell model

Next, we assessed the relative percentage of stem cell markers in tumors excised from the CAM xenografts. Eight independent UM-SCC-1 primary tumors were pooled to insure sufficient cells for stem cell analysis. Flow analysis with the aldefluor substrate and the DEAB inhibitor showed that 18.97 % of the total cell population reacted with the aldefluor substrate and were human cells and 81.03 % consisted of chick (aldefluor fluorescence negative) cells (Fig. 2). Of the human cell population when the ALDH inhibitor DEAB is removed, 8.17 % were ALDH$^{high}$ (also known as the stem cell or side population [26]) and 81.29 % were CD44$^{high}$ (Fig. 3). These results are consistent with what we have previously observed with CSC populations in UM-SCC-1 cells excised from a mouse model [26, 27]. Together, these results indicate that tumors grown in the CAM assay continue to generate HNSCC CSCs at rates similar to those observed in the murine model, thus offering an alternative to murine xenografts as an in vivo approach to study CSCs in HNSCC.

### WNT974 disrupts UM-SCC cell line xenograft growth and metastasis

After establishing the CAM model using several of the genetically characterized UM-SCC cell lines [14], we sought to test the effect of WNT974 on the growth and metastatic ability of cell lines of varying *NOTCH1* mutation status and in vitro pharmacodynamic response to WNT974: UM-SCC-11A (*NOTCH1* mutant, PD responder), UM-SCC-25 (*NOTCH1* frameshift mutant, PD responder), UM-SCC-1 (*NOTCH1* wildtype, PD responder), and UM-SCC-14A (*NOTCH1* wildtype, PD non-responder). Tumor weight analysis shown in Fig. 4 revealed a statistically significant decrease in primary tumor weight between treated and untreated embryos in UM-SCC-11A ($p = 1.0 \times 10^{-7}$), UM-SCC-1 ($p = 0.002$), and UM-SCC-25 ($p = 0.0076$), the three cell lines that previously showed in vitro pharmacodynamic responses to WNT974 [14]. There was no difference in tumor weights between treated and untreated embryos in UM-SCC-14A, which correspondingly was a non-PD responder. Furthermore, qPCR analysis of organs harvested from developing chicks for human ALU DNA revealed a statistically significant reduction in liver metastases in UM-SCC-11A ($p = 2.5 \times 10^{-5}$) and UM-SCC-25 ($p = 0.02$) (Fig. 5). Together the data demonstrates that WNT974 can effectively disrupt xenograft tumor growth and liver metastasis of several UM-SCC cell lines.

### Discussion

We and others have used the CAM assay for a variety of studies [24, 26, 27]. Here we confirmed the value of CAM assays as short term xenograft models of HNSCC proliferation and metastatic behavior in vivo with a variety of UM-SCC cell lines. We show that nine different UM-SCC cell lines form tumors and distant metastasis in this system. In fact, the high rates of observed tumors and metastases demonstrate the utility of the chick CAM assay for in vivo study of HNSCC tumor behavior as well as the potential for an expanded use of this preclinical model for studying response to drug therapy in head and neck cancer. Our results support the value of this model in screening tumors with different genomic compositions for response to new drug therapies, which could help expedite the preclinical phase of drug development, as well as to help identify patients who are most likely to respond to new therapies. This study demonstrates the generation of cancer stem cells within primary tumors grown in the CAM assay. Flow cytometric analysis of tumor cells detected CD44$^{high}$ and ALDH$^{high}$ cells at similar rates to those observed in murine model HNSCC tumors. Our ability to detect CSCs on tumor cells grown in the CAM assay provides opportunities for use of this model in the study of HNSCC CSC

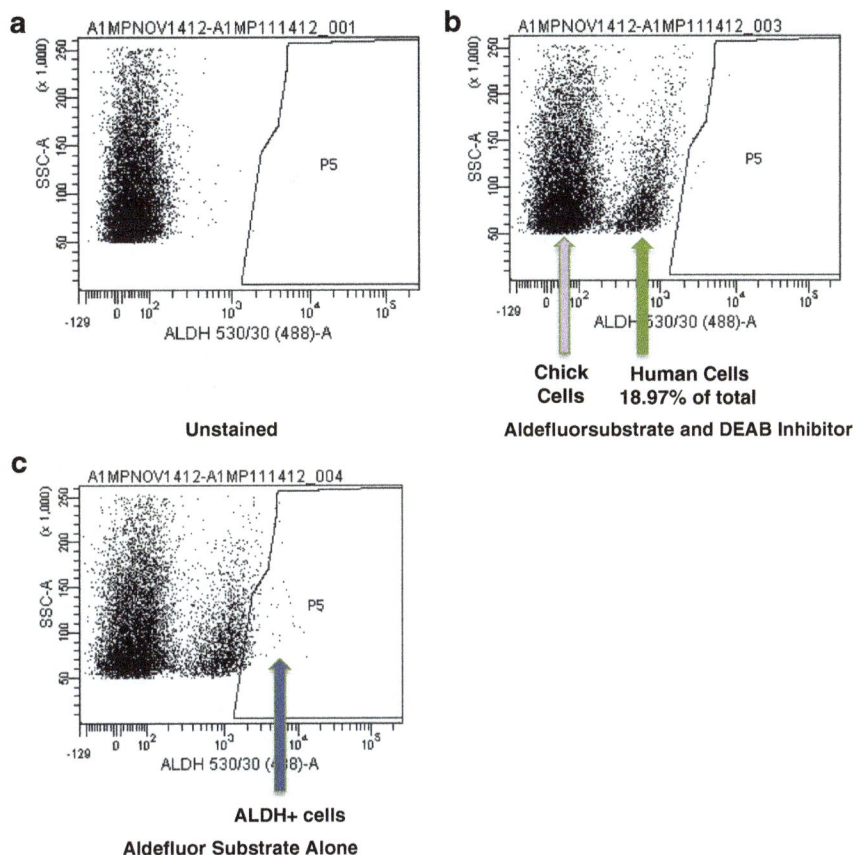

**Fig. 2** Analysis of ALDH positive cells in UM-SCC-1 CAM xenografts. **a** Flow cytometry of unstained sample of UM-SCC-1 primary tumor cells grown in the CAM assay. **b** Flow cytometry of UM-SCC-1 CAM xenograft tumor cells stained with Aldefluor substrate and DEAB inhibitor. The Aldefluor substrate only reacts with the mammalian ALDH enzyme, so inclusion of the substrate will allow the human cells to shift forward while the chick cells will show no shift from the unstained sample. **c** Removal of the DEAB inhibitor results in a right-shift of the ALDH+ population. 1.55 % of the total cell population is ALDH+, but only 18.97 % of the total cell population is human cells. Therefore, 8.17 % of the UM-SCC-1 cells in the CAM xenograft were analyzed to be ALDH+

populations, behavior, and response to drug therapies. The CAM model has several advantages as an adjunct to murine xenografts [24]. The CAM model is relatively inexpensive, can be completed in approximately a 16 day window from egg delivery until harvest and is sensitive to metastatic spread.

In addition to evaluating CAM assays as a model of therapeutic response, we explored the interaction between the Wnt and Notch signaling pathways in HNSCC, specifically in the context of the anti-cancer effects of Wnt pathway inhibition in tumors with different types of Notch pathway mutation. Given the previously proposed inhibitory effect of the Notch pathway on Wnt signaling [19, 20], it is possible that tumors that harbor mutations in Notch1 have increased Wnt signaling and are therefore more susceptible to Wnt pathway inhibition. This is also supported by the early in vitro study of

WNT974, which revealed an enriched rate of response to WNT974 among head and neck cancer cell lines with Notch1 loss-of-function (LOF) mutations, suggesting that Notch1 mutation status may play a role in responsiveness to Wnt pathway inhibition. However, it is also possible that Wnt gain of function mutations, which were not tested for in the cell lines used in this study, could be the independent driving force in tumorigenesis in the responder cell lines, resulting in the observed decreased tumor growth and metastasis following Wnt pathway inhibition in three of the four cell lines tested. Lack of sufficient statistical power due to the limited number of HNSCC cell lines tested did not allow for correlation of sensitivity of WNT974 in the CAM model to Notch 1 mutations status. However, the study provides strong, early evidence for a potential role of WNT974 in the treatment of patients with HNSCC as a significant therapeutic

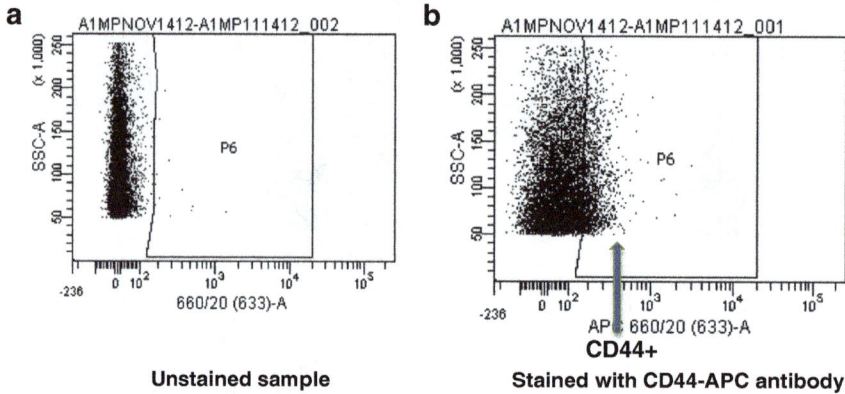

**Fig. 3** Analysis of CD44 positive cells in UM-SCC-1 CAM xenografts. **a** Flow cytometry results of unstained sample of UM-SCC-1 primary tumor cells grown in the CAM assay. **b** Flow cytometry results of UM-SCC-1 primary tumor cells stained with CD44-APC antibody. 15.44 % of the total cell population is CD44+, but only 18.97 % of the total cell population is human cells. Therefore 81.39 % of the UM-SCC-1 cells in the CAM xenograft are CD44+

response in the CAM assay was seen with three of the four tumor cell lines tested. Future experiments will analyze the effects of WNT974 in the context of additional biomarkers as well as in combination with other agents in order to predict and improve clinical response.

## Conclusion
HNSCC cell line xenograft growth, cancer stem cell distribution, metastasis and therapeutic response can be effectively assessed in CAM assays in a manner consistent with mouse xenograft assays. This allows for an expeditious means to screen the efficacy of new therapeutic agents across a large number of head and neck tumors such that more time consuming mouse xenograft models can be focused on the precision medicine protocols most likely to advance to clinical trials. Therefore, we expect that implementation of this model will significantly reduce the pre-clinical phase of drug development timelines.

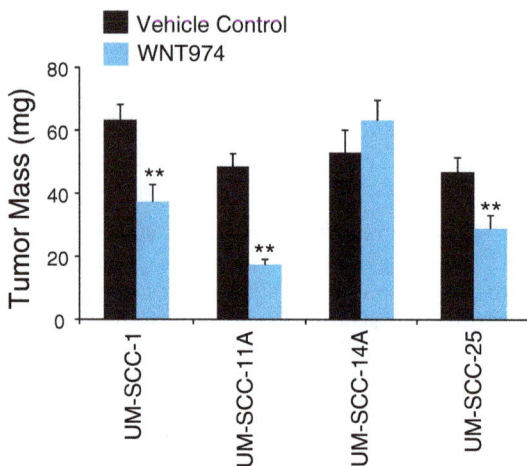

**Fig. 4** WNT974 blocks UM-SCC-1, -11A and -25, but not -14A, CAM xenograft growth. UM-SCC cell lines were implanted on CAM models and treated with 1 μM WNT974 or vehicle control (DMSO) every other day for eight days. At the conclusion of the experiment, tumors were harvested from the CAM and weighed. We assessed 22, 33, 24 and 27 viable animals UM-SCC-1, -11A, -25 and -14A, respectively, with half receiving vehicle control and the rest WNT974. Averages of all groups are shown along with standard error. ** $P < 0.05$

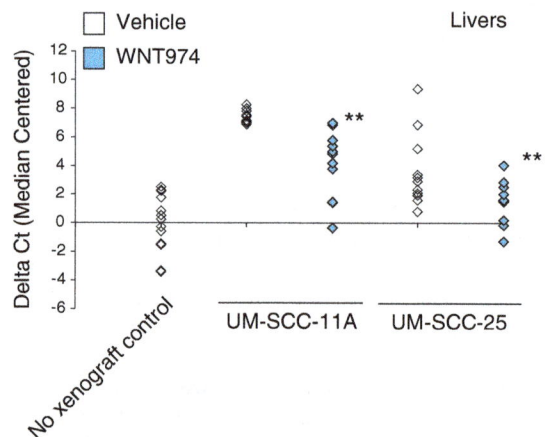

**Fig. 5** WNT974 blocks liver metastasis of UM-SCC-11A and UM-SCC-25 CAM xenografts. Livers from UM-SCC-11A and -25 CAM xenografts (from Fig. 4) were harvested at the conclusion of the experiment and assessed for human ALU DNA sequences by qPCR. WNT974 was administered every other day to a final concentration of 1 μM. Livers from non-xenografted animals were used as a negative control and Ct difference from the median centered average of normal livers is shown. All qPCR assays were run in quadruplicate. ** $P < 0.05$

## Competing interests

Drs. Harris, Liu and Che are employees of Novartis Global Research Foundation and are members of the team that developed WNT974. This drug has progressed to clinical trials including a trial involving head and neck cancer patients. Dr. Carey was the recipient of a grant from Novartis Global Research Foundation to help fund xenograft studies in mice.

## Authors' contributions

SFR participated in the design, carried out experiments, prepared the draft of the paper and approved the final manuscript. TEC, JLH, JL, MEPP, CRB, JCB, conceived the plan and participated in the design of the study, revised and approved the manuscript and provided funding fro the study. MPG, CMK, JHO, MVS, assisted with experiments and read and approved the final manuscript. JC provided advice and experitice and read and approved the manuscript. ELB provided assistance with experimental design and statistical analysis, read and approved the manuscript. All authors read and approved the final manuscript.

## Acknowledgements

Supported by NIH training grant Advanced Research Training in Otolaryngology NIH-NIDCD T32 DC05356, NIH NIDCR R01 DE019126, Head and Neck SPORE Grant NIH-NCI P50 CA 097248, NIH NIDCD P30 DC05188, Patricia Korigan Head and Neck Cancer Research Fund.

## Author details

[1]Department of Otolaryngology/Head Neck Surgery, University of Michigan School of Medicine, Ann Arbor, MI 48109-5616, USA. [2]Comprehensive Cancer Center, University of Michigan School of Medicine, Ann Arbor, MI 48109-5616, USA. [3]Cancer Center Biostatistics Core, University of Michigan School of Medicine, Ann Arbor, MI 48109-5616, USA. [4]Genomics Institute of the Novartis Research Foundation, 10675 John Jay Hopkins Drive, San Diego, CA 92121, USA. [5]Department of Otolaryngology/Head Neck Surgery, Stanford University, Stanford, CA 94305, USA. [6]Wayne State University School of Medicine, Detroit, MI 48201, USA.

## References

1. Ferlay J et al. Estimates of worldwide burden of cancer in 2008: GLOBOCAN 2008. Int J Cancer. 2010;127:2893–917.
2. Allen CT, Law JH, Dunn GP, Uppaluri R. Emerging insights into head and neck cancer metastasis. Head Neck. 2013;35:1669–78.
3. Siegel RL, Miller KD, Jemal A. Cancer statistics, 2015. CA Cancer J Clin. 2015;65:5–29.
4. Lin SS, Massa ST, Varvares MA. Improved overall survival and mortality in head and neck cancer with adjuvant concurrent chemoradiotherapy in national databases. Head Neck. 2016;38:208–15.
5. Partridge M. Head and neck cancer and precancer: can we use molecular genetics to make better predictions? Ann R Coll Surg Engl. 1999;81:1–11.
6. Clevers H, Nusse R. Wnt/beta-catenin signaling and disease. Cell. 2012;149:1192–205.
7. Yang F, Zeng Q, Yu G, Li S, Wang CY. Wnt/beta-catenin signaling inhibits death receptor-mediated apoptosis and promotes invasive growth of HNSCC. Cell Signal. 2006;18:679–87.
8. Reya T, Clevers H. Wnt signalling in stem cells and cancer. Nature. 2005;434:843–50.
9. Komiya Y, Habas R. Wnt signal transduction pathways. Organogenesis. 2008;4:68–75.
10. Logan CY, Nusse R. The Wnt signaling pathway in development and disease. Annu Rev Cell Dev Biol. 2004;20:781–810.
11. Moon RT, Bowerman B, Boutros M, Perrimon N. The promise and perils of Wnt signaling through beta-catenin. Science. 2002;296:1644–6.
12. McCarthy N. Tumorigenesis: WNT branches out. Nat Rev Cancer. 2013;13:80.
13. Anastas JN, Moon RT. WNT signalling pathways as therapeutic targets in cancer. Nat Rev Cancer. 2013;13:11–26.
14. PS Liu J, Hsieh M, Ng N, Sun F, Wang T, Kasibhatla S, Schuller AG, G Li AG, Cheng D, Li J, Tompkins C, Pferdekamper A, Steffy A, Cheng J, Kowal C, Phung V, Guo G, Wang Y, Graham M, Flynn S, Brenner JC, Li C, Villarroel MC, Schultz PG, Wu X, McNamara P, Sellers WR, Petruzzelli L, Borale AL, Martin Seidel HM, Mclaughlin ME, Che J, Carey TE, Vanasse G, Harris JL. Targeting Wnt-driven cancer through inhibition of Porcupine by LGK974. Proc Natl Acad Sci USA. 2013;110(50):20224–9.
15. Agrawal N et al. Exome sequencing of head and neck squamous cell carcinoma reveals inactivating mutations in NOTCH1. Science. 2011;333:1154–7.
16. Stransky N et al. The mutational landscape of head and neck squamous cell carcinoma. Science. 2011;333:1157–60.
17. Nicolas M et al. Notch1 functions as a tumor suppressor in mouse skin. Nat Genet. 2003;33:416–21.
18. Pickering CR et al. Integrative genomic characterization of oral squamous cell carcinoma identifies frequent somatic drivers. Cancer discovery. 2013;3:770–81.
19. Klaus A, Birchmeier W. Wnt signalling and its impact on development and cancer. Nat Rev Cancer. 2008;8:387–98.
20. Wilson A, Radtke F. Multiple functions of Notch signaling in self-renewing organs and cancer. FEBS Lett. 2006;580:2860–8.
21. Valdes TI, Kreutzer D, Moussy F. The chick chorioallantoic membrane as a novel in vivo model for the testing of biomaterials. J Biomed Mater Res. 2002;62:273–82.
22. Lokman NA, Elder AS, Ricciardelli C, Oehler MK. Chick Chorioallantoic Membrane (CAM) assay as an in vivo model to study the effect of newly identified molecules on ovarian cancer invasion and metastasis. Int J Mol Sci. 2012;13:9959–70.
23. Giannopoulou E et al. X-rays modulate extracellular matrix in vivo. Int J Cancer. 2001;94:690–8.
24. Brenner JC et al. Mechanistic rationale for inhibition of poly(ADP-ribose) polymerase in ETS gene fusion-positive prostate cancer. Cancer Cell. 2011;19:664–78.
25. Brenner JC et al. Genotyping of 73 UM-SCC head and neck squamous cell carcinoma cell lines. Head Neck. 2010;32:417–26.
26. Van Tubergen EA et al. Inactivation or loss of TTP promotes invasion in head and neck cancer via transcript stabilization and secretion of MMP9, MMP2, and IL-6. Clin Cancer Res. 2013;19:1169–79.
27. Hagedorn M et al. Accessing key steps of human tumor progression in vivo by using an avian embryo model. Proc Natl Acad Sci U S A. 2005;102:1643–8.

# 21

# Can preoperative thyroglobulin antibody levels be used as a marker for well differentiated thyroid cancer?

S. Hosseini[1], R. J. Payne[2], F. Zawawi[2,3], A. Mlynarek[2], M. P. Hier[2], M. Tamilia[4] and V. I. Forest[2*]

## Abstract

**Background:** It has been reported that thyroglobulin antibody are more frequently elevated in patients with thyroid cancercompared to general population. This study aims at evaluating whether preoperative thyroglobulin antibody (TgAb) levels increase the likelihood that a thyroid nodule is malignant.

**Methods:** A retrospective review of 586 patients who underwent thyroidectomy was conducted. Demographic data, TgAb levels, and final histopathology were recorded. Patients were divided into two groups: TgAb positive (defined as TgAb ≥ 30 IU/ml) and TgAb low/negative (defined as TgAb < 30).

**Results:** Preoperative TgAb levels were available in 405 patients. There were 353 (87 %) patients in the TgAblow/negative group (malignancy rate: 50.42 %) and 52 (13 %) patients in the TgAb positive group (malignancy rate: 65.38 %). The sensitivity, specificity, positive predictive value and negative predictive value of TgAb ≥ 30 IU/ml for thyroid malignancy were 16.04 %, 90.67 %, 65.38 % and 49.58 %, respectively. The relative risk of having a malignant thyroid nodule when the TgAb titers were≥30 IU/ml was 1.30 (CI1.04-1.62) and the odds ratio was 1.86 (CI 1.01-3.41). Both the Pearson chi-square test (p = 0.024) and Fisher's exact test (p = 0.017) yielded statistical significance between the two groups.

**Conclusions:** In this study, patients with preoperative TgAb ≥ 30 IU/ml had a higher rate of malignancy when compared topatients with TgAb < 30 IU/ml. This suggests that an elevated TgAb level may indicate that a thyroid nodule is at an increased risk for malignancy.

## Background

Thyroid nodules are commonly encountered in the general population. It is estimated that there is a 5 to 10 % lifetime risk of having a thyroid nodule [1]. Among all thyroid nodules, about 5 % are cancerous independently of their size [2]. With the steady rise in the detection rate of thyroid nodules, there has been increased interest to identify parameters that can be used as risk factors and predictors of thyroid cancer [3–5].

As a matter of fact, in an attempt to identify other risk factors to help with risk stratification, serum thyroglobulin (Tg) and their antibodies have been studied. Previous reports have shown a relationship between elevated measurements of Tg and well-differentiated thyroid

carcinoma (WDTC). Tg has been recognized as an established tumor marker for thyroid cancer [6–9]. However, serum thyroglobulin antibody (TgAb) levels may interact with Tg and give a lower serum Tg value. In fact, Tg complexed with TgAb cannot be detected by the currently available immunometric assay methods, which impairs in those cases the clinical utility of Tg as a prognostic factor for WDTC. However, this has lead to another question on the potential significance of TgAb in risk stratification of thyroid nodule.

Depending on the population studied and the assay used, TgAb levels are elevated in approximately 20 % of patients with WDTC, as compared to 10 % of individuals in the general population [10]. Also, high titers of TgAb are present in the serum of most patients with chronic lymphocytic thyroiditis (CLT). In 2010, Kim et al. reported for the first time that a positive TgAb test was an independent predictor of thyroid nodule

* Correspondence: viforest@yahoo.ca
[2]Department of Otolaryngology – Head and Neck Surgery, McGill University, Montreal, QC, Canada
Full list of author information is available at the end of the article

malignancy, regardless of the presence of CLT [11]. Subsequently, other reports showed conflicting results. The aim of the present study is to assess whether higher levels of preoperative TgAb correlate with an increased likelihood of a thyroid nodule being malignant.

## Methods

This study is a retrospective review of 586 patients who underwent a thyroidectomy by a single surgeon at the McGill University teaching hospitals between January 2012 and December 2013. Our investigation obtained ethics approval by the McGill University Health Center Research Ethics Board and the Jewish General Hospital Research Ethics Office.

The inclusion criteria were age > 18 years old, hemi or total thyroidectomy, and available preoperative TgAb measurements and final histopathology reports. Patients with final diagnoses other than WDTC were excluded from the study. The histopathology analysis was done according to the World Health Organization Classification of Thyroid Tumors. CLT was identified on histopathological analysis. Data collated included patients' demographic data, final histopathology reports, and preoperative TgAb measurements.

Patients were divided into two groups based on TgAb titers: TgAb positive group, defined as TgAb ≥30 IU/ml, and TgAb low/negative group, defined as TgAb <30 IU/mL. TgAb levels were measured using the Immulite 2000 anti-TgAb assays (Siemens, Llanberis, United Kingdom).

Patients with an incidental finding of micropapillary thyroid carcinoma without extrathyroidal extension (ETE) and/or lymph node (LN) positivity were recorded as having benign pathology. These carcinomas were categorized as such since they present an indolent behavior and a favorable prognosis, which suggest their resemblance to benign carcinomas [12]. Micropapillary carcinomas with unfavorable histopathological features, such as ETE and/or LN positivity, behave more aggressively and are hence more appropriately managed as malignant carcinomas [12].

Sensitivity, specificity, positive predictive value, negative predictive value, relative risk and odds ratio of TgAb ≥30 IU/ml as a diagnostic test for thyroid malignancy were calculated. The data was statistically analyzed using SPSS 20.0. Pearson chi-square and Fisher's exact test were used to identify difference between groups. A $p$ value of 0.05 or less was considered statistically significant.

## Results

### Clinical characteristics

Among the 586 patients who underwent thyroid surgery during the study period, 181 were excluded from the study: 174 had incomplete data (TgAb value or final histopathology not available), 6 had medullary carcinoma

and 1 had anaplastic carcinoma. Among those with incomplete data, 157 patients had unrecorded TgAb values but available pathology reports, showing a rate of malignancy of 68.8 % (108/157) in this subgroup of patients. A total of 405 patients were included in this study. There were 329 females (81 %) and 76 (19 %) males, giving a female to male ratio of approximately 4:1. In the TgAb positive group, 92 % (48/52) of the patients were women in comparison to 80 % (282/353) in the TgAb negative group ($p = 0.031$). The mean age in the TgAb positive group was 45 years compared to 50 years in the TgAb negative group ($p = 0.013$).

There were 212 (52 %) patients with WDTC: 182 (86 %) of which had papillary carcinoma, 16 (7 %) had micropapillary carcinoma with ETE and/or LN positivity, and 14 (7 %) had follicular carcinoma. There were 193 (48 %) patients with benign pathology, of which 68 (35 %) had micropapillary carcinoma without ETE and/or LN positivity. The flow chart of this study is shown in Fig. 1. The patient characteristics are presented in Table 1.

Among the 405 patients, 52 (13 %) were found to have TgAb levels ≥30 IU/mL, while the remaining 353 (87 %) had TgAb values <30 IU/mL. The TgAb values ranged from <20 (lowest value detected by the assay used) to 3362. A total of 340 (84 %) patients had values <20 while the median and mean TgAb values of the remaining patients were 96 and 412 (standard deviation 739). In the malignant group, 175 (83 %) patients had TgAb values <20 vs. 165 (85 %) in the benign group, while the median and mean TgAb values of the remaining patients were 108 vs. 53 and 751 (standard deviation 1920) vs. 313 (standard deviation 479) respectively.

There were 34 out of the 52 patients in the positive TgAb group who were diagnosed with WDTC, compared to 178 of the 353 patients in the low/negative TgAb group, resulting in a malignancy rate of 65 % vs. 50 %, respectively ($p = 0.05$). In other words, overall, 16 % of patients with WDTC had positive TgAb levels, compared to 9 % of the patients with a benign pathology (Table 1). The prevalence of malignancy according to TgAb levels is presented in Fig. 2. It is worth noting that within the benign group, 7.4 % of patients with micropapillary carcinoma without ETE and/or LN positivity had TgAb values ≥30 (5 out of 68) compared to 10.4 % (13 out of 125) of patients with other benign pathologies.

Overall, the final histopathology reports revealed the presence of CLT in 98 out of 405 patients (24.2 %). An approximately equal proportion of patients in both the malignant and benign groups presented with CLT (24.5 % vs. 23.8 % respectively). In the TgAb positive group, 50 % of patients with malignant disease had CLT. Similarly, 50 % of patients in the benign group harboured CLT in their thyroids. About 20 % of patients in the TgAb negative group had CLT, with once again an

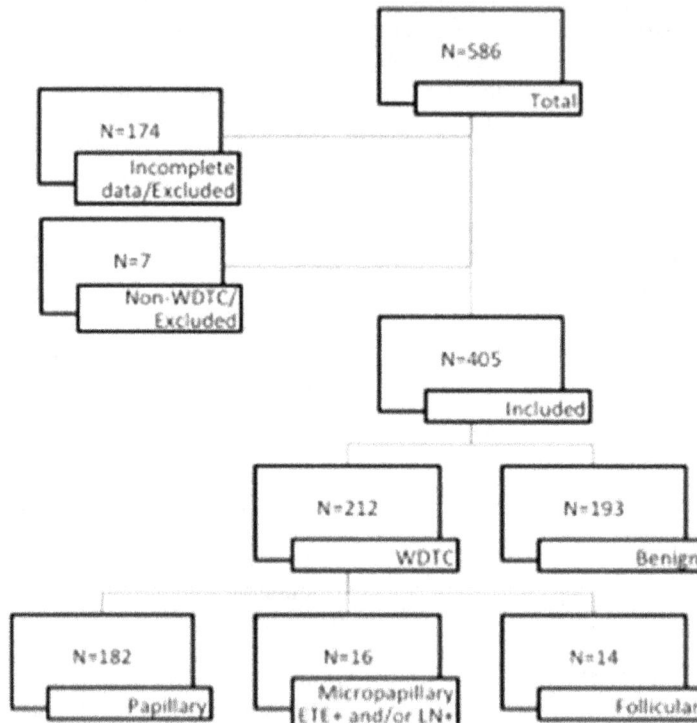

**Fig. 1** Flow chart of diagnosis

approximately equal proportion of patients in the malignant and benign groups (19.7 % vs. 21.1 % respectively). These results are shown in Table 2.

### Statistical analysis

The sensitivity, specificity, positive predictive value and negative predictive value of TgAb $\geq$30 IU/ml as a predictive parameter of thyroid malignancy were 16.04 % (CI 11.37-21.68), 90.67 % (CI 85.66-94.38), 65.38 % (CI 50.91-78.03) and 49.58 % (CI 44.24-54.92), respectively. Both the Pearson chi-square test ($p = 0.024$) and Fisher's exact test ($p = 0.017$) yielded statistical significance between the two groups.

### Discussion

This study demonstrates that the prevalence of WDTC was higher in patients with positive TgAb, compared to

**Table 1** Patient characteristics of the sample ($N = 405$)

|                         | Benign ($N = 193$) | Malignant ($N = 212$) | p-value |
|-------------------------|--------------------|-----------------------|---------|
| Age (years)             | 49.53 ± 13.94      | 49.25 ± 13.87         | NS      |
| Gender, no. female (%)  | 164 (84.97)        | 165 (77.83)           | NS      |
| TgAb ≥ 30 IU/mL, no. (%) | 18 (9.33)         | 34 (16.04)            | 0.024   |

Data represents mean ± standard deviation or number (percentage)
NS not significant

patients with low/negative TgAb. Our results suggest that a TgAb count $\geq$30 IU/ml may be specific for WDTC, although a lower count should not be used to rule out malignancy. In accordance with our data, other authors have reported that elevated TgAb levels could be an indicator that a thyroid nodule is at increased risk for malignancy. As mentioned earlier, Kim et al. were the first to report that a positive TgAb test was an independent predictor of thyroid nodule malignancy, regardless of the presence of CLT. A more recent study conducted by Grani et al. showed that an isolated TgAb positivity could be a mild risk factor for thyroid cancer, as opposed to Hashimoto's thyroiditis, which did not correlate positively with malignant pathology [13].

Our study shows that in the TgAb positive group, there is a significantly higher proportion of women and patients were slightly younger compared to those in the TgAb negative group. Demographics and levels of TgAb were examined in the National Health and Nutrition Examination Survey (NHANES III), a large study that was conducted on the American population between 1988 and 1994 [14]. They reported that TgAb were more prevalent in women than in men. However, in this cohort, levels of TgAb were increasing with age when comparing youth vs adults vs elderly patients. We compared age according to the mean age of both groups which

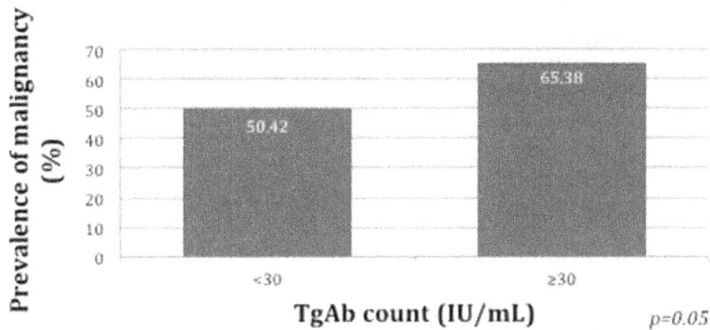

**Fig. 2** Prevalence of malignancy according to TgAb levels

could explain the difference in this finding. The age groups were separated differently than our series of patients. Nevertheless, it is relevant to note that they lie in the same age category, as increasing concentrations with age in the NHANES III study was only significant when comparing groups with greater age difference (i.e. youth vs. adults vs. elderly).

Our results show that 50 % of TgAb positive patients had CLT compared to 20 % of TgAb negative patients. An association between the presence of TgAb and CLT has also been reported in the literature [15, 16]. However, we did not find a significant correlation between CLT and WDTC, as prevalence of CLT was the same for benign and malignant pathologies. This is in agreement with the literature. In fact, a population-based fine-needle aspiration biopsy study [17] and two large prospective studies with a 10-year follow-up [18, 19] did not find an association between CLT and WDTC. Currently, in the literature, there is uncertainty on whether CLT is a cause, a consequence or simply, histologically accompanying a malignancy, as both share some common pathways in molecular genetic pathology. It is also difficult to differentiate histologically between peritumoral lymphocytic infiltrations and true CLT [20–26]. However, most believe that pathologic processes of autoimmune thyroid disease have to be independent from the ones of tumorogenesis to explain the increased prevalence of CLT in TgAb positive patients.

**Table 2** Prevalence of specimens showing chronic lymphocytic thyroiditis according to TgAb group and final pathology

Number of specimens with CLT/total number of specimens (%)

|  | Benign | Malignant | Total |
|---|---|---|---|
| TgAb ≥ 30 | 9/18 (50) | 17/34 (50) | 26/52 (50) |
| TgAb < 30 | 37/175 (21.1) | 35/178 (19.7) | 72/353 (20.4) |
| Total | 46/193 (23.8) | 52/212 (24.5) | 98/405 (24.2) |

*CLT* Chronic lymphocytic thyroiditis

In the aforementioned studies by Kim et al. [11] and Grani et al. [13], the patient's final diagnostic outcome was established following FNAC, with only a minority of diagnoses confirmed by histological follow-up. One limitation of using FNAC as a diagnostic tool is that the cytological features observed in the sample obtained are not necessarily representative of the entire thyroid tissue and cannot consequently offer a definitive diagnosis. An alternative to this problem consists of using the final pathology report obtained after surgical excision, which is the only diagnostically conclusive method. However, the latter also presents limitations, namely the bias caused by the selection of patients with high suspicion of thyroid cancer, and hence requiring thyroidectomy. In order to balance this selection bias, our study focused on the comparison between a TgAb positive and a TgAb negative group. Moreover, selecting a sample of surgical candidates was especially relevant in the context where risk assessment algorithms are particularly needed for patients in whom surgery is considered a treatment option. It is worth noting that another source of potential selection bias stems from the relatively high malignancy rate (68.8 %) in patients excluded from the study due to unavailable TgAb values.

Finally, it is important to mention that in the current literature there is no defined threshold of what is considered an elevated TgAb titer in WDTC. Most studies published set their cut-off values according to the recommendations of the assay kit provided by the manufacturer, which are calculated for its use in the diagnosis of CLT. When used for that purpose, the cut-offs are set higher as it is believed that higher titers of TgAb are needed to interfere with Tg levels in patients with CLT compared to WDTC [27]. In fact, two studies suggested that up to 20 % of samples may be misclassified as TgAb negative when the manufacturer's cut-off levels are used, as they are set too high [28, 29]. Since the manufacturer of the assay we used recommended a cut-off of 40 IU/

mL, we lowered it to 30 IU/mL in an effort to capture more patients with potentially interfering TgAb values. This implies that a threshold of 30 IU/mL may not be transferable to centres using a different anti-TgAb assay with variable manufacturer's recommendations. The reason for establishing the threshold to 30 and not to some other value below 40 relates to the statistical analysis of the test; a value of 30 offered the highest specificity among values showing statistical significance between the two groups.

Another limitation of our study is that it is retrospective. On one hand, this approach allowed us to accumulate data for a large number of cases; on the other hand, it limited our access to complete information for a number of patients. Nevertheless, we believe that the impact on the validity of our results is minimal as our results are concordant with other reports published in the literature. The results of the current study show that patients with elevated TgAb levels have a significantly higher rate of malignancy compared to patients with lower levels. However, this needs to be interpreted in the context of the aforementioned limitations. As such, incorporating TgAb levels measurement in the preoperative risk assessment of patients presenting with thyroid nodules could be helpful to predict malignancy when used with other variables. Nevertheless, an isolated TgAb test alone is not powerful enough and should not influence decision-making. Our results need confirmation from larger, prospective studies to better clarify the potential role of serum TgAb levels in the prediction of thyroid malignancy.

## Conclusions

Incorporating TgAb levels measurement in the preoperative risk assessment of patients presenting withthyroid nodules could be helpful to predict malignancy when used with other variables. Nevertheless, an isolated TgAb test alone is not powerful enough and should not influence decision-making. Our results need confirmation from larger, prospective studies to better clarify the potential role of serum TgAb levels in theprediction of thyroid malignancy.

### Competing interests
The authors declare that they have no competing interests.

### Authors' contributions
SH, and FW carried out the data collection, statistical analysis and drafted the manuscript. All authors read and approved the final manuscript.

### Author details
[1]Faculty of Medicine, McGill University, Montreal, QC, Canada. [2]Department of Otolaryngology – Head and Neck Surgery, McGill University, Montreal, QC, Canada. [3]Department Otolaryngology - Head and Neck Surgery, King Abdulaziz University, Jeddah, Saudi Arabia. [4]Division of Endocrinology, Jewish General Hospital, McGill University, Montreal, QC, Canada.

### References
1.  Mazzaferri EL. Management of a solitary thyroid nodule. N Engl J Med. 1993; 328(8):553–9.
2.  Hegedus L. Clinical practice. The thyroid nodule. N Engl J Med. 2004;351(17): 1764–71.
3.  Yassa L, Cibas ES, Benson CB, Frates MC, Doubilet PM, Gawande AA, Moore FD Jr, Kim BW, Nose V, Marqusee E, Larsen PR, Alexander EK. Long-term assessment of a multidisciplinary approach to thyroid nodule diagnostic evaluation. Cancer. 2007;111:508–16.
4.  Hayat MJ, Howlader N, Reichman ME, Edwards BK. Cancer statistics, trends, and multiple primary cancer analyses from the Surveillance, Epidemiology, and End Results (SEER) program. Oncologist. 2007;12:20–37.
5.  Brander A, Viikinkoski P, Tuuhea J, Voutilainen L, Kivisaari L. Clinical versus ultrasound examination of the thyroid gland in common clinical practice. J Clin Ultrasound. 1992;20:37–42.
6.  Scheffler P, Forest VI, Leboeuf R, Florea AV, Tamilia M, Sands NB, et al. Serum thyroglobulin improves the sensitivity of the McGill thyroid nodule score for well-differentiated thyroid cancer. Thyroid. 2014;24(5):852-7.
7.  Sands NB, Karls S, Rivera J, Tamilia M, Hier MP, Black MJ, Gologan O, Payne RJ. Preoperative serum thyroglobulin as an adjunct to fine-needle aspiration in predicting well-differentiated thyroid cancer. J Otolaryngol Head Neck Surg. 2010;39:669–73.
8.  Hocevar M, Auersperg M. Role of serum thyroglobulin in the pre-operative evaluation of follicular thyroid tumours. Eur J Surg Oncol. 1998;24:553–7.
9.  Lee EK, Chung KW, Min HS, Kim TS, Kim TH, Ryu JS, Jung YS, Kim SK, Lee YJ. Preoperative serum thyroglobulin as a useful predictive marker to differentiate follicular thyroid cancer from benign nodules in indeterminate nodules. J Korean Med Sci. 2012;27:1014–8.
10. Spencer CA. Clinical review: Clinical utility of thyroglobulin antibody (TgAb) measurements for patients with differentiated thyroid cancers (DTC). J Clin Endocrinol Metab. 2011;96(12):3615–27.
11. Kim ES, Lim DJ, Baek KH, Lee JM, Kim MK, Kwon HS, et al. Thyroglobulin antibody is associated with increased cancer risk in thyroid nodules. Thyroid. 2010;20(8):885–91.
12. Ardito G, Revelli L, Giustozzi E, Salvatori M, Fadda G, Ardito F, et al. Aggressive papillary thyroid microcarcinoma: prognostic factors and therapeutic strategy. Clin Nucl Med. 2013;38(1):25–8.
13. Grani G, Calvanese A, Carbotta G, D'Alessandri M, Nesca A, Bianchini M, et al. Thyroid autoimmunity and risk of malignancy in thyroid nodules submitted to fine-needle aspiration cytology. Head Neck. 2013;24(5):852-7.
14. Hollowell JG, Staehling NW, Flanders WD, Hannon WH, Gunter EW, Spencer CA, et al. Serum TSH, T(4), and thyroid antibodies in the United States population (1988 to 1994): National Health and Nutrition Examination Survey (NHANES III). J Clin Endocrinol Metab. 2002;87(2):489–99.
15. Toyoda N, Nishikawa M, Iwasaka T. Anti-thyroglobulin antibodies. Nihon Rinsho. 1999;57(8):1810–4.
16. Farwell AP, Braverman LE. Inflammatory thyroid disorders. Otolaryngol Clin North Am. 1996;29(4):541–56.
17. Jankovic B, Le KT, Hershman JM. Clinical Review: Hashimoto's thyroiditis and papillary thyroid carcinoma: is there a correlation? J Clin Endocrinol Metab. 2013;98(2):474–82.
18. Crile G. Struma lymphomatosa and carcinoma of the thyroid. Surg Gynecol Obstet. 1978;147:350–2.
19. Holm LE, Blomgren H, Lo"whagen T. Cancer risks in patients with chronic lymphocytic thyroiditis. N Engl J Med. 1985;312:601–4.
20. Wirtschafter A, Schmidt R, Rosen D, Kundu N, Santoro M, Fusco A, Multhaupt H, Atkins JP, Rosen MR, Keane WM, Rothstein JL. Expression of the RET/PTC fusion gene as a marker for papillary carcinoma in Hashimoto's thyroiditis. Laryngoscope. 1997;107:95–100.
21. Arif S, Blanes A, Diaz-Cano SJ. Hashimoto's thyroiditis shares features with early papillary thyroid carcinoma. Histopathology. 2002;41:357–62.
22. Unger P, Ewart M, Wang BY, Gan L, Kohtz DS, Burstein DE. Expression of p63 in papillary thyroid carcinoma and in Hashimoto's thyroiditis: a pathobiologic link. Hum Pathol. 2003;34:764–9.
23. Larson SD, Jackson LN, Riall TS, Uchida T, Thomas RP, Qiu S, Evers BM. Increased incidence of well-differentiated thyroid cancer associated with Hashimoto thyroiditis and the role of the PI3k/Akt pathway. J Am Coll Surg. 2007;204:764–75.
24. Kang DY, Kim KH, Kim JM, Kim SH, Kim JY, Baik HW, Kim YS. High prevalence of RET, RAS, and ERK expression in Hashimoto's thyroiditis and in papillary thyroid carcinoma in the Korean population. Thyroid. 2007;17:1031–8.

25.  Antonaci A, Consorti F, Mardente S, Giovannone G. Clinical and biological
     relationship between chronic lymphocytic thyroiditis and papillary thyroid
     carcinoma. Oncol Res. 2009;17:495–503.
26.  Muzza M, Degl'Innocenti D, Colombo C, Perrino M, Ravasi E, Rossi S, Cirello
     V, Beck-Peccoz P, Borrello MG, Fugazzola L. The tight relationship between
     papillary thyroid cancer, autoimmunity and inflammation: clinical and
     molecular studies. Clin Endocrinol (Oxf). 2010;72:702–8.
27.  Verburg FA, Luster M, Cupini C, Chiovato L, Duntas L, Elisei R, et al.
     Implications of thyroglobulin antibody positivity in patients with
     differentiated thyroid cancer: a clinical position statement. Thyroid. 2013;
     23(10):1211–25.
28.  Spencer C, Petrovic I, Fatemi S. Current thyroglobulin autoantibody (TgAb)
     assays often fail to detect interfering TgAb that can result in the reporting
     of falsely low/undetectable serum Tg IMA values for patients with
     differentiated thyroid cancer. J Clin Endocrinol Metab. 2011;96:1283–91.
29.  Cubero JM, Rodriguez-Espinosa J, Gelpi C, Estorch M, Corcoy R.
     Thyroglobulin autoantibody levels below the cut-off for positivity can
     interfere with thyroglobulin measurement. Thyroid. 2003;13:659–61.

# 22

# Xanthogranuloma in the heavily irradiated low neck in a patient with head and neck cancer

Lisa Singer[1], Sarah M. Calkins[2], Andrew E. Horvai[2], William R. Ryan[3] and Sue S. Yom[1,3*]

## Abstract

**Background:** Head and neck cancer is often managed with a combination of surgery, radiation therapy, and chemotherapy, and skin toxicity is not uncommon. Xanthogranuloma is a pathological finding resulting from an inflammatory reaction that has not been previously reported following head and neck radiation therapy.

**Case presentation:** A patient with squamous cell carcinoma of the oropharynx, treated with definitive chemoradiation and hyperthermia, presented at eight-month follow-up with an in-field cutaneous lesion in the low neck, initially concerning for recurrent tumor.
Biopsy showed xanthogranuloma and the patient underwent complete resection with congruent surgical pathology. The patient remained free of malignancy but continued to experience wound healing difficulties at the resection site which resolved with specialized wound care and hyperbaric oxygen.

**Conclusions:** Skin toxicity is not uncommon in patients with head and neck cancer treated with radiation therapy. Awareness of unusual pathologic sequelae, such as xanthogranuloma, is needed to provide patient counseling while continuing appropriate surveillance for recurrent malignancy.

**Keywords:** Xanthogranuloma, Radiation therapy, Head and neck cancer, Skin, Toxicity

## Background

For patients with locally advanced head and neck cancer, the use of radiation therapy with concurrent chemotherapy is supported by multiple randomized trials [1]. This treatment can produce both acute and late toxicity to normal tissues [2]. Known late toxicities to the skin include permanent skin tanning, telangiectasias, necrosis, and fibrosis.

We report a case of a patient with head and neck cancer treated with radiation therapy who later presented with xanthogranuloma arising within the radiation field. Xanthogranuloma is a histopathological diagnosis, referring to a lesion comprised of abundant histiocytes, often displaying foamy cytoplasm and associated foreign body giant cells [3]. Juvenile xanthogranulomatosis (JXG) is a

clinical diagnosis first described in the 1950s, referring to children with one or more of these lesions [4]. JXG is thought to be a benign disorder, although ocular involvement may impact 0.5 % of patients with skin involvement [4]. Xanthogranulomas have been described in adults in association with multiple possible risk factors, including trauma, infection, and malignancy. Xanthogranuloma has been reported in a patient treated with radiation therapy for breast cancer, but it has not been previously reported in the English literature following head and neck irradiation [5]. To increase awareness of this potential late effect of chemoradiation, we present the case and review relevant related literature.

## Case presentation

At the age of 45, a patient with a 30-pack year history of tobacco use and no significant past medical history presented to our institution with pathology-proven AJCC Stage IVA, T3 (lingual epiglottis extension), N2c (bilateral lymph node involvement), M0 squamous cell

* Correspondence: yoms@radonc.ucsf.edu
[1]Department of Radiation Oncology, University of California, San Francisco, 1600 Divisadero St, Suite H-1031, San Francisco, CA 94143 - 1708, USA
[3]Department of Otolaryngology, University of California, San Francisco, 1600 Divisadero St, Suite H-1031, San Francisco, CA 94143 - 1708, USA
Full list of author information is available at the end of the article

carcinoma of the left base of tongue. Notably, he had history of a palpable left upper neck mass three years prior, but fine needle aspiration (FNA) at that time was non-diagnostic. The neck mass recurred and he initially pursued treatment with homeopathic therapy. The mass increased in size, leading him to seek further medical attention and ultrasound showed a very large left supraclavicular mass and a right submandibular mass. FNA of the left neck mass showed p16-overexpressing squamous cell carcinoma. Positron emission tomography with computed tomography (PET/CT) showed a mass involving the left tonsillar pillar and extending to the piriform sinus, with increased avidity on FDG-PET and measuring over 3 cm in longest diameter. He was also noted to have FDG-avid suspicious lymph nodes involving the right level IIA, left level IIA and left level IV. A left parapharyngeal lymph node was also concerning. At the time of the initial radiation oncology consult he endorsed weight loss, left neck pain, dysgeusia, decreased appetite, and tracheal pressure without shortness of breath. He had received no treatment for the left oropharyngeal cancer except for treatment with hyperthermia in ten fractions at an outside facility.

On exam, he was found to have Karnofsky Performance Status of 80, vital signs within normal limits, and a greater than 6 cm left-sided lymph node conglomerate and palpable left level II lymph node and right level II/III lymph nodes, with slight tracheal deviation to right. Concurrent cisplatin-based chemoradiation was advised and the patient consented to treatment.

**Treatment**
The patient was treated at our institution with intensity-modulated radiation therapy, 70.88 Gy in 34 fractions, prescribed to the 88 % isodose line, targeting the left oropharynx and bilateral neck with 6 MV photons, with concurrent hyperthermia given twice a week to the massive nodal mass as well as cisplatin.

His treatment course was complicated by intractable nausea and vomiting following the first cycle of cisplatin. Due to these symptoms, as well as purulent drainage from the left neck mass following radiation, he was hospitalized. There was no evidence of infection identified during hospitalization but there was a golf-ball-sized area of skin rupture in the left low neck emitting pus and drainage that was attributed to tumor necrosis. His chemotherapy was switched to weekly administration. Over the course of treatment, he also developed grade 2 oral mucositis and dry desquamation of other parts of the skin. Due to a clinically evident decrease in tumor size, a repeat radiation planning CT was obtained and a new radiation plan was generated for use during the last ten fractions. The patient did not require a feeding tube during

treatment, although for the month following completion of radiation therapy, he elected to receive frequent intravenous hydration.

**Post-treatment surveillance**
At the six month follow-up appointment, magnetic resonance imaging (MRI) of the head and neck showed treatment response of the primary tumor and bilateral neck. On interval physical exam, he had residual right level II lymphadenopathy and stiffness in the left neck with erythematous and hypo-pigmented areas. There were no palpable base of tongue lesions. At 3 month follow-up, PET/CT showed that the right level II lymph node was not FDG-avid. At repeat MRI two months later, the right level II lymph node was stable and the patient appeared to have no evidence of disease although on exam, telangiectasias were noted in the skin at the left supraclavicular region.

At follow-up eight months after completion of chemoradiation, he was found to have a 1.5x1.5 cm irregularly shaped, reddish-purplish-colored lesion extruding out from the skin in level IV of the left neck, with surrounding deep red ecchymosis. This new mass was located in the area of the rupture through skin. MRI at that time showed small left level 3, 5a, and 5b lymphadenopathy underlying the area. The cutaneous left neck lesion was concerning for cancer recurrence and he was referred for biopsy. The lesion is shown in Fig. 1.

**Cytopathology**
FNA with three passes was performed. Aspirate material was abundantly cellular and composed of numerous foamy histiocytes and a sparse inflammatory infiltrate within a background of lipid debris. No epithelial cells were noted on aspirate smears or cell block material. Additionally, a pankeratin immunohistochemical stain was performed and was negative, further arguing against an epithelial component.

CT of the chest was also obtained, which revealed no metastases. The patient was referred to otolaryngology-head and neck surgery for management of the left neck lympadenopathy. Flexible fiberoptic nasopharyngolaryngoscopy was normal. A left level IV lesion was again visible and palpable on exam, with surrounding skin intact but with associated erythema. Punch biopsy of the cutaneous lesion was performed showing dystrophic xanthomatosis and resection was advised. MRI was re-reviewed and it was determined that there was no clear sign of cancer persistence or recurrence within the deep neck.

**Resection of xanthogranuloma**
At nine months following completion of chemoradiation, the patient elected for gross resection of the left neck mass. The mass was over 4 cm in size, and transfer of

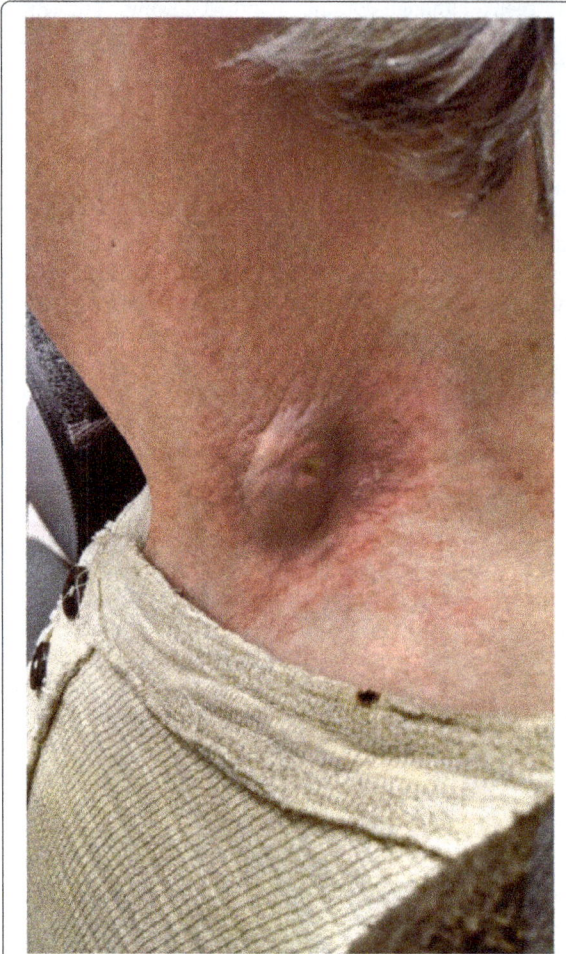

Fig. 1 Left low neck lesion in patient treated with chemoradiation for head and neck cancer

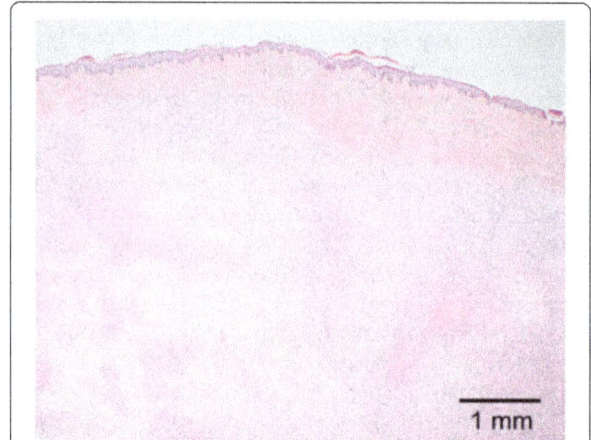

Fig. 2 Histologic section showing dense population of foamy histiocytes (xanthoma cells), occasional multinucleate giant cells, and scattered interspersed lymphocytes involving the deep dermis and subcutis

of immunostaining for S100-protein and SOX10 argued against the possibility of melanoma. Overall, the findings were consistent with dystrophic xanthomatosis (also known as dystrophic xanthogranulomatosis).

### Surveillance

MRI seven weeks after resection showed no evidence of disease. Due to the patient's history of lymphocytopenia pre-dating initiation of chemotherapy and possible association between the development of xanthogranulomas and hematological malignancy, the patient was re-evaluated by the hematology service [6]. The prior low lymphocyte count was thought to be spurious and no evidence for a lymphoproliferative disorder was identified. At three months following the resection, the patient was found to

adjacent skin that had not been radiated was required to close the defect.

### Surgical pathology

Gross examination revealed a yellow, firm, oval subcutaneous mass measuring 2.1 x 1.6 x 1.0 cm. Histologic sections revealed a dense population of foamy histiocytes (xanthoma cells), occasional multinucleate giant cells and scattered interspersed lymphocytes (Figs. 2 and 3) involving the deep dermis and superficial subcutis. In some areas, these cells were found to surround degenerating collagen and nuclear debris (Fig. 4). No obvious epithelial cells or carcinoma were identified on H&E sections and a keratin immunostain was negative, further arguing against a component of metastatic carcinoma. The foamy cells were positive for CD68, supporting a histiocyte lineage (Fig. 5). Histochemical stains were negative for acid-fast and fungal microorganisms, arguing against an infectious component. Lack

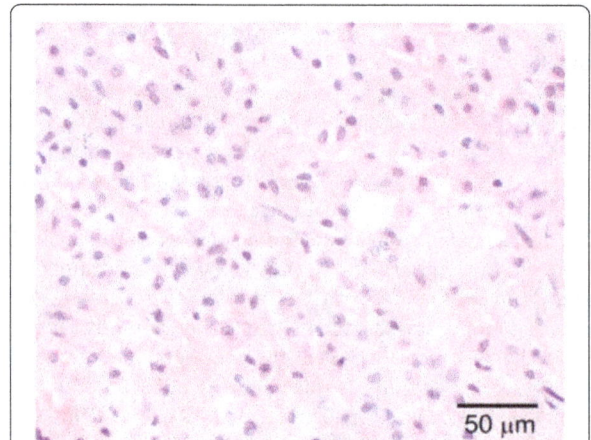

Fig. 3 Histologic section showing foamy histiocytes, multinucleate giant cells, and interspersed lymphocytes

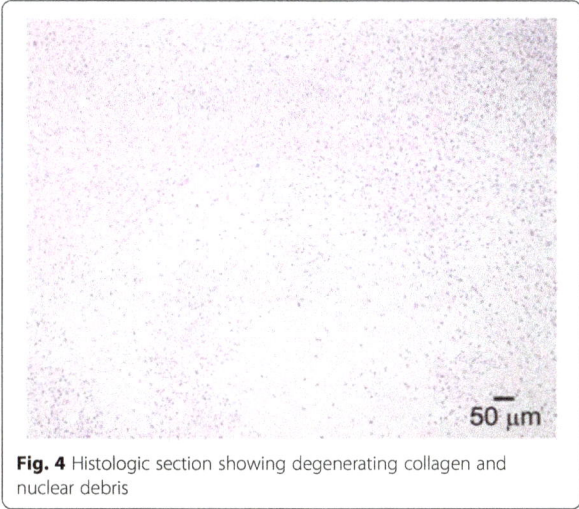

**Fig. 4** Histologic section showing degenerating collagen and nuclear debris

have mild erythema of the left neck with an open lesion at the post-operative site (Fig. 6). Medical grade honey and foam dressing were prescribed, with continued follow-up to monitor wound healing. At 14 months from chemoradiotherapy completion and 6 months from lesion excision, the patient had no sign of cancer recurrence but continued to experience wound healing difficulties. It was decided to administer a month of hyperbaric oxygen treatments and collagenase dressings. By the next followup 3 months later, the skin had finally closed, leaving residual fibrosis and telangiectasia (Fig. 7).

## Conclusions

At eight months following completion of chemoradiation for a locoregionally advanced head and neck cancer, a patient was to found to develop a xanthogranuloma within

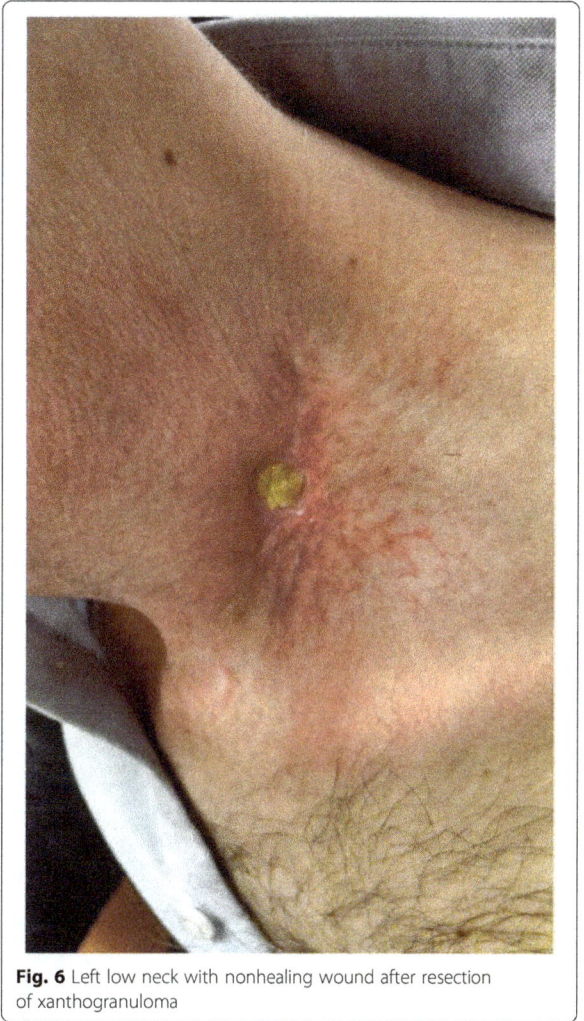

**Fig. 6** Left low neck with nonhealing wound after resection of xanthogranuloma

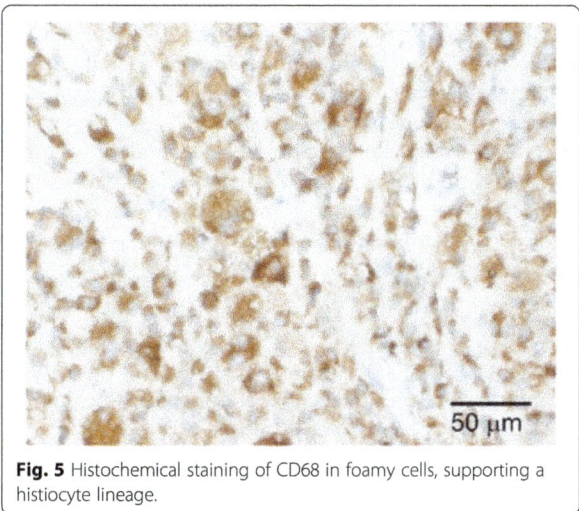

**Fig. 5** Histochemical staining of CD68 in foamy cells, supporting a histiocyte lineage.

the radiation field. The xanthogranuloma arose in a location where the skin had ruptured over a large nodal mass during the course of treatment. This represents a late radiation toxicity that has not yet been reported in the English literature in a patient with head and neck cancer. Assessment of patient and treatment-related factors may improve understanding of this toxicity.

A recent consensus report discussed factors contributing to skin toxicity in patients with head and neck cancer treated with chemoradiation [7]. Host factors contributing to toxicity include nutritional status, sun exposure, and smoking, as well as comorbidities such as lupus, diabetes, or hypertension. While this patient did not have known comorbidities, he did have a history of smoking. His nutritional status was reasonably maintained during treatment. Treatment-related factors cited in the consensus report included skin dose and fraction size >2 Gy per fraction, as well as the use of bolus and

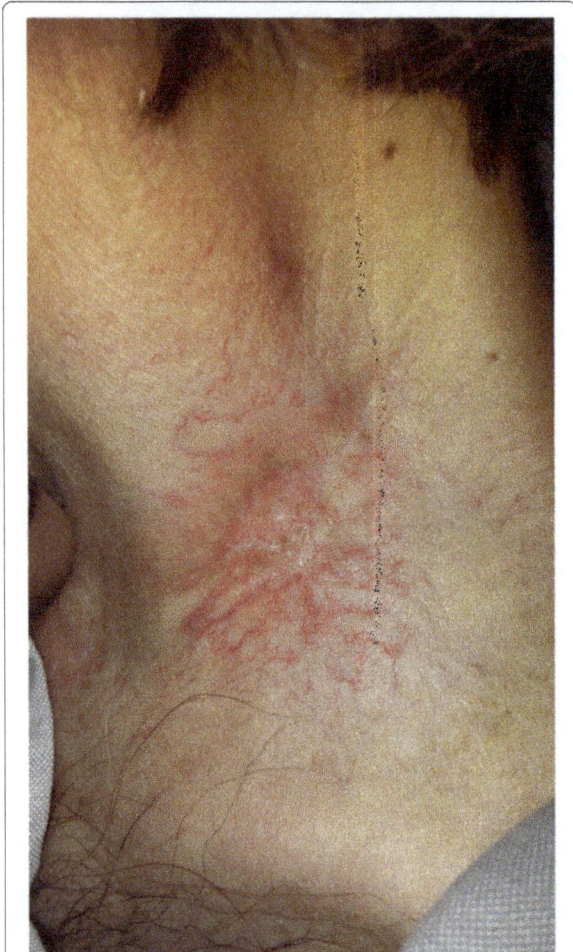

**Fig. 7** Resolution of left low neck wound after xanthogranuloma resection

(dry desquamation in >50 % of skin surface area vs <50 % in the areas not treated with hyperthermia). Late effects were similar with and without hyperthermia, although one case of RTOG/EORTC grade 4 subcutaneous necrosis was identified within the hyperthermia field. In a single-institution study randomizing patients with superficial tumors to radiation with or without hyperthermia, the incidence of thermal burns was increased with hyperthermia [11]. In summary, this information suggests that the radio-sensitizing effects of hyperthermia may put patients at higher risk for toxicity and should be monitored carefully.

Xanthogranuloma has been reported in a patient receiving breast radiation [5]. In this case report, the lesion was identified 12 months following completion of breast radiation therapy. The authors speculated that due to the time course, radiation likely played a role. Unlike the xanthogranuloma in our patient, this lesion was 4 mm in maximum diameter and was able to be excised with punch biopsy. Both the breast cancer patient and our patient received radiation therapy and chemotherapy, although, as per standard of care, the treatments were not concurrent in the breast cancer patient. Our patient, like the breast cancer patient, presented with xanthogranuloma as a delayed late effect. However, in our patient, the tumor rupture through the skin during treatment likely contributed to chronically impaired integrity of the tissues in that region with a much more exuberant presentation of xanthogranuloma. We hypothesize that the necrosis and pus ignited a chronic inflammatory response arising preferentially in that location, releasing a macrophage flood that enabled development of xanthogranuloma.

While patients in the literature have been treated with chemoradiation and hyperthermia for head and neck cancer and have not developed xanthogranuloma, our patient is unique in that he received neoadjuvant hyperthermia at an outside facility prior to initiating definitive treatment at our institution. It is possible that the xanthogranuloma development was encouraged in part due to an interaction between this patient's immune response and the intensive radio-sensitization resulting from concurrent cisplatin and localized hyperthemia. In any case, awareness of acute and late skin toxicities, including xanthogranuloma, can help direct the workup, which can be confusing given the over-riding concern for malignant recurrence.

**Consent**

Written informed consent was obtained from the patient for publication of this report and any accompanying images. The patient was given access to this report.

**Competing Interests**

The authors declare that they have no competing interests.

radio-sensitizing therapies. Due to the extensive nodal disease in the low left neck, the skin dose was high and this increased the risk for toxicity. This patient was also treated with two radio-sensitizing therapies in the area: cisplatin and hyperthermia.

Prior studies on the use of radiation, chemotherapy, and hyperthermia in patients with head and neck cancer have not identified the skin toxicity that we describe in this case report. In a study of 40 patients followed for a median of 9 months, two Grade 1 burns were identified [8]. In a retrospective study of radiation with or without hyperthermia, acute toxicity was similar and late toxicity was higher in the combined treatment group, with two patients diagnosed with bone necrosis [9]. A Phase I-II study on the use of concurrent cisplatin, hyperthermia and radiation [10] showed that acute skin toxicity was slightly higher with the use of hyperthermia than without

**Authors' contributions**
LS collected the data and drafted the manuscript. SMC and AEH carried out the histochemical studies and provided the figures. WRR provided surgical clinical data. SSY conceived of the study, directed its design and coordination, and obtained the patient photographs and consent. All authors read and approved the final manuscript.

**Author details**
[1]Department of Radiation Oncology, University of California, San Francisco, 1600 Divisadero St, Suite H-1031, San Francisco, CA 94143 - 1708, USA. [2]Department of Pathology, University of California, San Francisco, San Francisco, CA, USA. [3]Department of Otolaryngology, University of California, San Francisco, 1600 Divisadero St, Suite H-1031, San Francisco, CA 94143 - 1708, USA.

**References**
1. Pignon J-P, le Maître A, Maillard E, et al. Meta-analysis of chemotherapy in head and neck cancer (MACH-NC): an update on 93 randomised trials and 17,346 patients. Radiother Oncol. 2009;92:4–14.
2. Wong RKS, Bensadoun RJ, Boers-Doets CB, et al. Clinical practice guidelines for the prevention and treatment of acute and late radiation reactions from the MASCC Skin Toxicity Study Group. Support Care Cancer. 2013;21:2933–48.
3. Chisolm SS, Schulman JM, Fox LP. Adult Xanthogranuloma, Reticulohistiocytosis, and Rosai-Dorfman Disease. Dermatol Clin. 2015;33:465–73.
4. Pajaziti L, Hapçiu SR, Pajaziti A. Juvenile xanthogranuloma: a case report and review of the literature. BMC Res Notes. 2014;7:174.
5. Cohen PR, Prieto VG. Radiation port xanthogranuloma: solitary xanthogranuloma occurring within the irradiated skin of a breast cancer patient-report and review of cutaneous neoplasms developing at the site of radiotherapy. J Cutan Pathol. 2010;37:891–4.
6. Shoo BA, Shinkai K, McCalmont TH, et al. Xanthogranulomas associated with hematologic malignancy in adulthood. J Am Acad Dermatol. 2008;59:488–93.
7. Russi EG, Moretto F, Rampino M, et al. Acute skin toxicity management in head and neck cancer patients treated with radiotherapy and chemotherapy or EGFR inhibitors: Literature review and consensus. Crit Rev Oncol Hematol. 2015;96:167–82.
8. Huilgol NG, Gupta S, Dixit R. Chemoradiation with hyperthermia in the treatment of head and neck cancer. Int J Hyperthermia. 2010;26:21–5.
9. Valdagni R, Amichetti M. Report of long-term follow-up in a randomized trial comparing radiation therapy and radiation therapy plus hyperthermia to metastatic lymph nodes in stage IV head and neck patients. Radiat Oncol Biol. 1994;28:163–9.
10. Amichetti M, Graiff C, Fellin G, et al. Cisplatin, hyperthermia, and radiation (trimodal therapy) in patients with locally advanced head and neck tumors: a phase I-II study. Int J Radiat Oncol Biol Phys. 1993;26:801–7.
11. Jones EL, Oleson JR, Prosnitz LR, et al. Randomized trial of hyperthermia and radiation for superficial tumors. J Clin Oncol. 2005;23:3079–85.

# 23

# A retrospective review in the management of T3 laryngeal squamous cell carcinoma: an expanding indication for transoral laser microsurgery

A. Butler*, M. H. Rigby, J. Scott, J. Trites, R. Hart and S. M. Taylor

## Abstract

**Background:** The purpose of this study was to evaluate the functional and oncological outcomes of patients treated for T3 laryngeal squamous cell carcinoma. Specifically comparing transoral laser microsurgery and radiotherapy/chemoradiotherapy treatment modalities.

**Method:** A retrospective review of patients treated for T3 laryngeal SCC between 2002 and 2010 was undertaken.

**Results:** Forty-nine patients were included. 15 cases were glottic, (9 treated with TLM, 6 with RT/CRT), 33 supraglottic (6 treated with TLM, 27 with RT/CRT) and 1 subglottic subsite (treated with RT/CRT). There was no statistical difference between treatment groups for 24 month locoregional control (72.3 %), overall survival (glottis 86.7 %, supraglottic 70.4 %) and disease specific survival (glottic 93.3 % and supraglottic 74.1 %). Overall laryngeal preservation (84.9 %) was also similar in both groups.

**Conclusion:** Our institution is expanding the application of TLM to selected patients with T3 laryngeal carcinoma. Oncological outcomes have not been jeopardized by this approach and the treatment is well tolerated by patients with few complications.

**Keywords:** Laryngeal, Carcinoma, Transoral, Laser, Glottic

## Background

Laryngeal cancer is the second most frequent head and neck cancer. The overwhelming majority of these cancers are squamous cell carcinomas. These cancers are associated with both tobacco and alcohol use and, while this is changing, have historically occurred predominantly in males. For the 2010 Canadian population, laryngeal cancer had an estimated incidence rate of 2.0/100 000 person*years for males and 0.9/100 000 person*years in females [1]. U.S data has demonstrated that over the past 30 years, laryngeal cancer has the distinction of being one of the few cancers of the head and neck that has shown a decrease in survival [2, 3].

Transoral laser microsurgery (TLM), originally introduced in 1972 by Jako and Strong [1], has consistently been shown to have good oncological and functional

outcomes in patients with early glottic cancer. Steiner et al,. reported oncological and functional results in the treatment of T3 laryngeal tumours equivalent to radiotherapy (RT)/chemoradiotherapy(CRT) and open laryngeal surgery, which expanded the indications for TLM in laryngeal cancer [2]. Despite this, the management of T3 glottic carcinoma remains controversial. Most commonly, such tumours are treated with radical radiotherapy with adjuvant chemotherapy, open partial resection, or total laryngectomy.

Although recent studies support a possible role for a primary surgical approach, few centers such as the QEII Health Sciences Centre in Halifax, Nova Scotia have incorporated the use of TLM in the management of T3 glottic tumours [2]. The purpose of this paper is to review all T3 laryngeal squamous cell carcinomas (SCC) treated at the QEII Health Sciences Centre in Halifax, Nova Scotia, and to compare those patients

* Correspondence: drangelabutler@gmail.com
Dalhousie University, Halifax, Canada

treated with TLM to those managed with radiotherapy/chemoradiotherapy.

## Method

Data was obtained from the senior authors prospective database of malignancies treated with TLM at the QEII Health Sciences Centre in Halifax, Nova Scotia. Our institutional research ethics board approved the collection of information within the database. The details of this database have been previously described [4]. It has been prospectively maintained since 2005, and data prior to 2005 included retrospectively.

Inclusion criteria included all patients who underwent TLM or RT/CRT with curative intent for previously untreated T3 laryngeal SCC between January 2002 and December 2010. Exclusion criteria included all other sub-sites and stages, and recurrent T3 glottic SCC.

A retrospective cohort analysis was performed including a descriptive analysis of demographics and oncological outcomes. Demographics recorded included age, gender and smoking status. ANOVA test for difference in means and the Fisher Exact test were performed to identify any differences between the two therapeutic groups. Tumours were staged according to TNM American Joint Committee on Cancer (AJCC) guidelines [5]. Tumours excised with TLM were staged pathologically. Treatment modality and date of treatment commencement were recorded. Any treatment morbidity or complications were identified. Survival analysis using Kaplan Meier curve was performed, assessing local, regional and distant metastatic control, disease free survival, disease specific survival, overall survival and laryngeal preservation. Two year outcomes were recorded as 5 year data was not yet available.

All patients were treated with either transoral laser microsurgery +/- adjunctive radiation therapy (TLM), chemoradiation (CRT) or radiation therapy (RT) alone. Allocation to treatment modality was not randomized and was based on patient preference and recommendation of the site Head and Neck Oncology Tumour Board. Not all patients were considered eligible for all treatment modalities. Patients undergoing radiation alone either refused chemotherapy, or had a medical contraindication. Transoral laser surgery was performed using a tumour splitting technique with a $CO_2$ laser. Frozen sections were performed intraoperatively, and positive margins post-operatively were re-resected. Radiation therapy was performed using intensity modulated radiation therapy with 70 Gy with standard fractionation. Concurrent chemotherapy consisted of Cisplatinum with or without 5-fluorouracil given on weeks 1, 4 and 7 concurrently with radiation.

Functional outcomes of voice and swallowing were documented as assessed at the last follow up review,

using Voice Handicap Index (VHI) 10 and Functional Outcome Swallowing Study (FOSS) respectively. No scores were available prior to treatment commencement. Results were analysed using the Wilcoxon significance rank test.

## Results

Forty-nine patients met the inclusion criteria of the study. Fifteen (30.6 %) were treated with TLM and the remaining 34 (69.4 %) were treated with RT/CRT. No patients underwent open laryngeal surgery for primary treatment. 15 cases were glottic, (9 treated with TLM, 6 with RT/CRT), 33 supraglottic (6 treated with TLM, 27 with RT/CRT) and 1 subglottic subsite (treated with RT/CRT). Table 1.

Thirty-eight patients (77.6 %) were male, with no difference in gender distribution between the two treatment groups (p-value 0.5). The mean age was 69.1 years (61.1 years TLM, 66.5 years RT/CRT, age difference between treatment groups $p$ value 0.39). Mean follow-up duration for those treated with TLM was 29 months, and 41 months for those treated with RT/CRT. Thirty-three patients were staged as N0, eight as N1 and eight as N2. No patients presented with distant metastasis. The majority of patients with nodal metastasis received RT/CRT (17) as primary treatment rather than TLM (3). Seven (46.7 %) of TLM patients underwent adjuvant RT. None received adjuvant chemotherapy. Twenty-four (77.4 %) patients who underwent RT received concurrent chemotherapy. There were no statistically significant differences in the parameters of age, gender, smoking status, nodal status and date of initial treatment between treatment modalities. Table 2.

### Locoregional control

Thirteen patients in the study group developed a locoregional recurrence (26.5 %). The Kaplan-Meier estimates for 24 month locoregional control was 72.3 % in the entire cohort. There was no difference between the treatment groups (72 % TLM, 71.6 % RT/CRT $p$ value 0.94) Fig. 1.

In patients with glottic cancer, the Kaplan Meier estimate for locoregional control was 86.7 %. Two patients in the glottic group developed locoregional recurrence (12.5 %). Although they were both treated with TLM, this was not statistically significant compared to those

**Table 1** Treatment according to subsite

| Primary treatment modality | TLM | | | RT | | Total |
|---|---|---|---|---|---|---|
| Adjuvent treatment | | RT | CT | | CT | |
| Glottic | 9 | 4 | 0 | 6 | 4 | 15 |
| Supraglottic | 6 | 3 | 2 | 27 | 20 | 33 |
| Subglottic | | | | 1 | | 1 |

**Table 2** Patient age, gender, nodal staging, smoking status and date of treatment according to treatment

|  | All | TLM | RT | CRT | p |
|---|---|---|---|---|---|
| Number | 49 | 15 | 10 | 24 | - |
| Age |  |  |  |  | 0.39[a] |
| Mean | 63.1 | 61.1 | 66.5 | 63.0 |  |
| (SD) | (9.6) | (11.2) | (7.5) | (9.4) |  |
| Gender |  |  |  |  | 0.50[b] |
| Female | 11 | 3 | 1 | 7 |  |
| Male | 38 | 12 | 9 | 17 |  |
| (% Male) | (78 %) | (80 %) | (90 %) | (71 %) |  |
| Nodal stage |  |  |  |  | 0.36[b] |
| 0–I | 41 | 14 | 9 | 18 |  |
| II–III | 8 | 1 | 1 | 6 |  |
| (%II–III) | (16 %) | (7 %) | (10 %) | (25 %) |  |
| Smoking |  |  |  |  | 0.67[b] |
| No | 16 | 5 | 5 | 7 |  |
| Yes | 10 | 4 | 1 | 5 |  |
| Unknown | 23 | 6 | 4 | 12 |  |
| (% Yes[c]) | (37 %) | (44 %) | (17 %) | (42 %) |  |
| Date of initial treatment |  |  |  |  | 0.30[b] |
| 2002–06 | 24 | 5 | 5 | 14 |  |
| 2007–11 | 25 | 10 | 5 | 10 |  |
| (% 2007–11) | (51 %) | (67 %) | (50 %) | (42 %) |  |

[a]ANOVA F-test for means TLM, RT, CRT
[b]Fisher exact test for table TLM, RT, CRT
[c]% of those with known smoking status

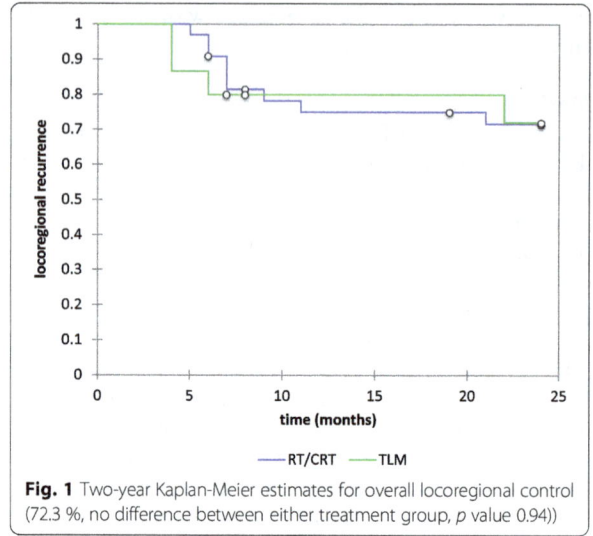

**Fig. 1** Two-year Kaplan-Meier estimates for overall locoregional control (72.3 %, no difference between either treatment group, p value 0.94))

Overall disease specific survival was 81.4 % and was also similar for those treated with TLM (86.2 %), and those treated with RT/CRT (79.4), (p value 0.60) Fig. 3. Glottic DSS was 93.3 % and supraglottic DSS was 74.1 %. Again neither group showed a statistically significant difference between treatment regimens (p value 0.41 and 0.75 respectively).

**Laryngeal preservation**
Overall laryngeal preservation rates (84.9 %) trended towards being greater in the TLM group (93 vs 81 %), but this was not statistically significant. (p value 0.35) Fig. 4.

treated with RT/CRT (p value 0.98) Both patients were managed with a salvage laryngectomy.

The Kaplan Meier estimate for locoregional control in patients with supraglottic cancer was 64.5 %, with no statistically significant difference between treatment groups (p value 0.98). Of the 11 patients (33.3 %) with recurrence, 2 were treated with TLM (33.3 %) and 9 with RT/CRT (33.3 %). Both patients treated with TLM who developed recurrence, were successfully treated with subsequent radiotherapy. Those patients with recurrence treated initially with RT/CRT, 2 were managed successfully with TLM, 1 was treated palliatively, and the remaining patients underwent salvage total laryngectomy.

**Survival**
Of the 49 patients, 12 (24.5 %) died within 24 months. Of these, 9(18.3 %) deaths were disease-related. Kaplan-Meier estimates showed 2 year overall survival was 75 % and again similar between the two treatment groups with 73.3 %% in the TLM group and 75.8 % RT/CRT group (p value 0.8) Fig. 2. Glottic overall survival was 86.7 % while supraglottic overall survival was 70.4 %. Neither group showed a statistical difference between treatment regimens.

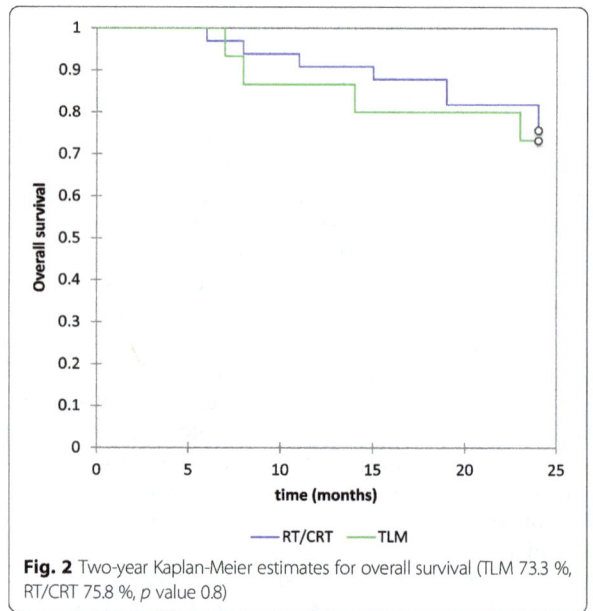

**Fig. 2** Two-year Kaplan-Meier estimates for overall survival (TLM 73.3 %, RT/CRT 75.8 %, p value 0.8)

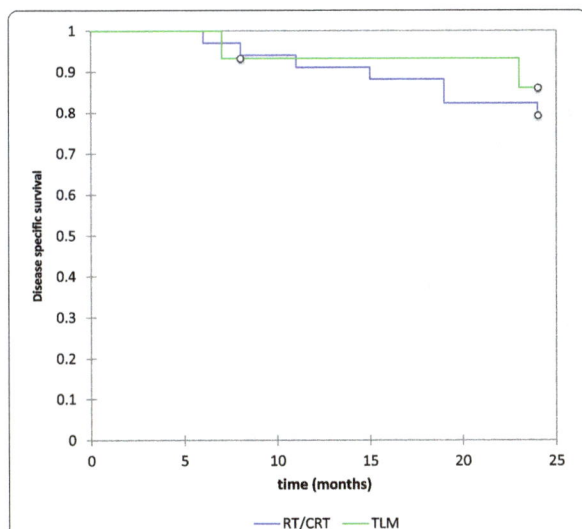

**Fig. 3** Two-year Kaplan-Meier estimates for overall disease specific survival (81.4 %, no difference between either treatment group, *p* value 0.60)

Glottic laryngeal preservation was 86.7 % and supraglottic laryngeal preservation 83.9 %. Although there was not a statistical difference between TLM and RT/CRT in either subsite, it is worth noting that no patients treated with TLM in the supraglottic group required a salvage laryngectomy.

### Post-operative complications and functional results

Voice Handicap Index (VHI) and Functional Outcome Swallow Scale (FOSS) scores were available in only a limited number of patients. For glottic cases, the median function outcomes at last post-treatment visit trended towards worse voice scores (VHI 10) for those treated

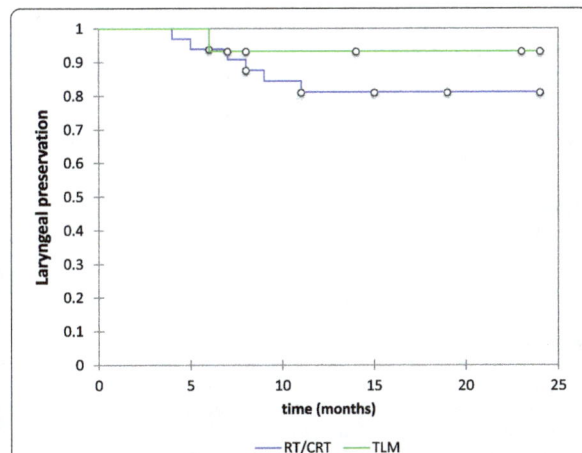

**Fig. 4** Two-year Kaplan-Meier estimates for overall laryngeal preservation (84.9 %, no difference between either treatment group, *p* value 0.35)

with TLM (15 TLM, 11 RT/CRT) but this was not statistically significant. However, for supraglottic cases, VHI trended towards better in those treated with TLM (9 TLM, 11.5 RT/CRT). Median FOSS scores were identical.

In the TLM glottic group one patient developed a small post-operative hemorrhage, which did not require any intervention. No patients required temporary or permanent tracheostomy, and none required nasogastric feeding. One patient in the RT/CRT group required nasogastric nutrition and three patients were unable to tolerate chemotherapy and the treatment discontinued.

### Discussion

Following the Department of Veterans Affairs Laryngeal Cancer Group trial the management of laryngeal cancer shifted towards chemoradiation [6]. During the 1990's it was noted by Hoffman et al. that with the increased use of CRT, the 5-year survival for T3N0M0 laryngeal cancer had declined [7]. More recently, there continues to be much debate regarding best treatment practices for advanced laryngeal tumours, in particular a move back towards primary surgical treatment.

Total laryngectomy (TL) is frequently used to treat T3 glottic carcinoma with or without (chemo) radiotherapy. Although good oncological results are achieved with TL, the operation has obvious functional sequelae. Published 5-year locoregional control and overall survival range from 69 to 87 % and 53 to 56 % respectively [8–10]. Open partial laryngectomy also has good locoregional control and overall survival with 5-year rates between 73 and 83 % and 71 to75% respectively [11, 12]. In this study, our locoregional control and overall survival for T3 glottic carcinomas treated with TLM are similar to that of open laryngeal procedures, with locoregional control of 87 % and 2 year overall survival of 68 %.

Radiotherapy alone in the absence of chemotherapy has been shown to have poorer outcomes. Chemotherapy, however, is contraindicated in patients with poorer general health. In patients who therefore have a favourable tumour location, yet in whom chemotherapy is a contraindication, TLM is without question a reasonable surgical option.

As this was not a randomized study, those patients selected for TLM may have had favourable anatomy and tumour location. Because of this fact, a direct comparison of the two groups should be interpreted cautiously. However, management with TLM did not appear to jeopardize oncological outcomes in those selected for this minimally invasive approach.

The low numbers within groups make the study underpowered to detect clinically significant differences between treatments. However, adequate sample size for this study to power the log rank test this to be able to detect the difference between a 5-year survival of 0.8 to

0.7 are would require over 1000 cases, and would be difficult to obtain this sample size outside of a national database.

The cases in this trial were not selected for treatment by patient and tumour characteristics and were not randomized. There are two potential differences in the characteristics of persons between treatment modalities that, while not statistically significant, are concerning with respect to the comparability of treatment groups. The first is the increased mean age of those undergoing radiation therapy alone. This would be expected as age greater then 70–75 is a relative contraindication to CRT. This is the cutoff that has been excluded from most CRT trials, and there is a higher rate of significant morbidity associated with CRT in those over 70–75. The second is the fact that 75 % of all N2 and N3 disease was treated by CRT. N2 or N3 disease upstages T3 laryngeal cancer to stage IVa and IVb respectively. This relative overrepresentation of more advanced disease in the CRT group may underestimate the efficacy of this modality when compared to TLM and RT groups.

Although this study showed reasonably low complication rates in those receiving chemoradiotherapy, chemotherapy in addition to the radiotherapy is known to have associated significant toxicity with mucositis, leukopenia and a 2 % increase in early deaths secondary to acute toxicity [13–15]. As complications were not prospectively recorded, mucositis and leukopenia were not accurately documented in this study and it is likely that compared to surgical complications, they were underreported.

When locoregional recurrence does occur in patients treated with TLM, options for management include further TLM, RT/CRT or open partial or total laryngectomy. For patients treated primarily with RT/CRT, although salvage surgery is possible the rate of complications in particular pharyngocutaneous fistula, the need for microvascular or regional flaps, complexity of surgery and the overall cost of prolonged hospital stay significantly increase [16, 17]. Complications of salvage treatment were not specifically reviewed in this study. Anecdotal evidence suggests complications from salvage surgery are likely to be less if radiotherapy can be avoided.

Over the study period, the senior authors selection of patients for TLM has changed. As surgical experience in TLM increased for early glottic carcinoma and expertise has developed, so too was there an increase in the T3 cases treated with TLM. Bernal-Sorekelsen et al. reported that for locally advanced tumours, a significant difference in the experience of the surgeon altered the complication rate, in particular bleeding and aspiration pneumonia [18]. They recommended for TLM "beginners" even when experienced in external approaches, to accumulate a significant experience with early staged

tumors before attempting to treat advanced cases in this manner.

It has been the experience of the senior author, and also discussed in the literature, that T3 glottic tumours with vocal cord fixation are more likely to develop local recurrence [19]. Cord fixation may be due to a number of factors, including cricoarytenoid joint involvement, muscle infiltration or paraglottic space involvement. Whilst true cord fixation is both a poorer prognostic factor for TLM and more likely to result in post-operative aspiration, paraglottic involvement does not carry such a poor prognosis. Therefore careful pre-operative image review and clinical assessment of the patient is imperative. As noted by Vilaseca et all, pre-epiglottic space involvement is associated with a better prognosis for TLM, as the pre-epiglottic space can be easily exposed and wider margins achieved with good functional outcomes. It is our opinion that the same can be said for isolated paraglottic space invasion in T3 glottic cancer.

## Conclusion

The use of transoral laser microsurgery for advanced laryngeal cancer is controversial. With over a decade of increasing experience with TLM for early glottic cancer, our institution is expanding the application of TLM to selected T3 glottic carcinoma. Oncological outcomes are not jeopardized by this approach and the treatment is well tolerated by patients with few complications. The data reported herein supports the ongoing use of TLM for selected T3 glottic cancers at our centre.

**Abbreviations**
CRT, chemoradiotherapy; FOSS, functional outcome swallow study; RT, radiotherapy; SCC, squamous cell carcinoma; TLM, transoral laser microsurgery; U.S, United States; VHI, voice handicap index

**Acknowledgements**
No acknowledgements to be made. No funding was obtained for the study.

**Authors' contributions**
AB drafted the manuscript and contributed to statistical analysis. MR and JS collated the data and contributed to statistical analysis. RH and JT helped draft and edit the manuscript. MT conceived the study and was the primary operating surgeon in the surgical cases. All authors read and confirmed the script.

**Competing interests**
The authors declare that they have no competing interests.

**References**
1.  Strong MS, Jacko GJ. Laser surgery in the larynx. Early clinical experience with continuous CO2 laser. Ann Otol Rhinol Laryngol. 1972;81:791–8.
2.  Canis M, Martin A, Ihlen F, Wolff H, Kron M, Matthias C, Steiner W. Transoral laser microsurgery in treatment of pT2 and pT3 glottic laryngeal squamous cell carcinoma-results of 391 patients. Head Neck. 2014;36(6):859–66.
3.  Canis M, Ihler F, Martin A, Wolff H, Mathias C, Steiner W. Results of 226 patients with T3 laryngeal carcinoma after treatment with transoral laser microsurgery. Head Neck. 2014;36:652-9. doi:10.1002/hed.23338.

4.  Rigby M, Reynolds L, Hart R, Trites J, Brown T, Taylor SM. T2 glottic carcinoma: analysis of recurrences in 36 cases undergoing primary transoral laser microsurgery resection. J Otolaryngol Head Neck Surg. 2012;41:S1.

5.  Edge SB, Amercian Joint Committee on Caner. AJCC cancer staging manual. 7th ed. New York: Springer; 2010.

6.  VA Laryngeal Cancer Study Group. Induction chemotherapy plus radiation compared with surgery plus radiation in patients with advanced laryngeal cancer. The Department of Veterans Affairs Laryngeal Cancer Study Group. N ENgl J Med. 1991;324:1685–90.

7.  Hoffman HT, Porter K, Karnell LH, et al. Laryngeal caner in the United States: changes in demographics, patterns of care, and survival. Laryngoscope. 2006;116:1–13.

8.  Razack MS, Maipang T, Sako K, Bakamjian V, Shedd DP. Management of advanced glottic carcinomas. Am J Surg. 1989;158:318–20.

9.  Bryant GP, Poulsen MG, Tripcony L, DIckie GJ. Treatment decisions in T3N0M0 glottic carcinoma. Int J Radiation Oncol Bio Phys. 1995;31:285–93.

10. Foote RL, Olsen KD, Buskirk SJ, Stanley RJ, Suman VJ. Laryngectomy alone for T3 glottic cancer. Head Neck. 1994;16:406–12.

11. Biller HF, Lawson W. Partial laryngectomy for vocal cord cancer marked limitation or fixation of the vocal cord. Laryngoscope. 1986;96:61–4.

12. Vega SF, Scola B, Vega MF, Martinez T, Scola E. Laryngeal vertical partial surgery. Surgical techniques. Oncological and functional results. Article in Italian. Acta Otorhinolaryngol Ital. 1996;16:272–80.

13. Brizel DM, Albers ME, Fisher SR, et al. Hyperfractionated irradiation with or without concurrent chemoradiotherapy for locally advanced head and neck cancer. N Engl J Med. 1998;338:1798–804.

14. Jeremic B, Shibamoto T, Milicic B, et al. Hyperfractionated radiation therapy with or without concurrent low dose daily cisplatin in locally advanced squamous cell carcinoma of the head and neck: a prospective randomized trial. J Clin Oncol. 2000;18:1458–64.

15. Adelstein DJ, Adams GI LY, et al. An intergroup phase III comparison of standard radiation therapy and two schedules of concurrent chemoradiotherapy in patients with unresectable squamous cell head and neck cancer. J Clin Oncol. 2004;22:4665–73.

16. Scotton WJ, Nixon IJ, Pezier TF, et al. Time interval between primary radiotherapy and salvage laryngectomy: a predictor of pharyngocutaneous fistula formation. Eur Arch Otorhinolaryngol. 2013 Oct. (Epub ahead of print).

17. Ganley I, Patel S, Matsuo J, et al. Post operative complications of salvage total laryngectomy. Cancer. 2005;103(10):2071–81.

18. Vilaseca I, Bernal-Sprekelsen M, Blanch J. Transoral laser microsurgery for T3 laryngeal tumours: prognostic factors. Head Neck. 2010;32:929–38.

19. Bernal-Sprekelson M, Caballero-Borrego M. The learning curve in transoral laser microsurgery for malignant tumors of the larynx and hypophrynx: parameters for a leveled surgical approach. Eur Arch Otorhinolaryngology. 2013;270:623–8.

# 24

# The McGill Thyroid Nodule Score's (MTNS+) role in the investigation of thyroid nodules with benign ultrasound guided fine needle aspiration biopsies: a retrospective review

Sarah Khalife[1], Sarah Bouhabel[1], Veronique-Isabelle Forest[2], Michael P. Hier[2], Louise Rochon[3], Michael Tamilia[4] and Richard J. Payne[1,2*]

## Abstract

**Background:** Ultrasound guided fine needle aspiration (USFNA) biopsies of thyroid nodules sometimes create a decision-making dilemma for surgeons as they may yield falsely benign results. The McGill Thyroid Nodule Score + (MTNS+) was developed to aid in clinical guidance regarding the management of patients with these USFNA results. The aim of this study was to assess the MTNS+ as a clinical tool in patients with benign preoperative thyroid nodule USFNAs and to analyze the relationship between nodule size and malignancy in these patients.

**Methods:** We conducted a retrospective chart review of 1312 patients who underwent thyroidectomies between 2010 and 2015 at the McGill University Teaching Hospitals. Patients with Bethesda II (benign) USFNA results, calculated MTNS+, and nodule size evaluated on ultrasound were included in the study. The false-negative rate was calculated, and MTNS+ and nodule size were each compared to final pathology results. Binary logistic regression was used for statistical analysis.

**Results:** Of the 1312 patients, 101 met the inclusion criteria and together had an average MTNS+ score of 6.83, which corresponds to a predicted malignancy rate between 25 and 33 %. Final pathology revealed malignancy in 16 (15.8 %) subjects. The average MTNS+ of patients with malignant nodules on surgical pathology was 8.25, while that of patients with benign nodules was 6.56.
Patients with nodule size 1–1.9 cm (a) and 2–2.9 cm (b) each had an equal rate of malignancy of 2.97 % (n = 3), nodule size 3–3.9 cm (c) had a rate of 1.98 % (n = 2), and nodule size ≥4 cm (d) a rate of 7.92 % (n = 8).

**Conclusion:** The rate of malignancy (15.8 %) is higher than expected when reviewing the risk of malignancy in nodules considered as Bethesda class 2. On the other hand, the rate is lower than the 25–33 % predicted by the MTNS+. We also found a higher malignancy rate for nodules above 4 cm in size, but size was a poor predictor of malignancy when used alone. Therefore, while the MTNS+ may be helpful at helping to identify USFNAs that are incorrectly classified as benign, the percentage risk of malignancy is lower than expected.

**Keywords:** McGill Thyroid Nodule Score, Thyroid cancer, Ultrasound-guided fine needle aspiration biopsy, Benign nodule, Bethesda II, Nodule size

* Correspondence: rkpayne@sympatico.ca
[1]Department of Otolaryngology-Head and Neck Surgery, McGill University Health Centre, 1001 Boulevard Decarie, Montreal, QC, Canada
[2]Department of Otolaryngology-Head and Neck Surgery, Sir Mortimer B. Davis-Jewish General Hospital, McGill University, 3755 Côte Ste-Catherine Road, Montreal, QC, Canada
Full list of author information is available at the end of the article

## Background

The incidence of thyroid cancer has been significantly and rapidly increasing in Canada over the past 30 years [1, 2]. Ultrasound-guided fine needle aspiration (USFNA) biopsy is currently considered the gold standard for the assessment and management of thyroid nodules. While it is undeniable that USFNAs provide very important information as to the nature of the nodule, they may yield a falsely benign result in 5 % of cases [3, 4]. Given the potential health implications of misclassifying malignant thyroid nodules as benign, it is necessary to find a complementary clinical tool to evaluate the risk of malignancy and properly select patients who require surgery.

Previous studies [1, 5, 6] advocate the McGill Thyroid Nodule Score + (MTNS+), as a valuable scoring-system used to accurately determine a patient's overall risk of malignancy. The MTNS+ is based on 23 known thyroid cancer risk factors, which are tabulated and then assigned a percentage risk of malignancy (Table 1) [6].

**Table 1** McGill Thyroid Nodule Score Plus (MTNS+) Scoring Template

## McGill Thyroid Nodule Score +

### Clinical Parameters and Labs

| | | | |
|---|---|---|---|
| 1. Gender | Male | 1 | _____ |
| 2. Age | > 45 yr | 1 | _____ |
| 3. Palpable nodule | present | 1 | _____ |
| 4. TSH levels | TSH > 1.4mlU/L | 1 | _____ |
| 5. Serum Thyroglobulin (Tg) levels | Tg > 75ng/mL | 1 | _____ |
| | Tg > 187.5ng/mL | 2 | _____ |
| 6. Consistency | stone / bone hard | 2 | _____ |
| 7. Ionizing radiation exposure | present | 3 | _____ |
| 8. Family history of thyroid cancer | present | 3 | _____ |
| 9. Ethnicity (Filipino, Hawaii, Iceland) | present | 3 | _____ |

### Ultrasound & PET Scan

| | | | |
|---|---|---|---|
| 1. Echogenicity | hypoechoic | 1 | _____ |
| 2. Increased vascularity | present | 1 | _____ |
| 3. Shape | taller than wide | 1 | _____ |
| 4. Calcifications | coarse calcifications | 1 | _____ |
| | microcalcifications | 2 | _____ |
| 5. Enlarging | more than 10% | 1 | _____ |
| | more than 30% | 2 | _____ |
| 6. Lymphadenopathy | present | 2 | _____ |
| 7. Size | 2-2.9cm | 2 | _____ |
| | 3-3.9cm | 3 | _____ |
| | 4cm or greater | 4 | _____ |
| 8. PET scan focally positive | present | 4 | _____ |

### Cytology

| | | | |
|---|---|---|---|
| 1. Hürthle cell lesion | present | 2 | _____ |
| 2. Favour neoplasm | present | 3 | _____ |
| 3. Atypia (not reactive) | mild | 3 | _____ |
| | moderate | 4 | _____ |
| | severe / significant | 5 | _____ |
| 4. Suspicious for malignancy | present | 7 | _____ |
| 5. HBME-1 | present | 7 | _____ |
| 6. BRAF mutation (molecular analysis) | present | 7 | _____ |

Score Interpretation (Risk of Malignancy)
| | | |
|---|---|---|
| 0-1 – <5% | 7-8 – 33% | 15-18 – 79% |
| 2-3 – 14% | 9-11 – 65% | 19-22 – 92% |
| 4-6 – 25% | 12-14 – 71% | 23+ – >95% |

**Final Score:** _____

TSH Thyroid stimulating hormone. Tg Thyroglobulin. PET Positron emission tomography

This study aims to assess the accuracy of the MTNS+ in predicting the risk of malignancy of thyroid nodules with benign USFNAs. The association between nodule size and malignancy rate is also evaluated. Findings could reduce the proportion of missed malignancies and improve management of patients with thyroid nodules.

## Methods

Multi-center ethics review approval was obtained from Research Ethics Committees at the Jewish General Hospital (JGH) and the McGill University Health Centre (MUHC).

We conducted a retrospective chart review of 1312 patients who underwent thyroidectomies at the McGill University Teaching Hospitals between January 2010 and March 2015. 101 patients (7.7 %) met inclusion criteria that consisted of having Bethesda II (benign) USFNA biopsy results, pre-operative calculated MTNS+ scores and recorded nodule size on ultrasound. We excluded patients with unavailable pre-operative MTNS+, USFNA and nodule size results. All USFNA samples were obtained by endocrinologists, thyroid surgeons, or radiologists. Collected information on the MTNS+ was based on a scoring sheet that has been regularly filled out over many years when a patient consults the doctor. Positron emission tomography (PET) scan and BRAF mutation are the two MTNS+ variables that are not routinely measured.

MTNS+ and thyroid nodule size on ultrasound were each compared to final post-operative pathology classified as either benign or malignant. Papillary microcarcinomas with extrathyroidal extension (ETE) were considered malignant due to their unpredictable aggressive behaviour when associated with ETE [6, 7]. All other papillary microcarcinomas were considered benign, as they usually progress indolently [6, 7]. Using USFNA allowed us to ensure malignancy was assigned to the ipsilateral nodule that was biopsied, thus avoiding falsely assigning malignancy to benign nodules in patients with multinodular thyroid glands. The malignancy rate, the mean MTNS+, and the standard deviations were calculated for the group of patients with Bethesda II cytology, as well as within each subgroup: malignant and benign on surgical pathology results. Statistical analysis was done using Binary Logistic Regression for MTNS+ when compared to malignancy rates. Nodule size was separated into four categories: a) 1–1.9 cm, b) 2–2.9 cm, c) 3–3.9 cm, and d) ≥4 cm. Malignancy rates were calculated for each category and a receiver operating characteristic (ROC) curve was also computed for malignancy and nodule size as a continuous variable. Bivariate regression analysis and Spearman's correlations were run to compare MTNS+ and nodule size.

## Results

Of the 1312 charts reviewed, 101 patients (7.7 %) met inclusion criteria. Patient age ranged from 23 to 85, with a mean of 52 years old. There was a 6-fold female predominance with a male to female ratio of 14:87. Final pathology revealed malignancy in 16 subjects (15.8 %), while 85 (84.2 %) were benign. One of the 16 patients included in the malignant group had a microcarcinoma with ETE on final pathology. In this selected patient population, MTNS+ scores ranged from 1 to 18, with a mean value and standard deviation (SD) of 6.83 ± 2.31.

### MTNS+ and malignancy

Benign and malignant rates and densities for each MTNS+ are presented in Table 2 and Fig. 1, respectively. Amongst the 101 patients included in the study, all malignant nodules had an MTNS+ equal to or above 5, while benign nodules had MTNS+ values as low as 1. Average MTNS+ of patients with malignant pathology (8.25 ± 2.86 [95 % CI 6.72, 9.78]) was higher than MTNS+ of patients in the benign group (6.56 ± 2.11 [95 % CI 6.11, 7.02]) (Table 3). The MTNS+ mean difference between malignant and benign groups was 1.69 with 95 % confidence interval (CI) [0.11, 3.26].

**Table 2** Distribution of benign USFNA MTNS+ scores and their associated surgical pathology diagnosis

| MTNS | Total (n) | Benign n (%) | Malignant n (%) |
|---|---|---|---|
| 1 | 1 | 1 (1.0) | 0 (0.0) |
| 2 | 1 | 1 (1.0) | 0 (0.0) |
| 3 | 0 | 0 (0.0) | 0 (0.0) |
| 4 | 9 | 9 (8.9) | 0 (0.0) |
| 5 | 21 | 20 (19.8) | 1 (1.0) |
| 6 | 14 | 13 (12.9) | 1 (1.0) |
| 7 | 20 | 15 (14.9) | 5 (5.0) |
| 8 | 17 | 12 (11.9) | 5 (5.0) |
| 9 | 7 | 5 (5.0) | 2 (2.0) |
| 10 | 7 | 6 (5.9) | 1 (1.0) |
| 11 | 2 | 2 (2.0) | 0 (0.0) |
| 12 | 0 | 0 (0.0) | 0 (0.0) |
| 13 | 1 | 1 (1.0) | 0 (0.0) |
| 14 | 0 | 0 (0.0) | 0 (0.0) |
| 15 | 0 | 0 (0.0) | 0 (0.0) |
| 16 | 0 | 0 (0.0) | 0 (0.0) |
| 17 | 0 | 0 (0.0) | 0 (0.0) |
| 18 | 1 | 0 (0.0) | 1 (1.0) |
| Total | 101 | 85 (84.2) | 16 (15.8) |

*MTNS+* McGill Thyroid Nodule Score Plus. *USFNA* Ultrasound guided fine needle aspiration

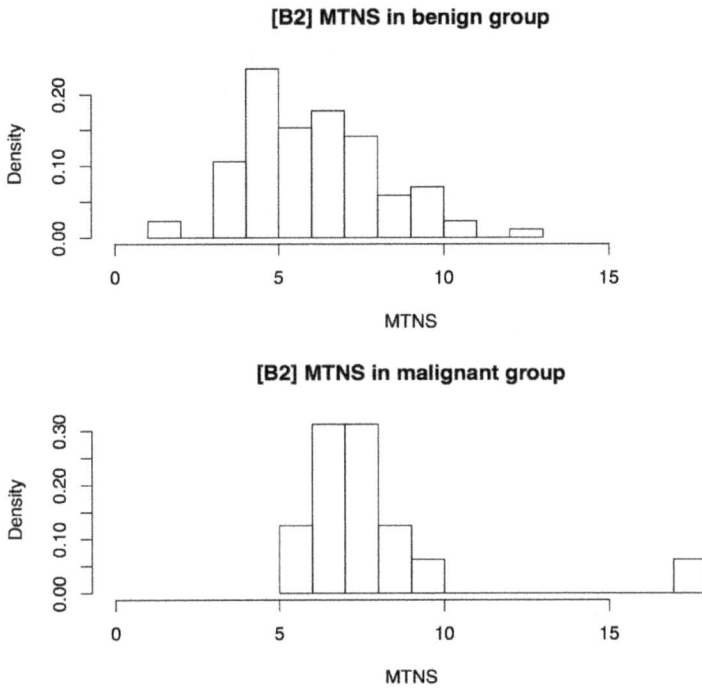

**Fig. 1** Frequency distribution of pre-operative MTNS+ in 101 thyroidectomy patients with Bethesda II USFNAs. Distribution of MTNS+ scores are displayed for thyroid nodules with: Top) Benign pathology on surgical biopsy, Bottom) Malignant pathology on surgical biopsy. MTNS+: McGill Thyroid Nodule Score Plus. USFNA: Ultrasound guided fine needle aspiration

A positive association between MTNS+ and malignancy was confirmed by logistic regression analysis with an odds ratio of 1.34 [95 % CI 1.05, 1.71].

### MTNS+ and nodule size
Largest nodule size on ultrasound ranged between 1 and 8.9 cm with a mean and standard deviation of 4.13 cm ±1.53. A positive correlation between MTNS+ and nodule size was shown by Spearman's correlation with an "r" coefficient value of 0.146 [95 % CI -0.05, 0.33]. The MTNS+ odds ratio was 1.52 [95 % CI 1.130, 2.044] when adjusted for nodule size through bivariate regression analysis. Patients with nodule size 1–1.9 cm had an OR of 16.2 [95 % CI 1.83, 143.427], those with nodule size 2–2.9 cm had an OR of 4.387 [95 % CI 0.806, 23.876], and nodule size 3–3.9 cm an OR of

0.341 [95 % CI 0.063, 1.832] when compared to nodules above 4 cm in size.

### Nodule size and malignancy
Benign and malignancy rates according to nodule size categories (cm) are presented in Table 4. Average nodule size was similar in patients with malignant and benign pathology (3.67 cm ±1.60, and 4.23 cm ±1.51, respectively). Patients with nodule size 1–1.9 cm (a) had a rate of malignancy of 2.97 % ($n = 3$), nodule size 2-2.9 cm (b) a rate of 2.97 % ($n = 3$), nodule size 3–3.9 cm (c) a rate of 1.98 % ($n = 2$), and nodule size ≥4 cm (d) a malignancy rate of 7.92 % ($n = 8$) (Fig. 2). ROC curve for nodule size and malignancy rate is presented in Fig. 3.

**Table 3** Distribution of MTNS+ scores within benign and malignant thyroid nodule categories confirmed on surgical pathology

| | Bethesda II Thyroid Nodules (N = 101) | | | | | | | | |
|---|---|---|---|---|---|---|---|---|---|
| | Benign (84.2 %) | | | | | Malignant (15.8 %) | | | |
| | N | Mean | StdDev | Min | Max | N | Mean | StdDev | Min | Max |
| MTNS | 85 | 6.56 | 2.11 | 1 | 13 | 16 | 8.25 | 2.86 | 5 | 18 |

*MTNS+* McGill Thyroid Nodule Score Plus. *StdDev* standard deviation

**Table 4** Association of benign USFNA nodule size and their corresponding surgical pathology diagnosis

| Nodule Size (cm) | Total n (%) | Benign n (%) | Malignant n (%) |
|---|---|---|---|
| a) 1–1.9 | 6 (5.94) | 3 (2.97) | 3 (2.97) |
| b) 2–2.9 | 9 (8.91) | 6 (5.94) | 3 (2.97) |
| c) 3–3.9 | 36 (35.64) | 34 (33.66) | 2 (1.98) |
| d) ≥4 | 50 (49.50) | 42 (41.58) | 8 (7.92) |
| Total | 101 (100) | 85 (84.16) | 16 (15.84) |

Nodule sizes were determined pre-operatively by ultrasound and were subdivided into categories a) 1–1.9 cm, b) 2–2.9 cm, c) 3–3.9 cm, d) ≥4 cm

*USFNA* Ultrasound guided fine needle aspiration

## Association Between Thyroid Nodule Size and Malignancy

Patients with malignant pathology (%)

| | 1–1.9 | 2–2.9 | 3–3.9 | >4 |
|---|---|---|---|---|
| ■ Benign | 2.97% | 5.94% | 33.66% | 41.58% |
| ■ Malignant | 2.97% | 2.97% | 1.98% | 7.92% |

Nodule Size (cm)

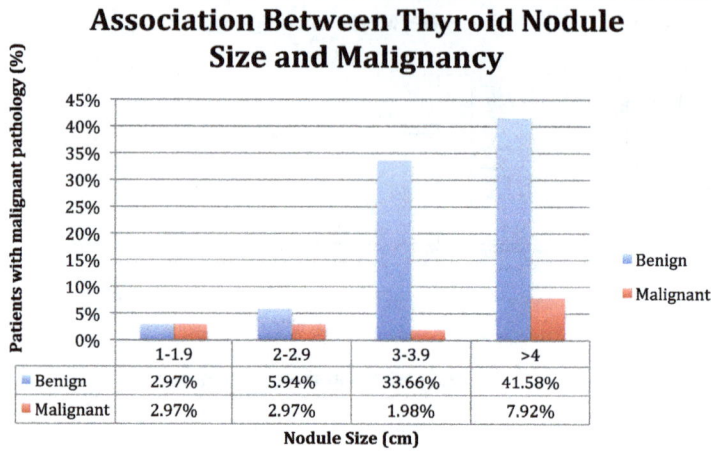

**Fig. 2** Association between thyroid nodule size and surgical pathology diagnosis in patients with benign USFNA biopsies. Nodule sizes on pre-operative ultrasounds were subdivided into categories a) 1–1.9 cm, b) 2–2.9 cm, c) 3–3.9 cm, d) ≥4 cm. USFNA: Ultrasound guided fine needle aspiration

## Discussion

Approximately 60 % of all performed USFNAs are Bethesda II (benign) on cytology [8] and should ideally result in a relief for patients, surgeons, and clinicians, in terms of treatment and prognosis. However, the 5 % false-negative rate of benign USFNAs [3, 9] cannot be disregarded. This is why the American Thyroid Association (ATA), the American Association of Clinical Endocrinologists (AACE) and the European Thyroid Association (ETA) suggest close observation of patients with follow-up ultrasounds 6–18 months later, and repeat USFNA if nodule growth is seen [3, 10].

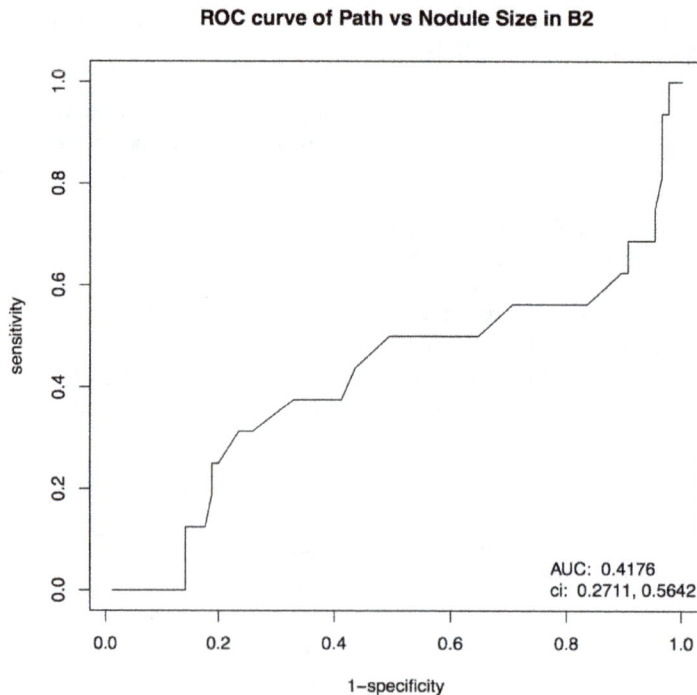

**ROC curve of Path vs Nodule Size in B2**

AUC: 0.4176
ci: 0.2711, 0.5642

**Fig. 3** Receiver operating characteristic curve for thyroid nodule size and risk of malignancy. Nodule size was determined by pre-operative ultrasound and malignancy was confirmed by post-operative pathology

Despite these recommendations, researchers continue to challenge the falsely benign rate stated by the Bethesda Classification [2, 9–11]. The 15.8 % rate of malignancy identified in our specific series is substantially higher than that predicted by Bethesda and ATA guidelines for benign USFNAs. Yet, it is consistent with the higher rates reported throughout literature, reaching values as high as 24.2 % [2, 5, 10–12]. This wide range may be explained in part by variations in technique, expertise and subjective interpreting differences between pathologists reading the slides and physicians performing ultrasounds and USFNAs in different institutions. Nevertheless, the difference remains significant. With this scientific scepticism, benign USFNA results will continue to pose a dilemma for the thyroid surgeon, particularly when known risk factors such as suspicious ultrasound findings or exposure to ionizing radiation are present.

Several studies recommend considering both cytology and suspicious ultrasound findings before making treatment decisions [10, 12]. Interestingly, Chernyavsky et al. found that a remarkable 90 % of falsely benign USFNAs (10.2 %) in their series had suspicious characteristics on ultrasound [10]. They go on to suggest repeat USFNA in these cases, in support of several other publications [10, 12, 13].

This is the reason that an evidence-based scoring system such as the MTNS+ assists in the pre-operative assessment of thyroid nodules. Its use could allow for earlier therapeutic decision-making. The MTNS+ has been shown to be an accurate tool for predicting the risk of malignancy [1, 6]. This 23-parameter summative tool (Table 1) proposed by Sands et al. and then modified in 2013 by Scheffler et al., was developed in order to help physicians formulate the management of thyroid nodules [1, 6]. It takes into consideration multiple evidence-based risk factors such as clinical factors (family history, exposure to radiation), worrisome ultrasound features, as well as cytology results. Combined into a single score, they enable a comprehensive identification of thyroid nodules that are more likely to harbour a malignant disease.

Our study succeeds in demonstrating that the MTNS+ can be helpful in patients with benign USFNAs, but not as precise as when assessing indeterminate nodules. The 101 patients with benign USFNA in our study had a mean MTNS+ of 6.83 (±2.31), a value that predicts a risk of malignancy between 25 and 33 % (Table 1). Although this predicted range overestimates the true 15.8 % rate found in our study (Tables 2 and 3), both values, in support of recent studies, prove to be significantly higher than the 0–5 % stated by the ATA guidelines and the Bethesda classification [3, 9]. This leads to the question of whether an additional USFNA parameter in which points are subtracted for patients with Bethesda II USFNA results

should be added to the MTNS+ in order to improve its accuracy. New studies are currently underway to answer this question.

With a statistically significant MTNS+ mean difference between malignant and benign nodules, it is clear that malignant nodules tend to have a higher MTNS+ score than benign nodules. In addition, the odds ratio of 1.34 suggests that for every increase in 1 point of MTNS+, there is an increase in 34 % in odds of malignancy for this patient population. When adjusted for nodule size in our bivariate regression analysis, the odds ratio for MTNS+ increases to 1.52 and remains statistically significant.

Williams et al., one of the only other Canadian-based studies, had also reported a falsely benign rate of 16 % [2]. Our equal malignancy rate supports their recommendation that physicians should consider the malignancy rate for the particular patient population being treated rather than solely relying on generalized literature values based on cytology [2]. At our institution it is uncommon for patients with benign USFNA's to undergo surgery. Only patients with a high index of suspicion using the MTNS+ had surgery and were included in this analysis. More specifically, this group of patients had either worrisome ultrasound characteristics or risk factors for thyroid cancer that were a cause for concern. The MTNS+ scoring system automatically calculates these variables and enables informed and improved communication with patients. Therefore, the decision was made to operate despite the USFNA results. Other factors that may have contributed in certain cases are the presence of anxiety, compressive symptoms, or if the patient feels that the risk is too high to leave the nodule there. As a result, the true malignancy rate of patients who did not undergo surgery remains unknown. Therefore, our study does not contradict the commonly quoted 0–3 % malignancy rate of benign USFNAs stated by the Bethesda Classification [9]. In addition, the selection bias when selecting thyroidectomy patients is inevitable in surgical studies. It may also differ from one institution to another since there is still no consensus and no universal algorithm used to increase suspicion index for patients with benign USFNAs.

Large nodule size has long been proposed as a risk factor for malignancy of thyroid nodules. This holds true for patients with benign USFNAs, as previous findings have shown falsely benign rates ranging from 10.4 to 17 % [14–17] in nodules larger than 3 or 4 cm, depending on the study. Our study only supports these findings for nodules above 4 cm in size, although the malignancy rate of 7.92 % was slightly lower than that found in other studies. Only 1.98 % of nodules between 3 and 3.9 cm were malignant, which is lower than that of smaller and larger nodules (Fig. 2). This could be explained by the small number of patients in each nodule size category. However, with a weak ROC curve (Fig. 3), and since 44.58 % of nodules were above 4 cm and benign on final pathology (Fig. 2), it is clear that nodule size is a poor predictor of malignancy when used alone for patients with benign USFNAs.

The major limitation of this study is the selection bias. All patients underwent thyroidectomy based on higher clinical suspicion of malignancy using the MTNS+. This leaves the true malignancy rate unknown for patients who did not undergo surgery. Unfortunately, this is the case for research involving surgical patients.

## Conclusion

With the uncertain malignancy rate of benign USFNAs, the multitude of possible risk factors and the presence of a spectrum of management alternatives (observation alone, to re-biopsy and even thyroidectomy), the ensuing discussion with the patient is often confusing, and leads to further anxiety. MTNS+ appeases this problem as it allows the physician to describe the risk of malignancy to the patient as an individualized percentage, thus simplifying communication [1]. While MTNS+ in patients with benign USFNAs plays a role in determining the management in patients with benign thyroid nodules, it is less powerful than USFNAs with indeterminate nodules.

### Abbreviations
USFNA: ultrasound guided fine needle aspiration; MTNS+: McGill Thyroid Nodule Score +; JGH: Jewish General Hospital; MUHC: McGill University Health Centre; ETE: extrathyroidal extension; ATA: American Thyroid Association; AACE: American Association of Clinical Endocrinologists; ETA: European Thyroid Association; PET: positron emission tomography.

### Competing interests
The authors declare that they have no competing interests.

### Authors' contributions
RP proposed the research topic and designed the study. SK reviewed the charts, completed the database, and performed initial data interpretation. These were revised by SB. SK authored the initial manuscript, which was subsequently reviewed and approved by SK, SB, RP, VF, MH, MT, LR. Result interpretation and important modifications were made by all authors to enable completion of this manuscript. All authors read and approved the final manuscript.

### Acknowledgements
We would like to acknowledge Dr. Lawrence Joseph for completing the statistical analyses of this study.

### Financial support/disclosures
Funding from the BioMed Central Membership of Canadian Society of Otolaryngology – Head and Neck Surgery.

### Author details
[1]Department of Otolaryngology-Head and Neck Surgery, McGill University Health Centre, 1001 Boulevard Decarie, Montreal, QC, Canada. [2]Department of Otolaryngology-Head and Neck Surgery, Sir Mortimer B. Davis-Jewish General Hospital, McGill University, 3755 Côte Ste-Catherine Road, Montreal, QC, Canada. [3]Department of Pathology, Sir Mortimer B. Davis-Jewish General Hospital, McGill University, 3755 Côte Ste-Catherine Road, Montreal, QC, Canada. [4]Department of Endocrinology and Metabolism, Sir Mortimer B. Davis-Jewish General Hospital, McGill University, 3755 Côte Ste-Catherine Road, Montreal, QC, Canada.

### References
1. Sands NB, Karls S, Amir A, Tamilia M, Gologan O, Rochon L, et al. McGill Thyroid Nodule Score (MTNS): "rating the risk," a novel predictive scheme for cancer risk determination. J Otolaryngol Head Neck Surg. 2011;40 Suppl 1:S1–13. Pubmed Abstract.
2. Williams BA, Bullock MJ, Trites JR, Taylor SM, Hart RD. Rates of thyroid malignancy by FNA diagnostic category. J Otolaryngol Head Neck Surg. 2013;42:61. doi:10.1186/1916-0216-42-61. PubMed Abstract | Publisher Full Text.
3. Cooper DS, Doherty GM, Haugen BR, Kloos RT, Lee SL, Mandel SJ, et al. Revised American thyroid association management guidelines for patients with thyroid nodules and differentiated thyroid cancer. Thyroid. 2009;19(11):1167–214. doi:10.1089/thy.2009.0110. Publisher Full Text.
4. Alexander EK, Heering JP, Benson CB, Frates MC, Doubilet PM, Cibas ES, et al. Assessment of nondiagnostic ultrasound-guided fine needle aspirations of thyroid nodules. J Clin Endocrinol Metab. 2002;87(11):4924–7. doi:10.1210/jc.2002-020865. PubMed Abstract | Publisher Full Text.
5. Varshney R, Forest VI, Mascarella MA, Zawawi F, Rochon L, Hier MP, et al. The Mcgill thyroid nodule score - does it help with indeterminate thyroid nodules? J Otolaryngol Head Neck Surg. 2015;44:2. doi:10.1186/s40463-015-0058-6. PubMed Abstract | Publisher Full Text.
6. Scheffler P, Forest VI, Leboeuf R, Florea AV, Tamilia M, Sands NB, et al. Serum thyroglobulin improves the sensitivity of the McGill Thyroid Nodule Score for well-differentiated thyroid cancer. Thyroid. 2014;24(5):852–7. doi:10.1089/thy.2013.0191. PubMed Abstract | Publisher Full Text.
7. Ardito G, Revelli L, Giustozzi E, Salvatori M, Fadda G, Ardito F, et al. Aggressive papillary thyroid microcarcinoma: prognostic factors and therapeutic strategy. Clin Nucl Med. 2013;38(1):25–8. doi:10.1097/RLU.0b013e318279bc65. PubMed Abstract | Publisher Full Text.
8. Ajmal S, Rapoport S, Ramirez Batlle H, Mazzaglia PJ. The natural history of the benign thyroid nodule: what is the appropriate follow-up strategy? J Am Coll Surg. 2015;220(6):987–92. doi:10.1016/j.jamcollsurg.2014.12.010. PubMed Abstract | Publisher Full Text.
9. Cibas ES, Ali SZ, Conference NCITFSotS. The Bethesda system for reporting thyroid cytopathology. Am J Clin Pathol. 2009;132(5):658–65. doi:10.1309/AJCPPHLWMI3JV4LA. PubMed Abstract | Publisher Full Text.
10. Chernyavsky VS, Shanker BA, Davidov T, Crystal JS, Eng O, Ibrahim K, et al. Is one benign fine needle aspiration enough? Ann Surg Oncol. 2012;19(5):1472–6. doi:10.1245/s10434-011-2079-3. PubMed Abstract | Publisher Full Text.
11. Deniwar A, Hambleton C, Thethi T, Moroz K, Kandil E. Examining the Bethesda criteria risk stratification of thyroid nodules. Pathol Res Pract. 2015;211(5):345–8. doi:10.1016/j.prp.2015.02.005. PubMed Abstract | Publisher Full Text.
12. Choi YJ, Jung I, Min SJ, Kim HJ, Kim JH, Kim S, et al. Thyroid nodule with benign cytology: is clinical follow-up enough? PLoS One. 2013;8(5), e63834. doi:10.1371/journal.pone.0063834. PubMed Abstract | Publisher Full Text.
13. Moon HJ, Kim EK, Kwak JY. Malignancy risk stratification in thyroid nodules with benign results on cytology: combination of thyroid imaging reporting and data system and Bethesda system. Ann Surg Oncol. 2014;21(6):1898–903. doi:10.1245/s10434-014-3556-2. PubMed Abstract | Publisher Full Text.
14. McCoy KL, Jabbour N, Ogilvie JB, Ohori NP, Carty SE, Yim JH. The incidence of cancer and rate of false-negative cytology in thyroid nodules greater than or equal to 4 cm in size. Surgery. 2007;142(6):837–44. doi:10.1016/j.surg.2007.08.012. discussion 44 e1-3. PubMed Abstract | Publisher Full Text.
15. Wharry LI, McCoy KL, Stang MT, Armstrong MJ, LeBeau SO, Tublin ME, et al. Thyroid nodules (>/=4 cm): can ultrasound and cytology reliably exclude cancer? World J Surg. 2014;38(3):614–21. doi:10.1007/s00268-013-2261-9. PubMed Abstract | Publisher Full Text.
16. Giles WH, Maclellan RA, Gawande AA, Ruan DT, Alexander EK, Moore Jr FD, et al. False negative cytology in large thyroid nodules. Ann Surg Oncol. 2015;22(1):152–7. doi:10.1245/s10434-014-3952-7. PubMed Abstract | Publisher Full Text.
17. Meko JB, Norton JA. Large cystic/solid thyroid nodules: a potential false-negative fine-needle aspiration. Surgery. 1995;118(6):996–1003. discussion -4. PubMed Abstract | Publisher Full Text.

# 25

# Exploring the psychological morbidity of waiting for sinus surgery using a mixed methods approach

Gordon Fung-Zak Tsang[1*], Carmen L. McKnight[2], Laura Minhui Kim[3] and John M. Lee[1,2*]

## Abstract

**Background:** Patients with chronic rhinosinusitis (CRS) often have to endure significant wait times for endoscopic sinus surgery (ESS). The pyschiatric impact of placement on a waitlist for ESS has not been explored.

**Methods:** Questionnaires measuring CRS symptom severity and health-related anxiety and stress (SNOT-22, HADS, WPAI-GH) were sent to patients diagnosed with CRS and currently on a waitlist for ESS. Fifteen representative waitlisted patients participated in one-on-one semi-structured interviews discussing their experience with their wait for ESS. A deductive thematic analysis was used to interpret the interview data using a quantitative driven mixed methods analysis.

**Results:** Participants waiting for ESS reported worsening clinical symptomatology during their waiting period. Participants reported waitlist and CRS impact on both work and social aspects of their lives. The HADS scale showed no overall significant level of depression or anxiety in the HADS screening questionnaire. The qualitative data describe the effects of the symptom burden of CRS.

**Conclusions:** Patients waitlisted for ESS did not demonstrate any significant level of psychiatric distress, however variability exists. The qualitative arm of this study elucidates how patients cope with their wait.

**Keywords:** Rhinology, Chronic rhinosinusitis, Anxiety, Depression, Mixed methods, Qualitative, Survey, HADS, WPAI, Waitlist, Endoscopic sinus surgery

## Background

Chronic rhinosinusitis (CRS) with or without nasal polyposis is an inflammatory condition involving the mucosa of the nose and paranasal sinuses affecting approximately 5–15 % of the Canadian population [1]. Although initial treatment is generally non-surgical, surgical intervention may be required and efficacious in patients who are refractory to maximal medical treatment in terms of symptom relief [1]. Due to persisting funding issues for elective surgeries in our health care system, the wait time for surgery for CRS is often lengthy, averaging 164 days in the province of Ontario [2]. There is significant institutional variability and in Toronto ranges between 93 and 413 days (at the time of the submission of this study) [2]. Patients are often

markedly symptomatic at the time of referral for surgery with previously demonstrated progression of Sinonasal Outcome Test 22 (SNOT-22) scores during their wait [3]. Thus, long wait times may significantly affect their psychological well-being and may lead to significant patient distress [4–13].

The current study explores the patient experience while waiting for ESS and the effect that wait times have on psychological morbidity and burden. A mixed methods approach was designed for this cross-sectional study. Questionnaires used include the SNOT-22, the Hospital Anxiety and Depression Scale (HADS), and the Work Productivity and Activity Impairment General Health (WPAI-GH) questionnaire. A qualitative component was used to help interpret and inform findings from the questionnaires and identify major contributors to psychological stressors.

* Correspondence: LeeJo@smh.ca
[1]Department of Otolaryngology-Head & Neck Surgery, University of Toronto, Toronto, ON, Canada
Full list of author information is available at the end of the article

## Methods

The study protocol was reviewed and approved by the central research ethics board (St. Michael's Hospital, Toronto, ON) prior to starting data collection and analysis.

### Patient population and data collection

Data was accrued from a cross-section through a cohort of patients currently on a single surgeon's (JL) waiting list for ESS for CRS during in 2014. The surgeon has a subspecialty focus in rhinology and anterior skull base surgery in a tertiary care hospital and there are approximately equal numbers of patients seen for primary and revision ESS for CRS. All patients were residents of Ontario, Canada. Inclusion criteria for participating patients on the waitlist include: documented diagnosis of CRS, patients underwent a trial of maximal medical therapy as outlined in current guidelines [1], ≥18 years of age, completed a consent to ESS for treatment of CRS (some consents included septoplasty as an adjunct procedure for obtaining adequate surgical access or when deemed required based on clinical symptoms), adequate fluency in English to provide informed consent and complete questionnaires, on waitlist for longer than 2 weeks. Exclusion criteria includes: patients who were pregnant or have been diagnosed with any of cystic fibrosis, immotile cilia syndrome, immunodeficiency syndrome, severe ongoing depression or drug addiction, or with medical reasons for delaying surgery. Additionally, we excluded patients who were urgently scheduled for ESS because of impending complications related to their illness (i.e. mucocele formation, significant skull base/orbital involvement). A chart review was performed on wait-listed patients producing a cohort of 68 patients who met study criteria (out of a total of 165 patients). An information sheet was mailed to all eligible participants inviting them to partake in a series of three questionnaires (SNOT-22, WPAI-GH, HADS).

During the chart review process, a sample of patients were purposefully chosen to provide a rich and meaningful representation of the experience of waiting for ESS. This sampling method is in keeping with qualitative studies [14]. The selected patients were then contacted by phone and asked to complete a series of three questionnaires and participate in a recorded, anonymous, one-on-one interview with the option of completing an in-person interview. The interview consisted of a verbal consent process followed by questions and were recorded on a digital recorder. The surgeon (JL) did not perform any of the interviews so as to minimize the risk of bias and also to allow participants to freely express their thoughts and feelings.

Participants in the quantitative study portion were asked to participate by completing three questionnaires only. A total of 26 participants completed the questionnaires in full. All questionnaires were completed as either a hard copy or online. Participants choosing to complete the

questionnaires online were emailed a unique identification code to input into a secured online survey website administered by Fluid Surveys (http://fluidsurveys.com/). The above selection process is summarized in Fig. 1.

### Demographic data

A chart review was performed for participating patients to ensure inclusion/exclusion criteria and to gather clinical and demographic data. A current "wait-time" was determined by calculating the number of days between the day their surgical consent was completed from the completion day of their questionnaires.

### Questionnaires

The SNOT-22 is a validated clinical tool used to objectively describe patient symptom from CRS burden and track clinical outcomes. It was used to help in the characterization of the patient population currently under study. The HADS tool is a 14 item self-implemented questionnaire that is divided into two sections, each designed to screen for states of anxiety and depression in the setting of a hospital medical outpatient clinic [15]. Each item is scored on a 4-point ordinal scale (range 0 to 3 with a higher score representing greater symptom severity) with a maximum total score of 21 in each depression and anxiety scales. The WPAI-GH questionnaire measures the impact of the patient's condition on both their work and non-work activities over a seven day recall period prior to its completion [16]. This general health questionnaire was chosen specifically for two reasons. Firstly, a specific version for CRS has not been validated. Secondly, CRS is often comorbid with other airway disorders (i.e., asthma) or upper airway infections and the disease processes can often interact. The questionnaire consists of six questions regarding the current state of

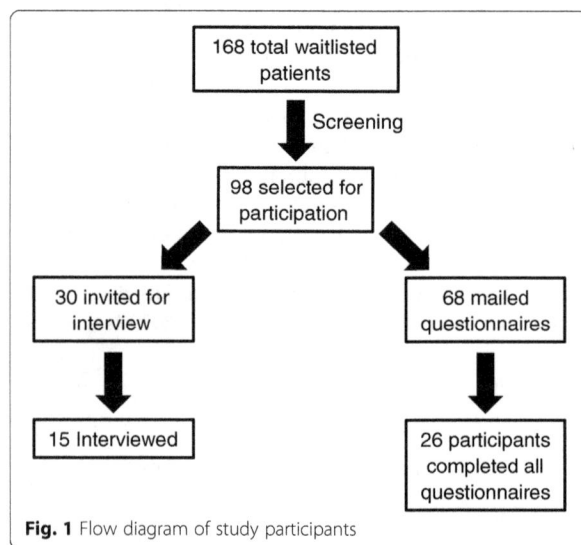

**Fig. 1** Flow diagram of study participants

employment, hours missed due to health problems, hours missed for other reasons, hours actually worked, and degree that health affected productivity in regular unpaid activities [17]. Four main outcomes are generated from the WPAI-GH and expressed in percentages: 1) percent work time missed due to health for those who were currently employed; 2) percent impairment while working due to health for those who were currently employed and actually worked in the past seven days; 3) percent overall work impairment due to health for those who were currently employed; and 4) percent activity impairment due to health for all respondents [17].

## Patient interviews

The interviews were all performed in a one-on-one format. A single interviewer performed all the interviews (GT) in a semi-structured format. An interview guide was developed by the authors and used during the interviews to extract important themes (Fig. 2). Follow up questions were asked by the interviewer to clarify or develop thoughts and ideas from patients as needed. Exploration or other themes took place only if the interviewee introduced them. No time limit was set for the interviews, but the average interview was approximately 15 min long. The recorded interviews were transcribed and coded by the interviewer (GT) and subsequently proofread for accuracy by a second reviewer independently. The interviews were analyzed by the two aforementioned reviewers using a deductive thematic analysis approach. Using this approach, the goal was to extract data to help explain the quantitative results from the surveys. For the purposes of the qualitative study, an a priori target minimum of 10 participant interviews was established. Given the research question, no more than 10 interviews were seen to be needed especially since a broad range of waitlisted participants were selected. A total of 15 interviews were completed to ensure information saturation. After the interviews, the participants were also requested to complete a set of questionnaires.

| Q1 | What has been your experience with being on a wait-list for sinus surgery? |
| Q2 | How long have you currently been waiting for sinus surgery (symptom onset/diagnosis/referral/consent)? |
| Q3 | What is your biggest concern regarding the wait for your surgery? |
| Q4 | Do you feel that your life has been affected by the wait? <yes> To Q5  <no> To Q6 |
| Q5 | How has the wait impacted your life? a. Has there been a change in your outlook in life? b. Do you feel that your life has been limited in any way by the wait? c. Any days missed form work or school due to your CRS? d. Are there any limitations on your social life because of your CRS? |
| Q6 | How did you feel when you learned that you would have to wait for surgery, and how has this changed/evolved throughout the waiting period? |
| Q7 | How has your level of anxiety been throughout the waiting period? |
| Q8 | What coping strategies have you used to deal with some of the changes you face with waiting for surgery? If available, what type of assistance would help improve your experience? |
| Q9 | In your opinion, what would be an appropriate maximum wait time for you or a person like with CRS waiting for sinus surgery? |

**Fig. 2** Interview Guide

## Data analysis

Standard summary statistics were calculated for all survey results. All statistical tests were 2-sided with $P$ values less than 0.05 deemed significant. Statistical analysis (linear regression) was performed on SPSS version 23.0.

## Results
### Demographics

A total of 26 patients completed the questionnaires, demographics data is shown in Table 1. The average age of participants surveyed was $50.7 \pm 12.5$ years of age. There were an approximately equal number of male and female participants (14 males and 12 females). The average wait time at the time of completion of the surveys was 216 with a range of 31–425 days in patients who volunteered to complete the study. Demographics data was compared between the qualitative and questionnaire groups of patients to ensure homogeneity between participants from the two groups. Sex, average age, wait times, and SNOT-22 scores in the qualitative group of patients were similar to that of the questionnaire only group and no statistical difference was found between these two groups ($P = 0.96$ for SNOT-22).

### SNOT-22

The average SNOT-22 score in this group was $60.8 \pm 23.9$, which is equivalent to scores seen in CRS patients [18]. The four most frequently reported worst symptoms on the SNOT-22 were nasal obstruction, lack of a good night's sleep, waking up tired, and loss of smell or taste. A comparison was made between the SNOT-22 score from the questionnaires and from a baseline SNOT-22 score done at the time of their consent for surgery. Their scores at the time of consent were an average of 51.8, demonstrating an increase in this cohort by a score of 9 during their present wait, using a paired $t$-test analysis ($p = 0.01$) (Fig. 3).

### HADS outcomes

The HADS tool allows for two-factor (anxiety and depression) analysis within a single clinical measurement tool [19]. The average score for the anxiety scale (HADS-

**Table 1** Patient demographics from the questionnaire group

| Characteristic | Average (SD) |
|---|---|
| All patients | $n = 26$ |
| Age | 50.7 (12.5) years |
| Male | $n = 14$ |
| Previous ESS | 12 |
| Wait time[a] | 216 (104) days |
| Median wait time | 255 days |

[a]As calculated by subtracting the time when the patient completed the questionnaires and when they consented for surgery

184        Head and Neck Surgery: Advances in Otolaryngology

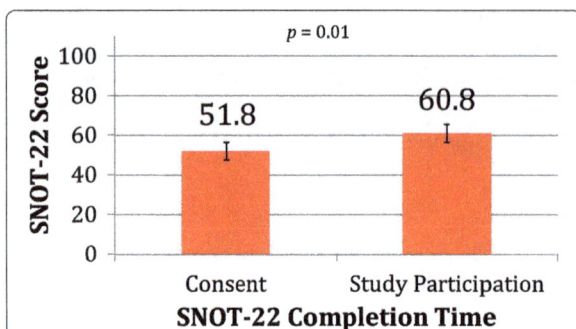

**Fig. 3** SNOT-22 score at time of consent compared to completion by same participants at the time of the study

A) was 7.1 ± 4.2 with nine people scoring 8 or higher. The depression scale (HADS-D) average was 7.6 ± 5.2 with thirteen people scoring 8 or higher. The total score average for the HADS was 14.7 ± 8.6. Scores of ≥8 the HADS-A and HADS-D scales suggest a high likelihood of clinically significant anxiety or depression, respectively. A score of >15 for the HADS scale increases the positive predictive value of the scales [15]. Its clinical utility has been evaluated in previous literature and has been shown to have good (specificity 80 %, sensitivity 90 %) validity as a screening measurement of generalized anxiety [20, 19]. No correlation found between the total HADS score and the length of wait experienced by patients ($R^2 < 0.1$) in our linear regression analysis.

**WPAI-GH outcomes**

According to the questionnaire, 18 of the 26 patients answered that they were working at the time of the study. At the time that the survey was administered, the workers reported absence from their jobs 4.8 ± 13.6 % as a result of their CRS related health issues. The questionnaire findings show that despite a relatively low amount of missed work days, the reported impairment was 34.4 ± 27.9 % with a range between 0 and 90 % as a result of their symptoms. A much greater degree of impairment was found in non-work related activities (i.e., recreational, household, etc.), 50.8 ± 20.5 % with a range between 0 and 90 %. Findings are summarized in Table 2.

**Table 2** WPAI-GH questionnaire results

| Patients who worked for pay | n = 18 | Mean (SD) % |
|---|---|---|
| Percent of work time missed due to health | 18 | 4.8 (13.6) |
| Percent impairment while working due to health | 18 | 34.4 (27.9) |
| Percent overall work impairment due to health | 18 | 36.4 (30.1) |
| Percent activity impairment due to health | 26 | 50.8 (29.5) |

**Qualitative interview results**

Deductive thematic analysis of the 15 interviews yielded the following recurring themes:

**There is a multifactorial contribution to patients' frustration with being on a lengthy wait list for surgical treatment for CRS**

Patients stated that despite expectations of a wait, it was longer than expected. Other unrelated health care experiences were used in several instances to reflect upon their experiences positively or negatively.

*"I wasn't surprised because I know that's how it is in Canada for most surgeries, but I didn't expect it to be this long for the wait. My friend went into another doctor for her tonsils on the same day I did and she got a call back a month later and was booked in for 3 months later. So I was expecting a shorter wait."*

*"Within the time I've been waiting for [sinus surgery], I've been diagnosed, treated, and I'm on the recovery road from a hip replacement surgery...that didn't take long at all."*

Fear of progression of CRS and the unpredictability of their symptoms was a source of personal feelings of anxiety, which was exacerbated by a longer wait.

*"I expected to wait because it wasn't an urgent situation. As I've said, I've lived with it for decades. If I have to wait a year, I was totally okay with that...If there was a situation where my health was at risk (i.e., cancer), I would be concerned and anxious. But in this case, none."*

**Having a predetermined date regardless of wait time for surgery was the only thing which was persistently described as something that would improve their experience while being on a wait list for surgery**

*"It would be helpful if I had a date for [this surgery], even if it's in the future at least I can plan on it. I guess other than that, it's the anxiety of not knowing when the surgery is. If they said it's a year from now and given me a date, that would have been helpful."*

**Symptoms did not contribute to patients feeling depressed**

Most patients in this cohort did not have difficulty coping with their illness when prompted, nor did they see the need to develop any specific coping strategies to help deal with the wait or their symptoms.

When asked specifically about feeling depressed, patients did not indicate that they felt depressed about their wait list situation specifically.

*"The bad days, I'm not depressed. I'm kind of sad. I have to go to work and sit there for 8 hours, have my nose plugged up and a stuffy forehead kind of experience. Nothing where I don't feel like waking up, nothing that bad."*

There was concern from a number of patients regarding whether there would be progression of their symptoms prior to surgery and the unpredictable nature of CRS exacerbations.

**Patients felt that they were significantly affected in their personal lives in social situations and at home by their CRS symptoms**

Seven patients described that their symptoms of CRS directly or indirectly affected their social situations. Patients did not generally avoid social situations but many were self-conscious about their symptoms and had to find ways to manage their symptoms and in some occasions avoided social encounters to avoid embarrassment.

*"I'm a little self-conscious about my nose continuing to run, the need to blow [my] nose, that kind of thing. I wouldn't say avoiding social situations but certainly... bring Kleenex everywhere I go. I'm aware, if I'm in a social situation, I'm constantly conscious of it. I don't want have a runny nose while I'm talking to somebody (laughs)."*

Two interviewees described an inability to get restful sleep as a factor that had an impact on their home and social activities.

*"I haven't let it impact my social life. The only thing is, you're not a 100 % there if you're kind of tired. Actually, I would say it has because...I go to bed really early because I'm tired. My friend and my husband all complain that I don't last past 9[pm], whereas before I would be awake until 1 or 2 at night. Because I don't sleep well, I get tired easily, especially towards the end of the day."*

Work productivity was impaired mostly from an inability to get a restful sleep. Work absences were only attributable to periods of acute exacerbations in CRS patients interviewed and were worse during certain times of the year.

*"If you don't sleep well, it affects your productivity and your focus at work. Also, it's disturbing to my husband. Sometimes, you know, when I wake up at night, he can tell. He says, "I can tell you didn't sleep well at all." Sometimes, I'll have to go to the living room, get some cushions and sleep in a really inclined position."*

A majority of patients described no particularly difficulty coping with their CRS in the context of a waitlist for the following reasons: dealing with a benign disease, strength of the physician-patient relationship, relief they were receiving appropriate treatment, and that they were adequately educated about the process and their disease

These were also factors that resulted in patients tolerating a prolonged wait despite being offered a referral by the primary surgeon to other sinus surgeons with shorter wait times. When asked, twelve of the interviewees in our study suggested that a six month wait should be the maximum amount of time to wait for CRS.

The interviewees described that they understood that CRS was not a life-threatening illness and mentioned that they were willing to accept some wait time for ESS in the face of a budget-restricted health care system.

**Discussion**

This is the first study to evaluate patient experience while on a wait list for elective surgery for CRS. Although a previous study has shown that CRS symptom severity correlates with a high HADS score at the time of clinical evaluation [21], what happens to these patients is unknown while they are waiting for surgery. Unfortunately, long wait times for ESS has become common as health care expenditures are increasingly restricted. Therefore, the question arose of whether simply waiting on a wait list for surgery independently had any measurable amounts of psychiatric distress.

Interestingly, many patients in our study reported overall less than expected levels of anxiety and depression as measured on HADS despite a high level of symptom severity as measured by the SNOT-22. This may seem contrary to a finding that pre-operative patients at the time of consent considered the potential wait time to be a significant concern before undergoing elective ESS [22]. Our qualitative research indicated that there were a number of factors allowing them to cope with their disease, thus likely limiting psychiatric distress. Notably, an important recurring theme was that patients felt relieved that a plan of treatment was established with their surgeon in the context of a disease that is chronic and will require ongoing medical therapy. The act of being placed on a waitlist may entirely be somewhat beneficial, regardless of wait time. However, it is important to re-emphasize to patients that surgery itself is not curative but the entire goal of ESS is to enable better long term management and control.

The results from the WPAI in our CRS population mirror those from Stankiewicz et al., examining the at the effect of CRS on work productivity [23]. Although there was minimal absenteeism from the workplace (4.8 % time absent from work) as a result of CRS symptoms, our findings demonstrate high levels of impairment with respect to workplace productivity (36.4 %) and non-work or social activities (50.8 %). Although patients were still able to perform necessary activities (i.e., work attendance), it was clear from our qualitative analysis that home lives and ability to interact socially were significantly impaired almost solely by CRS related symptoms.

ESS has now been established to clearly and effectively reduce CRS symptoms while improving quality of life, at least temporarily [22, 24]. Ours is the second study to demonstrate worsening of CRS symptoms (SNOT-22) during the pre-operative wait period. Smith et al. have previously shown both worsening SNOT-22 scores and increased medication usage while waiting for ESS [22]. The mechanism of worsening symptoms was unclear through our qualitative data. However, patients interviewed for our study described that the continued use and the potential for an increasing reliance on medications (particularly oral antibiotics and oral steroids) was an important contributor to their subjective levels of anxiety. Hypothetically, with increasing wait times for ESS, the combination of both progression of CRS symptoms and increasing reliance on systemic medications could push patients to clinically significant levels of psychological distress.

It is also important to note that there was considerable variability with respect to both SNOT-22 and HADS measurements in the tested population. This raises the question of whether there are smaller subsets of patients who are affected to a greater degree and whether these patients are suffering significant psychiatric morbidity from limited access to timely care. Identifying and triaging patients with a quick clinical screening tool for psychiatric distress such as the HADS may be beneficial for patient mental health and their disease from a health care resource point of view. Patients with higher levels of anxiety and depression tend to utilize more health care resources including antibiotics and physician visits [25].

## Conclusions

This study evaluates the functional and psychological impact on patients with CRS and who are currently on a waitlist for ESS. There was no correlation between the length of wait time and the degree of anxiety and depression among patients and overall, no significant levels of psychiatric distress were found. However, our study adds additional evidence that CRS symptoms can worsen while waiting for ESS and this may manifest itself in impairment in both work and social-related activities. With our qualitative analysis, we were better able to understand the patient experience while being on a waitlist for ESS. Overall, patients largely realized they had a benign chronic condition and felt reassured that they were getting appropriate treatment. The physician-patient relationship that was developed was also important in allowing patients to cope with longer wait times. Nonetheless, most patients felt that six months is the appropriate wait time for sinus surgery. There may be a

small subset of patients with more psychological distress that may benefit from having surgery sooner.

### Abbreviations
CRS, chronic rhinosinusitis; ESS, endoscopic sinus surgery; HADS, Hospital Anxiety and Depression Scale; SNOT-22, Sinonasal Outcome Test; WPAI-GH, Work Productivity and Activity Impairment-General Health Questionnaire

### Authors' contributions
GT is the primary author and participated in all aspects of the study. CM helped with REB submission review and data acquisition. LK participated in REB submission process and drafting the manuscript. JL conceived the study and was instrumental in the editing process. All authors read and approved the final manuscript.

### Competing interests
The authors declare that they have no competing interests.

### Author details
[1]Department of Otolaryngology-Head & Neck Surgery, University of Toronto, Toronto, ON, Canada. [2]Department of Otolaryngology-Head & Neck Surgery, St. Michael's Hospital, Toronto, ON, Canada. [3]Faculty of Medicine, University of Toronto, Toronto, ON, Canada.

### References
1. Desrosiers M, Evans GA, Keith PK, et al. Canadian clinical practice guidelines for acute and chronic rhinosinusitis. J Otolaryngol Head Neck Surg. 2011;40 Suppl 2:S99–193.
2. Ontario Ministry of Health and Long Term Care.[accessed April 6, 2015]; (http://www.ontariowaittimes.com/Surgerydi/en/PublicMain.aspx?Type=0)
3. Smith KA, Smith TL, Mace JC, Rudmik L. Endoscopic sinus surgery compared to continued medical therapy for patients with refractory chronic rhinosinusitis. Int Forum Allergy Rhinol. 2014;4(10):824–7.
4. Eskander A, Devins GM, Freeman J, et al. Waiting for thyroid surgery: a study of psychological morbidity and determinants of health associated with long wait times for thyroid surgery. Laryngoscope. 2013;123(2):541–7.
5. Gallagher R, McKinley S. Stressors and anxiety in patients undergoing coronary artery bypass surgery. Am J Crit Care. 2007;16(3):248–57.
6. Hodge W, Horsley T, Albiani D, et al. The consequences of waiting for cataract surgery: a systematic review. CMAJ. 2007;176(9):1285–90.
7. Oudhoff JP, Timmermans DR, Bijnen AB, van der Wal G. Waiting for elective general surgery: physical, psychological and social consequences. ANZ J Surg. 2004;74(5):361–7.
8. Oudhoff JP, Timmermans DR, Knol DL, et al. Waiting for elective general surgery: impact on health related quality of life and psychosocial consequences. BMC Public Health. 2007;7:164.
9. Oudhoff JP, Timmermans DR, Knol DL, et al. Waiting for elective surgery: effect on physical problems and postoperative recovery. ANZ J Surg. 2007;77(10):892–8.
10. Paterson WG, Barkun AN, Hopman WM, et al. Wait times for gastroenterology consultation in Canada: the patients' perspective. Can J Gastroenterol. 2010;24(1):28–32.
11. Sampalis J, Boukas S, Liberman M, et al. Impact of waiting time on the quality of life of patients awaiting coronary artery bypass grafting. CMAJ. 2001;165(4):429–33.
12. Sjöling RN, Agren RN, Olofsson N, et al. Waiting for surgery; living a life on hold–a continuous struggle against a faceless system. Int J Nurs Stud. 2005;42(5):539–47.
13. Nanayakkara JP, Igwe C, Roberts D, Hopkins C. The impact of mental health on chronic rhinosinusitis symptom scores. Eur Arch Otorhinolaryngol. 2013;270(4):1361–4.
14. Auerbach C and Silverstein LB. Qualitative Data: An introduction to coding and analysis. New York and London: NYU Press. 2003. 1st Edition.
15. Zigmond AS, Snaith RP. The hospital anxiety and depression scale. Acta Psychiatr Scand. 1983;67(6):361–70.

16. Reilly MC, Zbrozek AS, Dukes EM. The validity and reproducibility of a work productivity and activity impairment instrument. Pharmacoeconomics. 1993;4:353–65.
17. Reilly Associates Health Outcomes Research. (http://www.reillyassociates.net)
18. Hopkins C, Gillett S, Slack R, Lund VJ, Browne JP. Psychometric validity of the 22-item Sinonasal Outcome Test. Clin Otolaryngol. 2009;34(5):447–54.
19. Bjelland I, Dahl AA, Haug TT, Neckelmann D. The validity of the Hospital Anxiety and Depression Scale an updated literature review. J Psychosom Res. 2002;52:69–77.
20. Julian LJ. Measures of anxiety. Arthritis Care Res (Hoboken). 2011;63.
21. Tomoum MO, et al. Depression and anxiety in chronic rhinosinusitis. Int Forum Allergy Rhinol. 2015;5:674–81.
22. Yeung JC, et al. Preoperative concerns of patients undergoing endoscopic sinus surgery. Int Forum Allergy Rhinol. 2014;4(8):658–62.
23. Stankiewicz J, et al. Impact of chronic rhinosinusitis on work productivity through one-year follow-up after balloon dilatation of the ethmoid infundibulum. Int Forum Allergy Rhinol. 2011;1:38–45.
24. Smith TL, Batra PS, Seiden AM, Hannley M. Evidence supporting endoscopic sinus surgery in the management of adult chronic sinusitis: A systematic review. Am J Rhinol. 2005;19:537–43.
25. Wasan A, Fernandez E, Jamison RN, Bhattacharyya N. Association of anxiety and depression with reported disease severity in patients undergoing evaluation for chronic rhinosinusitis. Ann Otol Rhinol Laryngol. 2007;116(7):491–7.

# 26

# The surgical plane for lingual tonsillectomy

Eugene L. Son[1*], Michael P. Underbrink[1], Suimin Qiu[2] and Vicente A. Resto[1]

## Abstract

**Background:** The presence of a plane between the lingual tonsils and the underlying soft tissue has not been confirmed. The objective of this study is to ascertain the presence and the characteristics about this plane for surgical use.

**Methods:** Five cadaver heads were obtained for dissection of the lingual tonsils. Six permanent sections of previous tongue base biopsies were reviewed. Robot assisted lingual tonsillectomy was performed using the dissection technique from the cadaver dissection.

**Results:** In each of the 5 cadavers, an avascular plane was revealed deep to the lingual tonsils. Microscopic review of the tongue base biopsies revealed a clear demarcation between the lingual tonsils and the underlying minor salivary glands and muscle tissue. This area was relatively avascular. Using the technique described above, a lingual tonsillectomy using TORS was performed with similar findings from the cadaver dissections.

**Conclusions:** A surgical plane for lingual tonsillectomy exists and may prove to have a role with lingual tonsillectomy with TORS.

**Keywords:** Lingual tonsil, Surgical plane, Transoral robotic surgery, Lingual tonsillectomy

## Background

The base of tongue had once been a difficult area for surgery to perform on because of problems with exposure. With new innovations in endoscope technology, transoral laser microsurgery and transoral robotic surgery (TORS) with the da Vinci Surgical System manufactured by Intuitive Surgical, Inc., access to the tongue base has been made more feasible. In the base of tongue, the lingual tonsils are an important target for surgery. There are two main indications for lingual tonsillectomy.

The first indication is lingual tonsil hypertrophy (LTH), which can contribute to obstructive sleep apnea (OSA) in pediatric and adult patients. LTH among other functionally or fixed areas of obstruction in the upper aerodigestive tract are targets for sleep surgery. In pediatric patients, LTH can be primary or a secondary following a tonsillectomy and adenoidectomy [1].

The second indication is for squamous cell carcinoma of unknown primary (SCCUP) in the head and neck [2].

There has been an increase in the incidence of human papilloma virus (HPV) related oropharyngeal squamous cell carcinoma [3]. A large of number of SCCUP with negative clinical and radiographical evidence of a primary tumor are most commonly found to have primaries in the palatine and lingual tonsils. More recently, performing palatine tonsillectomy and lingual tonsillectomy has returned finding the primary tumor in 75–90 % allowing patients to receive a decreased amount of radiation lessening side effects [3, 4].

Lingual tonsillectomy techniques include cold dissection, electrocautery, coblation, carbon dioxide ($CO_2$) laser and microdebrider [5–9]. Many of these methods ablate or disrupt the microarchitecture of the lingual tonsils. In SCCUP, carpet resection of the lingual tonsils requires the desired tissue to be left intact for diagnosis under a microscope by a pathologist. Lingual tonsillectomy techniques have been described but no evidence of a surgical plane of dissection is available. Some have described the presence of a potential capsule and some have stated there is none. Joseph et al. described a layer of fibrous tissue that sometimes delineates this tissue

* Correspondence: eson85@gmail.com
[1]Department of Otolaryngology - Head and Neck Surgery, University of Texas Medical Branch, 301 University Boulevard, Galveston, TX 77555, USA
Full list of author information is available at the end of the article

from the tongue but no definite capsule [10]. Multiple authors in the early 20th century described a potential plane as "a basement membrane analogous to the capsule of the faucial tonsils" but not as delineated or developed as that tissue [11–14]. Dundar et al. describes the lingual tonsil having no capsule [5]. Lin and Koltai in their case series of coblation of lingual tonsillectomy in 26 pediatric patients describe no clear demarcation between the lingual tonsils and the tongue musculature, although the change in tissue quantities becomes readily apparent [1]. We believe that deep to the lingual tonsils, a relatively avascular plane made up of connective tissue exists. This potential surgical plane may be utilized in lingual tonsillectomy for the aforementioned indications.

## Methods

This study was approved by the institutional review board from the University of Texas Medical Branch. Five fresh cadaveric heads were procured for the purpose of this study. These cadavers were ages ranged from 86 years-old to 101 years-old including 2 females and 3 males.

### Cadaver dissection

The tongue from 5 cadaver heads were removed. Five complete dissections of the lingual tonsils were performed with scissors and forceps. First, a midline incision is made from the foramen cecum to the vallecula. An incision is also made immediately posterior to the circumvallate papilla. The anterior medial edge of a side of the lingual tonsils were grasped with forceps and then, dissection with the Iris scissors was performed in the lateral posterior direction until the lingual tonsils were removed en bloc on each side. Grossly, the muscle was identified as darker red in color and striations present. The dissection is carried to the border of the lateral pharyngeal wall and posteriorly to the edge of the vallecula. Care was take to remove the lymphoid tissue while keeping the underlying muscle intact. Digital photography was performed during the dissections.

### Histological sectioning

Six archived permanent sections of base of tongue biopsy specimens from the department of pathology at University of Texas Medical Branch were reviewed. Three cases with no malignancy detected and three cases with dysplasia were chosen for recording of digital photography under magnification. These specimens were from base of tongue biopsies from patients with SCCUP and had been fixed in formalin, processed for paraffin embedding and stained with hematoxylin and eosin. These specimens were reviewed for histological characterization of the lingual tonsils.

### Robot-assisted lingual tonsillectomy

A 52 year old male with SCCUP in the left neck underwent robot assisted lingual tonsillectomy as well as bilateral palatine tonsillectomy. A Fehy-Kastenbauer mouth gag was used for access to the tongue base. The da Vinci Surgical System was brought into the surgical field with visualization of the lingual tonsils. The 30-degree angled endoscope was placed in the midline, and the two working robotic arms were placed in the appropriate position. A Maryland dissector was used on the right arm and a monopolar cautery hook was used on the left arm for the left sided lingual tonsillectomy. The robot was then used to assist taking the lingual tonsil tissue down to the muscle layer, starting medially and dissecting laterally. A midline incision is made from the foramen cecum to anterior to the median glossoepiglottic fold. An incision is also made immediately posterior to the circumvallate papilla. The anterior medial edge of a side of the lingual tonsils were grasped and dissection was performed in the lateral posterior direction until the lingual tonsils were removed as one specimen for each side. Care was take to remove the lymphoid tissue keeping the underlying musculature intact. The specimens were then sent to the pathology department for histological review.

## Results and discussion

### Cadaver dissection

In all five cadaver dissections, the plane between the lingual tonsils and the underlying musculature was identified and used for excision of the lingual tonsils. There was a plane of dissection easily separating the lingual tonsils and the underlying tongue musculature. No grossly visible vessels nor nerves were encountered during the dissections (Fig. 1).

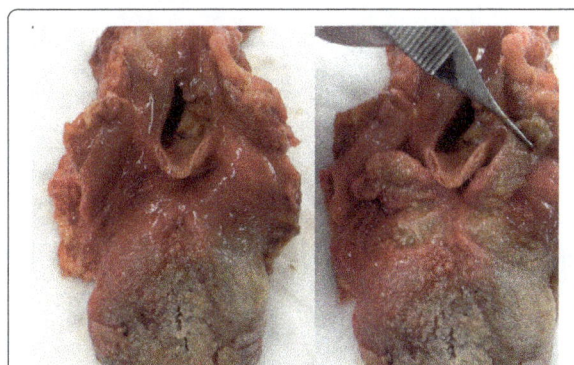

**Fig. 1** Gross dissection of lingual tonsils is shown. Left image shows the lingual tonsils before dissection and the right image shows the lingual tonsils dissected and reflected posteriorly

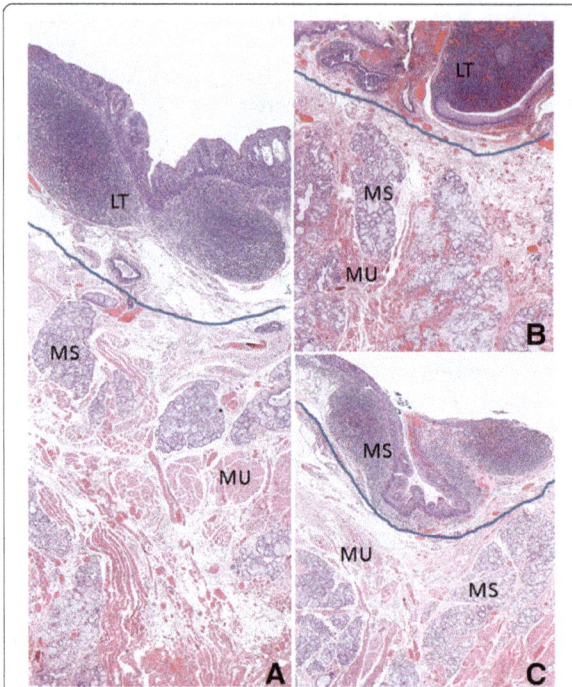

**Fig. 2** Permanent sections of base of tongue biopsies with benign pathology. Blue line demarcates surgical plane. Lingual tonsils (LT), minor salivary gland tissue (MS), muscle (MU) are labeled. Presence of submucosal edema exageratign plane in **a** compared to no edema in **b** (hypervascular) and **c**

## Histological sectioning

In these biopsies of the lingual tonsils, there was a relatively less vascular or avascular area between the lingual tonsil and the underlying minor salivary glands and muscle tissue in all cases (Figs. 2 and 3). Between the lingual tonsil and the submucosal muscular tissue at the base of the tongue a distinct space or line is demonstrated in both benign (Fig. 2) and premalignant (Fig. 3) cases. The space indicated by the drawn line is less vascular or avascular, by which the squamous mucosa with the lingual tonsil is distinct from the minor salivary gland and the muscle. The minor salivary gland and muscle is intimately admixed especially in the superficial portion of the muscle. Presence of submucosal edema (Fig. 2a) may exaggerate the space and presence of dysplasia associated with peritumoral lymphocytes infiltrate may obscure the space between the lingual tonsil and the underlying muscle as showed in Fig. 3c. However, in all conditions, dissection between two layers are feasible based on histological study.

## Robot-assisted lingual tonsillectomy

The procedure was performed uneventfully. No grossly visible vessels nor nerves were encountered during the dissections (Fig. 4). The patient had a normal postoperative course without any complications. Microscopic examination of this specimen showed microscopic foci of squamous cell carcinoma for which a random biopsy of the base of tongue would have missed.

The palatine tonsils have a well-described plan separating it from the surrounding oropharyngeal musculature. There

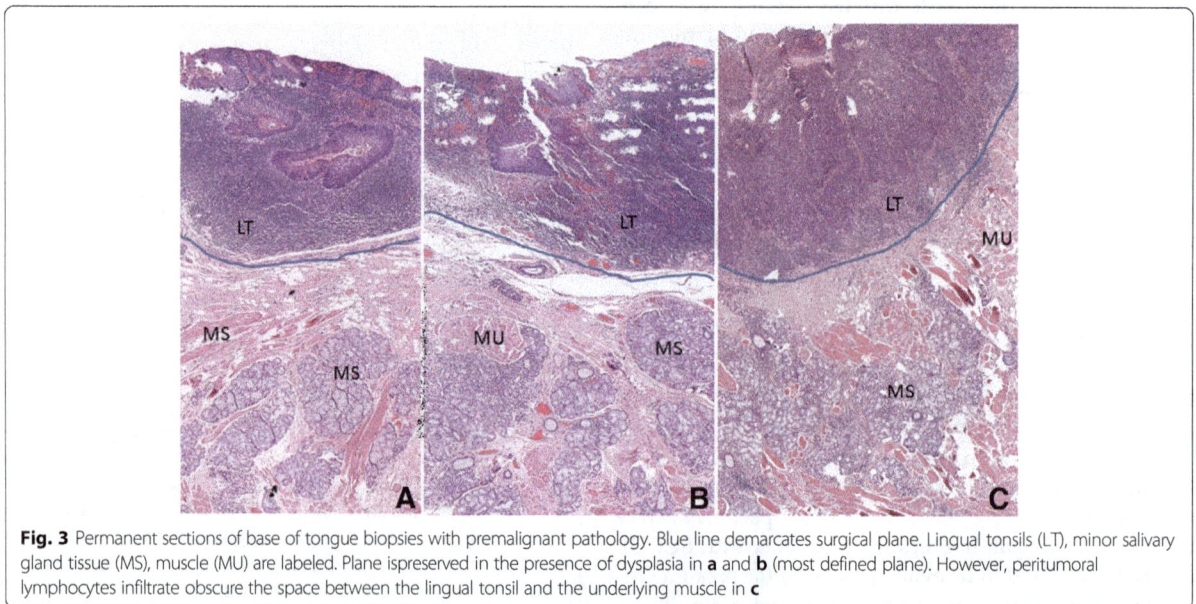

**Fig. 3** Permanent sections of base of tongue biopsies with premalignant pathology. Blue line demarcates surgical plane. Lingual tonsils (LT), minor salivary gland tissue (MS), musclle (MU) are labeled. Plane ispreserved in the presence of dysplasia in **a** and **b** (most defined plane). However, peritumoral lymphocytes infiltrate obscure the space between the lingual tonsil and the underlying muscle in **c**

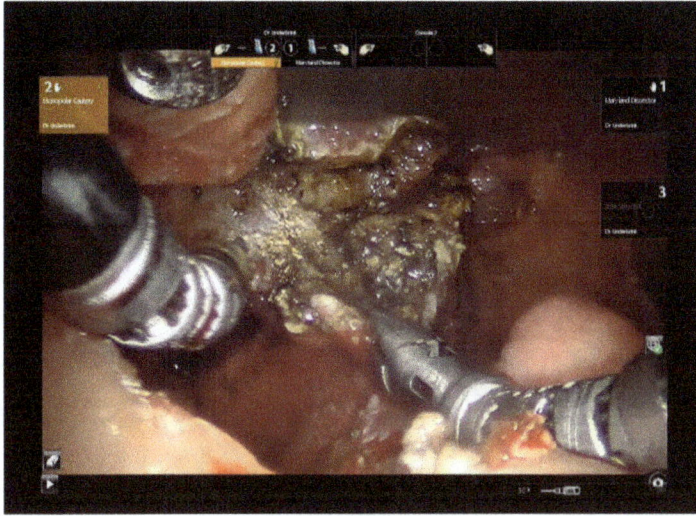

**Fig. 4** Intra-operative photography of lingual tonsillectomy during TORS. Lingual tonsil is grasped and reflected posteriorly

has been only speculation about the existence of a surgical plane for the lingual tonsils, being only described anecdotally in the current literature. In our study, we show a relatively avascular plane deep to the lingual tonsils in cadaver dissection, in histologic sections and in vivo.

In the five dissections performed, there was a space deep to the tonsils that gave less resistance in the force of dissection. In Fig. 1, there a is an uneven layer deep to this plane after dissection representing the minor salivary glands associated with the muscle layer as seen in the histological sections. In this plane, there were no grossly visible neurovascular structures appreciated for all specimens. There may be a feasible way for cold dissection of the tonsils using direct visualization or with robot assistance with a potential for decreased amount of cautery, minimal bleeding and decreased post-operative morbidity. This plane may also be utilized instead of ablative techniques such as in obstructive sleep apnea in pediatric patients to prevent secondary hypertrophy of the lingual tonsillar after tonsillectomy and adenoidectomy for obstructive sleep apnea.

Decreased use of cautery for dissection and hemostasis may provide better tissue diagnosis when lingual tonsillectomy is performed for elucidation of a diagnosis of an unknown head and neck primary tumor. In the case described, the diagnosis was made using a carpet resection of the lingual tonsils using our technique. Random biopsies of the base of tongue may miss a diagnosis making the consequential treatment different.

## Conclusions

The lingual tonsils have become more accessible in recent times for surgical intervention for diagnostic and treatment purposes. There is an avascular plane for dissection deep to the lingual tonsils and superficial to the underlying minor salivary glands and lingual musculature. This plane may be utilized in surgical resection in appropriate patients to potentially decrease post-operative morbidity and increase diagnostic yield. Further studies in human subjects with this plane utilized will need to be performed in the future.

**Abbreviations**

$CO_2$: carbon dioxide; HPV: human papilloma virus; LTH: lingual tonsil hypertrophy; OSA: obstructive sleep apnea; SCCUP: squamous cell carcinoma of unknown primary; TORS: transoral robotic surgery.

**Competing interests**

The authors declare that they have no competing interests.

**Authors' contributions**

ES performed the dissection, drafted and edited manuscript. MU performed the surgery and edited the manuscript. SQ prepared and interpreted the histology. VA conceived the study and edited the manuscript. All authors read and approved the final manuscript.

**Acknowledgement**

No other acknowledgments.

**Author details**

[1]Department of Otolaryngology - Head and Neck Surgery, University of Texas Medical Branch, 301 University Boulevard, Galveston, TX 77555, USA. [2]Department of Pathology, University of Texas Medical Branch, 301 University Boulevard, Galveston, TX 77555, USA.

**References**

1. Lin AC, Koltai PJ. Persistent pediatric obstructive sleep apnea and lingual tonsillectomy. Otolaryngol Head Neck Surg. 2009;141:81–5.
2. Mehta V et al. A new paradigm for the diagnosis and management of unknown primary tumors of the head and neck: A role for transoral robotic surgery. Laryngoscope. 2013;123:146–51.

3.  Forastiere AA et al. HPV-associated head and neck cancer: a virus-related cancer epidemic. Lancet Oncol. 2010;11:781–9.
4.  Nagel TH et al. Transoral laser microsurgery for the unknown primary: Role for lingual tonsillectomy. Head Neck. 2014;36(7):942–6.
5.  Dundar A et al. Lingual tonsil hypertrophy producing obstructive sleep apnea. Laryngoscope. 1996;106:1167–9.
6.  Abdel-Aziz M et al. Lingual tonsils hypertrophy; a cause of obstructive sleep apnea in children adenotonsillectomy: Operative problems and management. Int J Pediatr Otorhinolaryngol. 2011;75:1127–31.
7.  Robinson S et al. Lingual tonsillectomy using bipolar radiofrequency plasma excision. Otolaryngol Head Neck Surg. 2006;134:328–30.
8.  Bower CM. Lingual tonsillectomy. Oper Tech Otolaryngol. 2005;16:238–41.
9.  Kluszynski BA, Matt BH. Lingual tonsillectomy in a child with obstructive sleep apnea: a novel technique. Laryngoscope. 2006;116:668–9.
10. Joseph M, Reardon E, Goodman M. Lingual tonsillectomy: A treatment for inflammatory lesions of the lingual tonsil. Laryngoscope. 1984;94:179–84.
11. Cohen HB. The lingual tonsils: General considerations and its neglect. Laryngoscope. 1917;27:691–700.
12. Waugh JM. Lingual quinsy. Trans Am Acad Ophthalmol Otolaryngol. 1923;89:726–31.
13. Hoover WB. The treatment of the lingual tonsil and lateral pharyngeal bands of lymphoid tissue. Surg Clin North Am. 1934;14:1257–69.
14. Elfman LK. Lingual tonsils. Laryngoscope. 1949;59:1016–25.

# 27

# Detection of bacteria in middle ear effusions based on the presence of allergy: does allergy augment bacterial infection in the middle ear?

Woo Jin Kim[1], Byung-Guk Kim[1], Ki-Hong Chang[1] and Jeong-Hoon Oh[1,2]*

## Abstract

**Background:** Bacterial infection, Eustachian tube dysfunction, allergies, and immunologic factors are major causes of otitis media with effusion (OME). However, the exact pathogenesis of OME is still unclear. This study evaluated whether allergy influences bacterial growth in middle ear effusions.

**Materials:** Fifty-four samples were obtained from OME patients 3–10 years of age who underwent ventilation tube insertion and were divided into two groups based on the presence of allergy as determined using the multiple allergosorbent test (MAST). *Streptococcus pneumoniae*, *Haemophilus influenzae*, and *Moraxella catarrhalis* bacterial DNA in the middle ear effusions was analyzed using polymerase chain reaction. Overall detection rates and those for each species were compared between the two groups.

**Results:** Of the 54 middle ear effusion samples, 38 (70.4 %) contained bacterial DNA and 14 (36.8 %) of these contained DNA from multiple species. *S. pneumoniae* was detected in 27 samples (50 %), *H. influenzae* in 17 samples (31.4 %), and *M. catarrhalis* in 9 samples (16.6 %). There was no significant difference in the bacterial detection rates between the middle ear effusions of the MAST-positive and MAST-negative groups.

**Conclusion:** The rate of bacteria detection in middle ear effusions did not differ between allergic and non-allergic children.

**Keywords:** Middle ear effusion, Bacteria, Allergy

## Background

Otitis media with effusion (OME), fluid persisting in the middle ear cavity for more than 3 months, has been attributed to various causes [1]. Eustachian tube dysfunction is one of the most important factors in the development of this disease [2–4]. However, the exact pathogenic mechanism of OME is unclear. Eustachian tube dysfunction, including obstruction and abnormal patency, can be caused by extrinsic and intrinsic factors due to infection or allergy. The role of allergies in Eustachian tube dysfunction has been emphasized. The rate

of Eustachian tube function tympanometry abnormalities in a group of allergic rhinitis patients was higher than in healthy subjects [5]. These functional abnormalities may also be related to impairment of the mucociliary activity that facilitates reflow and aspiration of bacteria from the Eustachian tube [6]. The response to combined nasal instillation of bacteria and allergen in sensitized mice was more persistent than the response to either alone [7, 8]. Therefore, we hypothesized that the local allergic response in the middle ear can augment bacterial infection, which may lead to OME.

The most common organisms that cause OME are *Streptococcus pneumoniae*, *Haemophilus influenza*, and *Moraxella catarrhalis* [2, 6, 9, 10]. Although the presence of these bacteria DNA does not mean that bacterial infection is one of the main causes of OME, there is

* Correspondence: ojhent@catholic.ac.kr
[1]Department of Otorhinolaryngology-Head and Neck Surgery, College of Medicine, The Catholic University of Korea, Seoul, Korea
[2]Department of Otorhinolaryngology-Head and Neck Surgery, The Catholic University of Korea, 180 Wangsan-Ro, Dongdaemun-Gu, Seoul 130-709, South Korea

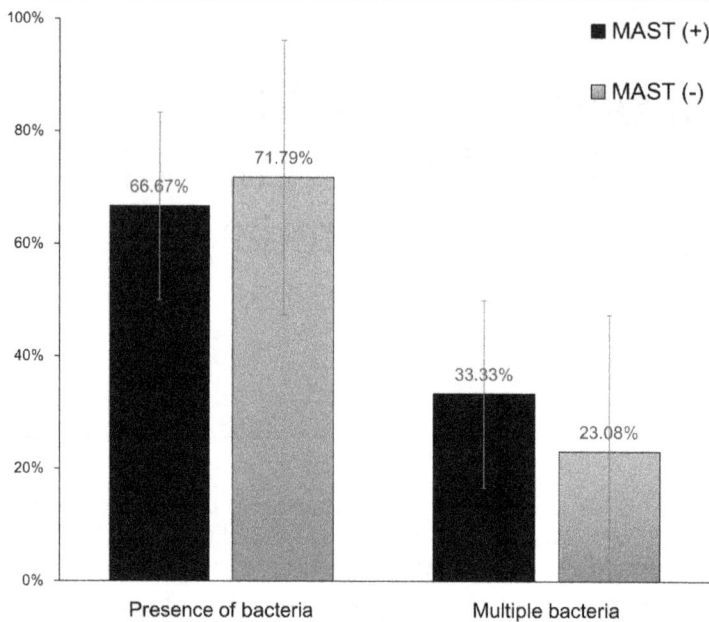

**Fig. 1** The rates of the overall detection of bacteria and detection of multiple bacteria in middle ear effusion using polymerase chain reaction in MAST-positive and -negative groups (MAST, multiple allergosorbent test)

increasing interest in the role of bacterial infection and associated inflammation as a cause of OME. Since respiratory infections and host immunity may be important in the pathophysiology of OME in children with Eustachian tube dysfunction, the presence of bacteria in OME can be affected by the patient's immune status. Therefore, this study evaluated the correlation between allergy and bacterial infection in the middle ear of OME patients.

In this study, the presence of bacterial infection in middle ear effusion (MEE) of the children younger than 12 years old was estimated from the detection rates of the bacterial pathogens *S. pneumoniae*, *H. influenzae*, and *M. catarrhalis* using polymerase chain reaction (PCR) and conventional culture methods. Among them, the detection rates of bacteria in the MEEs of patients with allergy according to the results of the multiple allergosorbent test (MAST) were compared with the rates in patients who did not have allergy.

## Methods

This study was approved by the institutional review board and the parents provided informed consent before participation. The enrolled subjects consisted of 34 consecutive pediatric patients (19 boys, 15 girls) under 12 years old, who admitted our clinic for the insertion of ventilating tube due to OME persisting for more than 3 months. The subjects were divided into two groups according to the presence of allergy. To determine the presence of allergy, blood samples were collected before the insertion of ventilating tube for the Korean panel of the multiple allergosorbent test chemiluminescent assay (MAST-CLA) (MAST Immunosystems, Mountain View, CA, USA). This assay consists of 35 different specific IgE antibodies with associated allergens from food, mold, pollen, and inhalant allergens that are most frequently positive in Koreans. The MAST-CLA was performed according to the' manufacturer's instructions. The amount of the produced chemiluminescence, which is proportional to the amount of allergen-specific IgE in the test serum, was measured in a densitometer; the results were interpreted as classes 0, 0/1, 1, 2, 3, or 4 based on the amount of light emitted, with classes 2 to 4 considered positive results. At the time of tube placement surgery, the external auditory canal was irrigated with 70 % alcohol and then the middle ear fluid was collected using a suction collector (Storz®, Germany). The collected fluid was stored immediately at −70 °C for subsequent analysis. The genomic DNA was extracted by mixing 50 μL of the stored middle ear effusion with 900 μL of cell lysis solution, followed by a 10 min centrifugation at 15,000 rpm at room temperature. DNA was extracted using PCR premix (Bioneer®, Daejeon, South Korea). For PCR, P6 protein was used as a primer for *Haemophilus influenzae*, PBP 2B for *Streptococcus pneumoniae*, and the M46 clone for *Moraxella catarrhalis*. Thirty-five cycles of 95 °C, 55 °C, and 70 °C were performed using a DNA thermal cycler. To detect the amplified product,

DNA was electrophoresed for 30 min in 2 % agarose gels. Specimens with consistent PCR results were used as positive controls and distilled water as a negative control.

The overall detection rate and that for each bacterial species was compared between the MAST-positive and -negative groups using the chi-square test.

## Results

Fifty-four ears of 34 children from 3–10 years old were enrolled in this study. Of the 54 ears, 15 were positive as determined by MAST, while the remaining 39 were negative. The mean ages of the children in the MAST-positive and -negative groups were $3.73 \pm 2.25$ years and $3.23 \pm 0.93$ years, respectively. The rate of bacteria detection using conventional culture methods was only 9.0 % (5/54) and the species cultured were *S. pneumoniae*, *S. epidermidis*, *S. capitis*, and α-hemolytic *Streptococcus*. The overall detection rate of bacterial DNA using PCR was 70.4 % (38 of 54 ears) (Table 1). In 14 of 38 ears (36.8 %), two or more bacterial species were detected in the same effusion sample. The overall detection rate of the bacteria did not differ significantly ($p > 0.05$) between the MAST-positive and -negative groups, nor did the detection rates of each bacterial species (Fig. 1). There was no significant difference in the detection rate of multiple bacteria between the two groups (Fig.1).

## Discussion

This study demonstrates that the children with evidence of allergy were equally likely as children without evidence of allergy to demonstrate evidence of bacterial infection in PCR tested MEE specimens. Although this study did not demonstrate a positive relationship between allergy and the bacterial infection in the pathogenesis of OME. However, numerous studies have indicated that allergic subjects are more susceptible to OME than non-allergic controls. The combination of allergic and bacterial stimulation can augment the development of OME. Labadie et al. showed that lipopolysaccharide (LPS)-induced OME, in which LPS simulated bacterial exposure, was more prominent in allergic rats [11]. Ebmeyer et al. found that the reaction to combined bacteria and allergen in sensitized mice was more persistent than the response to either alone and a reaction was absent in mast cell-deficient mice [12].

However, the exact mechanism of the relationship between the presence of bacteria in middle ear effusion and systemic immunity is still not clear. Theoretically, nasal obstruction due to an allergy can lead to an increase in negative pressure in the nasopharynx, resulting secondarily in decreased Eustachian tube patency, and disturbance of its ciliary epithelial function with subsequent increase in the negative pressure in the middle ear cavity. Several theories have been proposed to explain the Eustachian tube dysfunction caused by allergic inflammation, including retrograde spread of edema, poor mucociliary function, and venous engorgement and hypersecretion of mucus [3]. It has been suggested that the development of OME is the result of improperly functioning barriers (mucociliary system, immune system, and Eustachian tube) conferring resistance to bacteria [13]. The pathogenesis of OME is related primarily to Eustachian tube dysfunction, including obstruction, abnormal patency, and non-optimally functioning ciliated epithelium [3, 14]. These conditions can facilitate the aspiration of nasopharyngeal secretions containing pathogenic bacteria into the middle ear cavity, leading to the development of OME. The high prevalence of this condition in children reflects immaturity of function of both the immune system and the Eustachian tubes. The Eustachian tube of the infants has a smaller caliber and shorter length and joins the nasopharynx at a more acute angle in relation to the adults. All of these features predispose to dysfunction of the Eustachian tube and therefore increased risk of infection [15]. The negative finding of our study indicates that the anatomical immaturity of the Eustachian tube in children may plays a major role in the development of OME due to the bacterial infection rather than allergy. Chronic OME due to Eustachian tube dysfunction caused by allergy tends to occur much more frequently in adults than in children [3]. The analysis of differences of the detection rates among various age groups was not performed in this study. It would be helpful to distinguish the different pathogenesis of OME between children and adults.

There are several large literature reviews of the relationship of allergy to OME. Doyle concluded that allergy has been "reasonably well demonstrated" as a risk factor for otitis media." [16]; Tewfik and Mazer determined that Th2 mediated allergic inflammation was found in MEE in patients with OME [17]. In a prospective, cohort

**Table 1** The detection rates of major pathogenic bacteria in middle ear effusions using PCR in MAST-positive and -negative groups

| Bacterial species | No (%) of PCR-positive specimens in the MAST-positive group | No (%) of PCR-positive specimens in the MAST-negative group |
|---|---|---|
| *S. pneumoniae* | 6 (40.0 %) | 21 (53.9 %) |
| *H. influenzae* | 7 (46.7 %) | 10 (25.6 %) |
| *M. catarrhalis* | 3 (20.0 %) | 6 (15.4 %) |

*PCR* polymerase chain reaction; *MAST* multiple allergosorbent test

study of patients cared for in a private community prac-tice, all 89 OME patients proved to be atopic and spe-cific allergy immunotherapy resolved 85 % of OME [18]. Although, these results support the hypothesis that OME is an immune mediated allergic disease, evidence for direct causal relationship between OME and allergy have been lacking. Recent study showed that the preva-lence of allergic rhinitis was not different in 6- to 7-year-old children with OME and the reference group, sug-gesting a limited effect of allergy in the pathogenesis of OME in this age group [19]. Another study reported that no difference in Eustachian tube function was found in either the allergic rhinitis or control groups, which was interpreted as showing allergic rhinitis has little direct effect on Eustachian tube function [20].

One of the main reasons for the conflicting results re-garding the relationship of allergy and OME in the litera-tures may due to non-controlled study designs, including diagnostic criteria for allergy and differing populations [21]. The reported incidence of allergic rhinitis in OME ranges from 14 % to as high as 89 % [17, 22]. For the diag-nosis of allergy and determination of allergens, many pro-cedures can be used: skin tests, provocation tests, the radio-allergosorbent test (RAST), and MAST-CLA. In this study, the presence of allergy was defined using the MAST-CLA system, which is used to detect allergen-specific IgE antibodies using enzyme-linked anti-human IgE and a chemiluminescent assay, as reported previously [23]. This test avoids the use of radioactive reagents used in other in vitro tests and it permits the simultaneous quantitative measurement of specific IgE directed against 35 different allergens [24]. MAST-CLA sensitivity, specifi-city, and precision equal those of RAST and skin prick tests [25]. However, the MAST-CLA frequently shows concurrent positive results for multiple allergens in a sin-gle panel test; hence the clinicians can be confused as to whether the results should be interpreted as multiple aller-gens, cross-reactivity, or false positives. In this study, we used MAST-CLA results for detecting allergen-specific IgE antibodies, not for the determination of the specific al-lergens. Therefore, the definition of allergy in our study population was likely reliable. The criteria for the presence of allergy and the allergens affecting nasal allergy should be studied further, because current diagnostic tests pro-vide evidence only of an increased amount of specific IgE antibody in the skin or blood serum, which cannot be re-lated directly to nasal mucosa and Eustachian tube.

Another possible explanation for the negative correlation between the presence of allergy and OME is whether the middle ear mucosa is the target organ of the allergic inflam-mation. As mentioned above, the suggested mechanism of allergic involvement in OME is Eustachian dysfunction. However, not all allergic patients develop OME nor do all OME patients have allergies. Yeo et al. evaluated the

relationship of serum and effusion fluid immunoglobulin concentrations, with the presence of bacteria in effusion fluid determined by culture and PCR, and found no correl-ation between the immunoglobulin concentration in mid-dle ear effusion and the presence of bacteria in the effusion, while the serum immunoglobulin concentration was signifi-cantly related to the presence of effusion bacteria [26]. They suggested that the higher serum antibody concentration in bacteria-positive OME patients was due to a systemic im-mune reaction caused by inflammation in response to a local infection in the middle ear cavity. The relationship be-tween systemic immune reaction and local infection in middle ear effusion should be evaluated in further studies.

Bacteria detection rates of up to 94.5 % have been re-ported in middle ear effusions using PCR; we observed a 70.4 % overall detection rate. The detection of bacterial DNA by PCR does not imply the existence of metabolic-ally active bacteria, since PCR assays rely on the detection of genetic material regardless of the viability of the organ-ism. The discrepancy between the low detection rate of the bacteria using conventional culture and the high de-tection rate using PCR can be explained by the use of antibiotics before myringotomy and the insertion of venti-lating tubes, the involvement of biofilms in the progres-sion of infection, and intracellular infection persistence of bacteria in the middle ear mucosa [10, 27, 28].

## Conclusion
Bacteria were found in more than 70 % of the middle ear effusions, with more than one third showing multiple bacteria. The bacteria detection rates did not differ be-tween allergic and non-allergic children.

### Abbreviations
OME: otitis media with effusion; MEE: middle ear effusion; PCR: polymerase chain reaction; MAST: multiple allergosorbent test; RAST: radio-allergosorbent test.

### Competing interest
The authors declare that they have no competing interests.

### Authors' contributions
Study design, analysis, interpretation, drafting or revising of the paper involved all authors. Data collection and statistical analysis were performed by WJ Kim. All authors have given final approval of the version to be published and agree to be accountable for all aspects of the work.

### Acknowledgments
The authors thank the E.N.T. Fund of the Catholic University of Korea for providing funding to support this study.

### Funding
This study was supported by a grant of the E.N.T. Fund of the Catholic University of Korea made in the program year of 2015.

### References
1.   Kwon C, Lee HY, Kim MG, Boo SH, Yeo SG. Allergic diseases in children with otitis media with effusion. International Journal of pediatric otorhinolaryngology. 2013;77(2):158–61. doi:10.1016/j.ijporl.2012.09.039.

2.  Gok U, Bulut Y, Keles E, Yalcin S, Doymaz MZ. Bacteriological and PCR analysis of clinical material aspirated from otitis media with effusions. International journal of pediatric otorhinolaryngology. 2001;60(1):49–54.

3.  Pelikan Z. Role of nasal allergy in chronic secretory otitis media. Current allergy and asthma reports. 2009;9(2):107–13.

4.  Kariya S, Okano M, Hattori H, Sugata Y, Matsumoto R, Fukushima K, et al. TH1/TH2 and regulatory cytokines in adults with otitis media with effusion. Otology & neurotology : official publication of the American Otological Society, American Neurotology Society [and] European Academy of Otology and Neurotology. 2006;27(8):1089–93. doi:10.1097/01.mao.0000224087.93096.4d.

5.  Lazo-Saenz JG, Galvan-Aguilera AA, Martinez-Ordaz VA, Velasco-Rodriguez VM, Nieves-Renteria A, Rincon-Castaneda C. Eustachian tube dysfunction in allergic rhinitis. Otolaryngology–head and neck surgery : official journal of American Academy of Otolaryngology-Head and Neck Surgery. 2005;132(4):626–9. doi:10.1016/j.otohns.2005.01.029.

6.  Bluestone CD, Stephenson JS, Martin LM. Ten-year review of otitis media pathogens. Pediatr Infect Dis J. 1992;11(8 Suppl):S7–11.

7.  Blair C, Nelson M, Thompson K, Boonlayangoor S, Haney L, Gabr U, et al. Allergic inflammation enhances bacterial sinusitis in mice. The Journal of allergy and clinical immunology. 2001;108(3):424–9. doi:10.1067/mai.2001.117793.

8.  Naclerio R, Blair C, Yu X, Won Y-S, Gabr U, Baroody FM. Allergic rhinitis augments the response to a bacterial sinus infection in mice: A review of an animal model. American Journal of Rhinology. 2006;20(5):524–33. doi:10.2500/ajr.2006.20.2920.

9.  Park CW, Han JH, Jeong JH, Cho SH, Kang MJ, Tae K, et al. Detection rates of bacteria in chronic otitis media with effusion in children. Journal of Korean medical science. 2004;19(5):735–8.

10. Coates H, Thornton R, Langlands J, Filion P, Keil AD, Vijayasekaran S, et al. The role of chronic infection in children with otitis media with effusion: evidence for intracellular persistence of bacteria. Otolaryngology–head and neck surgery : official journal of American Academy of Otolaryngology-Head and Neck Surgery. 2008;138(6):778–81. doi:10.1016/j.otohns.2007.02.009.

11. Labadie RF, Jewett BS, Hart CF, Prazma J, Pillsbury 3rd HC. Allergy increases susceptibility to otitis media with effusion in a rat model. Second place–Resident Clinical Science Award 1998. Otolaryngology–head and neck surgery : official journal of American Academy of Otolaryngology-Head and Neck Surgery. 1999;121(6):687–92.

12. Ebmeyer J, Furukawa M, Pak K, Ebmeyer U, Sudhoff H, Broide D, et al. Role of mast cells in otitis media. The Journal of allergy and clinical immunology. 2005;116(5):1129–35. doi:10.1016/j.jaci.2005.07.026.

13. de Ru JA, Grote JJ. Otitis media with effusion: disease or defense? International journal of pediatric otorhinolaryngology. 2004;68(3):331–9. doi:10.1016/j.ijporl.2003.11.003.

14. Kouwen H, van Balen FA, Dejonckere PH. Functional tubal therapy for persistent otitis media with effusion in children: myth or evidence? International journal of pediatric otorhinolaryngology. 2005;69(7):943–51. doi:10.1016/j.ijporl.2005.02.015.

15. Revai K, Dobbs LA, Nair S, Patel JA, Grady JJ, Chonmaitree T. Incidence of acute otitis media and sinusitis complicating upper respiratory tract infection: the effect of age. Pediatrics. 2007;119(6):e1408–12. doi:10.1542/peds.2006-2881.

16. Doyle WJ. The link between allergic rhinitis and otitis media. Current opinion in allergy and clinical immunology. 2002;2(1):21–5.

17. Tewfik TL, Mazer B. The links between allergy and otitis media with effusion. Curr Opin Otolaryngol Head Neck Surg. 2006;14(3):187–90. doi:10.1097/01.moo.0000193190.24849.f0.

18. Hurst DS. Efficacy of allergy immunotherapy as a treatment for patients with chronic otitis media with effusion. International journal of pediatric otorhinolaryngology. 2008;72(8):1215–23. doi:10.1016/j.ijporl.2008.04.013.

19. Souter MA, Mills NA, Mahadevan M, Douglas G, Ellwood PE, Asher MI, et al. The prevalence of atopic symptoms in children with otitis media with effusion. Otolaryngology–head and neck surgery : official journal of American Academy of Otolaryngology-Head and Neck Surgery. 2009;141(1):104–7. doi:10.1016/j.otohns.2009.03.007.

20. Yeo SG, Park DC, Eun YG, Cha CI. The role of allergic rhinitis in the development of otitis media with effusion: effect on eustachian tube function. American journal of otolaryngology. 2007;28(3):148–52. doi:10.1016/j.amjoto.2006.07.011.

21. Chantzi FM, Kafetzis DA, Bairamis T, Avramidou C, Paleologou N, Grimani I, et al. IgE sensitization, respiratory allergy symptoms, and heritability independently increase the risk of otitis media with effusion. Allergy. 2006;61(3):332–6. doi:10.1111/j.1398-9995.2006.00971.x.

22. Miceli Sopo S, Zorzi G, Calvani Jr M. Should we screen every child with otitis media with effusion for allergic rhinitis? Arch Dis Child. 2004;89(3):287–8.

23. Ogino S, Bessho K, Harada T, Irifune M, Matsunaga T. Evaluation of allergen-specific IgE antibodies by MAST for the diagnosis of nasal allergy. Rhinology. 1993;31(1):27–31.

24. Scolozzi R, Vicentini L, Boccafogli A, Camerani A, Pradella R, Cavallini A, et al. Comparative evaluation of RAST and MAST-CLA for six allergens for the diagnosis of inhalant allergic disease in 232 patients. Clin Exp Allergy. 1992;22(2):227–31.

25. Finnerty JP, Summerell S, Holgate ST. Relationship between skin-prick tests, the multiple allergosorbent test and symptoms of allergic disease. Clin Exp Allergy. 1989;19(1):51–6.

26. Yeo SG, Park DC, Lee SK, Cha CI. Relationship between effusion bacteria and concentrations of immunoglobulin in serum and effusion fluid in otitis media with effusion patients. International journal of pediatric otorhinolaryngology. 2008;72(3):337–42. doi:10.1016/j.ijporl.2007.11.005.

27. Daniel M, Imtiaz-Umer S, Fergie N, Birchall JP, Bayston R. Bacterial involvement in otitis media with effusion. International journal of pediatric otorhinolaryngology. 2012;76(10):1416–22. doi:10.1016/j.ijporl.2012.06.013.

28. Fergie N, Bayston R, Pearson JP, Birchall JP. Is otitis media with effusion a biofilm infection? Clin Otolaryngol Allied Sci. 2004;29(1):38–46.

# 28

# Surgeon-performed ultrasound guided fine-needle aspirate biopsy with report of learning curve

Vinay T. Fernandes[1], Robert J. De Santis[2], Danny J. Enepekides[3] and Kevin M. Higgins[3]* (iD)

## Abstract

**Background:** Fine-needle aspiration biopsy has become the standard of care for the evaluation of thyroid nodules. More recently, the use of ultrasound guided fine-needle aspiration biopsy (UG-FNAB) has improved adequacy of sampling. Now there has been improved access to UG-FNAB as ultrasound technology has become more accessible. Here we review the adequacy rate and learning curve of a single surgeon starting at the adoption of UG-FNAB into surgical practice.

**Methods:** UG-FNABs performed at Sunnybrook Health Sciences Centre from 2010 to 2015 were reviewed retrospectively. Nodule characteristics were recorded along with cytopathology and final pathology reports. Chi-square analysis, followed by the reporting of odds ratios with confidence intervals, were used to assess the statistical significance and frequencies, respectively, of nodule characteristics amongst both diagnostic and non-diagnostic samples. A multiple regression analysis was conducted to determine if any nodule characteristic were predictive of adequacy of UG-FNABs. The learning curve was assessed by calculating the eventual adequacy rates across each year, and its statistical significance was measured using Fischer's Exact Test.

**Results:** In total 423 biopsies were reviewed in 289 patients. The average nodule size was 23.05 mm. When examining if each patient eventually received a diagnostic UG-FNAB, regardless of the number attempts, adequacy was seen to increase from 70.8 % in 2010 to, 81.0 % in 2011, 90.3 % in 2012, 85.7 % in 2013, 89.7 % in 2014, and 94.3 % in 2015 (Fischer's Exact Test, $p = 0.049$). Cystic ($x^2 = 19.70$, $p < 0.001$) nodules were found to yield higher rates of non-diagnostic samples, and their absence are predictive of obtaining an adequate biopsy as seen in a multiple regression analysis ($p < 0.001$) Adequacy of repeat biopsies following an initial non-diagnostic sample was 75.0 %.

**Conclusions:** Surgeons are capable of performing UG-FNAB with a learning curve noted to achieve standard adequacy rates. Cystic nodules are shown to yield more non-diagnostic samples in the surgeon's office.

**Keywords:** Ultrasound-guided fine-needle aspiration biopsy, Surgeon preformed, Thyroid nodules, Cystic lesions, Microcalcifications, Learning curve, Adequacy

* Correspondence: kevin.higgins@sunnybrook.ca
[3]Department of Otolaryngology–Head & Neck Surgery, University of Toronto, Sunnybrook Health Sciences Centre, 2075 Bayview Avenue, Suite M1 102, Toronto, ON M4N 3 M5, Canada
Full list of author information is available at the end of the article

## Background

Fine needle aspirates (FNA) are the standard of care for evaluating thyroid nodules. The use of FNA has decreased the percentage of surgical pathology specimens containing only benign thyroid tissue, and therefore decreased the amount of unnecessary operations. While historically these biopsies have been performed by palpation alone in the office, a shift toward biopsy under ultrasound guidance has increased the adequacy rate of biopsies to greater than 80 % [1–10]. With the increased availability of ultrasound technology in the office setting, head and neck surgeons and endocrinologists have begun incorporating the tool into their practice.

Office-based ultrasound and biopsy offers several potential benefits for patients. Although there is a paucity of evidence examining the patient experience, it is intuitive that patients who are able to undergo an ultrasound and biopsy at their surgeon's office following recommendation will wait less than those being referred to another clinic for biopsy. Furthermore, patients undergoing surveillance of thyroid nodules often have anxiety relating to the lack of diagnosis with the nodule. Many patients speak of the comfort they feel having their primary clinician perform the ultrasound surveillance and biopsy rather than a technologist or outside physician with whom they have no ongoing clinical relationship. For those previously biopsied benign nodules of large size, the surgeon's ability to survey them might reduce unnecessary surgery and further decrease the rate of benign pathology in surgical reports.

Previous studies have reported on the experience of radiologists as well as patient wait times for surgery and diagnostic accuracy for surgeon performed UG-FNABs. However, here we report the largest Canadian series of ultrasound-guided fine needle aspirate biopsies (UG-FNAB) conducted by surgeons.

## Methods

### Patients

Consecutive patient charts were reviewed from 2010 to 2015. Charts were collated from a list created by the Sunnybrook Health Sciences Centre (SHSC) otolaryngology office manager of patients catalogued as having undergone a thyroid biopsy with ultrasound guidance in the department. This search yielded 652 individual biopsies, which were then evaluated by a two reviewers. 229 charts were excluded: 38 had no ultrasound report available, 78 were not specifically thyroid biopsies, 28 were found to be duplicates, 39 had no cytology report available, and 46 were performed by a different practitioner. This project was approved by the Research Ethics Board of Sunnybrook Health Science Centre (ID 169–2013).

### Surgical technique

A Hitachi Aloka© ultrasound machine was used to perform a diagnostic ultrasound of both thyroid lobes and the lateral neck. The principal investigator conducted all UG-FNABs. Nodules with suspicious features were targeted according to ATA guidelines. The patient was placed in the supine position with a green towel placed for semi sterile technique. A 10 MHz probe identified the nodule, and using a 25 G needle nodules were targeted using primarily the capillary suction technique using multiple passes, and a combination of the short and long axis techniques.

### Data collection

Data extracted from patient charts included demographic information, FNA cytology reports and pathology reports. Adequacy of specimen and diagnosis was reported by the cytopathologist at SHSC according to the Bethesda system for reporting thyroid fine needle aspirate biopsy (FNAB). Nodule characteristics were drawn from the ultrasound procedure report.

### Analysis

Statistical analysis was completed with SPSS® (V20, IBM Corp ©). Statistical significance for all tests were set at $p < 0.05$. Chi-square analysis, followed by the reporting of odds ratios (OR) with confidence intervals (CI), was used to assess the statistical significance and measure of association, respectively, of nodule characteristics amongst both diagnostic and non-diagnostic samples. A multiple regression was conducted to determine if any nodule characteristic were predictive of adequacy of UG-FNABs. The learning curve was assessed by calculating the eventual adequacy rates across each year, and its statistical significance was measured using Fischer's Exact Test. The outcomes were recorded starting from the time at which the practice of using UG-FNAB was adopted into clinical practice. A comprehensive review of the North American and European English language literature was performed with the assistance of SHSC Librarians.

### Results

In total, 423 separate biopsies were examined in 289 individuals. Subject characteristics are noted in Table 1.

**Table 1** Subject characteristics

| | |
|---|---|
| Total patients *(n)* | 289 |
| Total UG-FNAB | 423 |
| Age | 55 (20–89) |
| Gender (M:F) | 77:212 |
| Nodule Size | 23.05 mm (3.9–100) σ = 14.04 |
| Adequacy | 86.9 % |

The overall eventual adequacy rate was 86.8 %, which means that 86.8 % of the patients across all years, regardless of the number of biopsies, received a diagnostic UG-FNAB. Figure 1 outlines the breakdown of cytopathology reports according to Bethesda classification. Amongst the non-diagnostic specimens, pathologists reported that 14 (14.6 %) were due to blood, 14 (14.6 %) were due to cyst contents, 36 (37.5 %) had no follicular cells, and 32 (33.3 %) were reported as having limited cellularity to make a diagnosis (Fig. 2).

There was no significant difference when adequacy was contrasted in terms of internal vascularity, echotecture, irregular margins, or microcalcifications in a chi-square analysis. However, cystic lesions (Fig. 3) ($\chi^2 = 19.70$, $p < 0.001$, OR = 3.21 CI: 1.89–5.43) were more commonly found amongst non-diagnostic specimens. Furthermore, a multivariate logistic regression was run to predict UG-FNAB adequacy from nodule size, cystic nature, echotexture, and the presence of microcalcifications. These variables statistically significantly predicted adequacy ($\chi^2 = 15.71$, $p = 0.003$, df = 4). However, Nagelkerke's $R^2$ of 0.091 shows that the independent variables were a poor model for prediction of adequacy. Moreoever, only one variable, cystic nature, added statistically significantly to the prediction, $p < 0.001$. The results from the multiple regression support those found in the chi-square analysis.

The learning curve was demonstrated sufficiently by measuring the proportion of patients per annum who eventually received a diagnostic UG-FNAB, regardless of the number attempts. Eventual adequacy (Fig. 4) was seen to increase from 70.8 % in 2010 to, 81.0 % in 2011,

90.3 % in 2012, 85.7 % in 2013, 89.7 % in 2014, and 94.3 % in 2015 (Fischer's Exact Test, $p = 0.032$). Amongst the UG-FNABs that were repeat biopsies following an initial non-diagnostic sample, the subsequent adequacy rate was 75.0 %, with an average of 12.4 days ($n = 16$) between initial and repeat biopsies across all years.

## Discussion

A review of surgeon-performed biopsies at Sunnybrook Health Sciences Centre has demonstrated an overall eventual adequacy rate of 86.9 %, with a clear learning curve experienced as the eventual adequacy rate improves each year, peaking at approximately 94.0 % in 2015. Our findings are consistent with the Canadian literature, which supports the association of cystic nodules were associated with non-diagnostic specimens [11] and shows that adequacy rates can approach 90 % [12]. Larger surgeon audits report overall adequacy rates of 70–92 % [1–4], while reports of radiologists, endocrinologists, and pathologists performing UG-FNABs suggest adequacy rates varying from 67 % to 94 % [5–10]. The current adequacy rate in our practice is comparable to those available in the literature.

Our institution uses the Bethesda system to report thyroid cytopathology [13]. The evidence reviewed at the Bethesda meeting suggested that non-diagnostic rates are between 2 and 20 %. Our data demonstrate that over time the adequacy rate will approach acceptable rates in a surgeon's office, showing evidence of a learning curve. To mitigate the impact of physician learning on patient safety early on, patients with unsatisfactory biopsies were

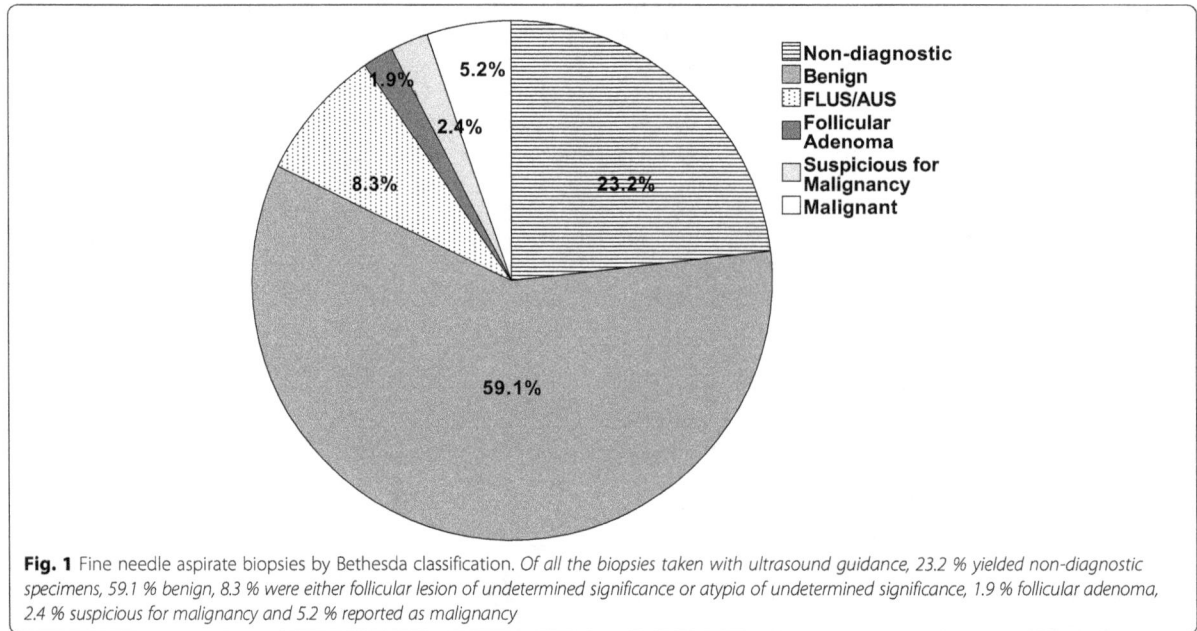

**Fig. 1** Fine needle aspirate biopsies by Bethesda classification. *Of all the biopsies taken with ultrasound guidance, 23.2 % yielded non-diagnostic specimens, 59.1 % benign, 8.3 % were either follicular lesion of undetermined significance or atypia of undetermined significance, 1.9 % follicular adenoma, 2.4 % suspicious for malignancy and 5.2 % reported as malignancy*

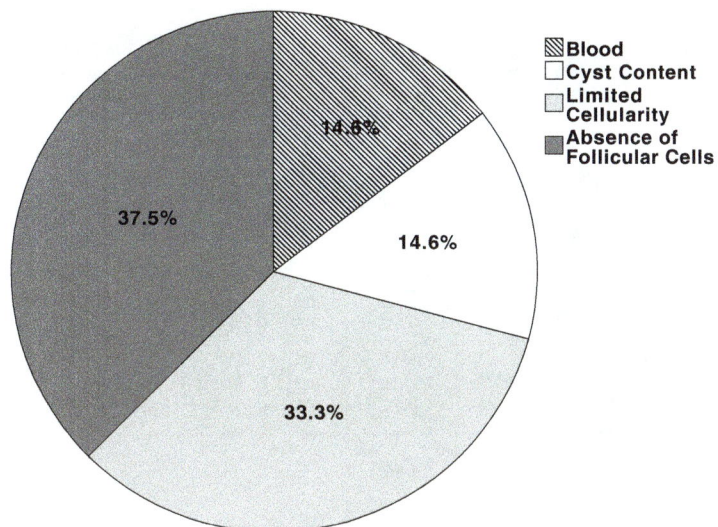

**Fig. 2** Breakdown of reason given for a specimen being non-diagnostic. *Of all the non-diagnostic biopsies, our cytopathologists commented that they were non-diagnostic for having blood (14.6 %), an absence of follicular cells (37.5 %), having cyst contents (14.6 %), or having limited cellularity (33.3 %)*

sent to radiology for repeat biopsy. As time went on and non-diagnostic rates diminished, this practice was abandoned. A review of repeat biopsies following non-diagnostic specimens in our centre demonstrated improved adequacy up to 75.0 % overall with a second biopsy. These figures are important, as the common practice to send a patient for a radiologist performed biopsy might increase the rate of lost-to follow up following non-diagnostic sampling, and certainly increases wait times. At our institution, rather than wait 4–6

weeks for a radiologist appointment, patients have the benefit of immediate biopsy at clinic visit. If repeat biopsy is sought during a clinic visit in which non-diagnostic results are reviewed, that repeat biopsy can be performed the same day.

Surgeon-performed ultrasound-guided fine needle aspirates has been adopted over the past decade in North America. As more and more physicians adopt the practice, it is necessary to obtain quality measures to ensure the procedure is performed adequately. One measure

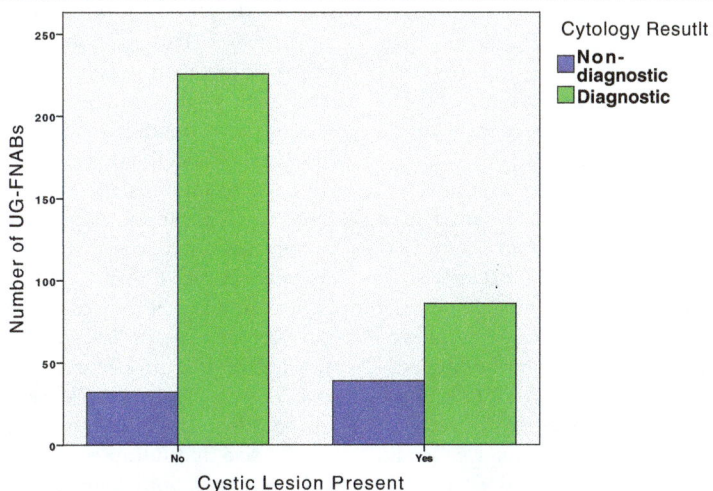

**Fig. 3** Distribution of diagnostic and non-diagnostic UG-FNABs by presence of cystic lesions. *This double bar graph represents the frequency of diagnostic and non-diagnostic UG-FNABs when cystic components are absent or present in the biopsied nodule. In total, 383 biopsies reported the cystic nature of the nodule; with 86 diagnostic and 39 non-diagnostic lesions with a cystic component; and 226 diagnostic and 32 non-diagnostic lesions without a cystic component*

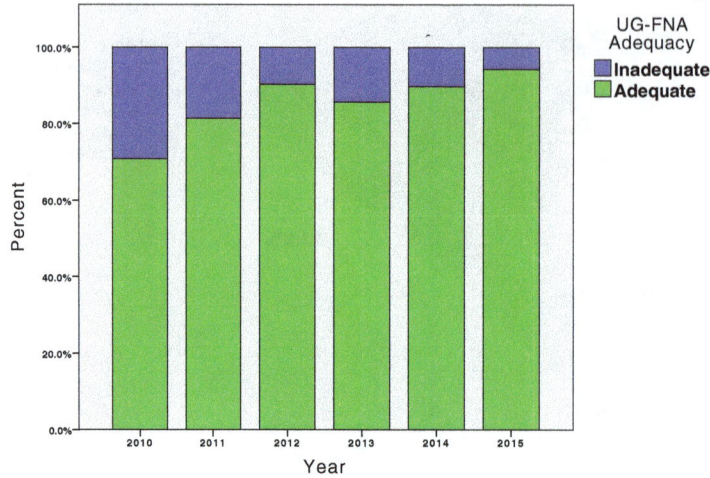

**Fig. 4** Eventual adequacy rate over time of all UG-FNABs divided by year. *This double bar graph represents the breakdown of patients who eventually received a diagnostic UG-FNAB, regardless of the number of biopsies, and those who never had a diagnostic UG-FNAB. The 289 patients were divided into the years they received their biopsy; with 17 diagnostic and 7 non-diagnostic in 2010; 47 diagnostic and 12 non-diagnostic in 2011; 56 diagnostic and 6 non-diagnostic in 2012; 30 diagnostic and 5 non-diagnostic in 2013; 35 diagnostic and 4 non-diagnostic in 2014; and 66 diagnostic and 4 non-diagnostic in 2015*

that must be understood in the adoption of a new procedure is the learning curve. The concept comes from the engineering industry; Wright described improving efficiency of production in his 1930's thesis as the skill of the workers increased [14]. While this concept is intuitive now with UG-FNABs, the number of biopsies needed to attain acceptable adequacy rates remains poorly answered. A South Korean comparison of an "experienced" versus "less-experienced" radiologist suggested no significant difference in adequacy rates to achieve 94 % [15]. However, not only had their experienced radiologist performed over 12,000 biopsies, their less experienced one had already performed at least 500. Mahoney reported astounding inadequacy rates of 0.4 % of thyroid biopsies, but admitted that they were within a 3-year interval after 15 years of experience [16].

In our assessment of learning curve, we analyzed adequacy within each calendar year, which resulted in a meaningful comparison. Published descriptions of UG-FNAB learning curve involve setting 100 patients [17], and similar case numbers have been described for the learning curve of other medical procedures. Surgical procedures are somewhat different, and many authors describe somewhere between 20 and 50 cases to achieve competency [18]. CT-guided FNA has been suggested to have a learning curve of only 40 cases, with DelGaudio reporting an improvement from 80 to 94 % adequacy [19].

A large proportion of the nodules biopsied had some portion of cystic content within them. The American Thyroid Association guidelines suggest that there is no indication for the biopsy of purely cystic nodules. In our

series, forty-five of the non-diagnostic specimens contained large cyst content. Some purely cystic nodules were aspirated for causing compression symptoms causing an overall adequacy rate for nodules described as cystic of 65.9 %. These aspirates recorded as cystic include large spongiform nodules, and so all were included in our non-diagnostic category. Controversy exists as to whether cystic content should be placed into a separate category on its own. In our study, cystic lesions were seen to more likely yield non-diagnostic results, likely because they have little to no follicular cells necessary for diagnosis. This relationship can help to explain why we have a less than perfect adequacy rate with UG-FNAB, even after a physician achieves expertise. Additionally, nodules with microcalcifications were more frequently observed in specimens that were diagnostic. Since the presence of microcalcifications is associated with papillary thyroid carcinoma, the above relationship reinforces that malignant nodules are generally being captured by UG-FNAB.

Once an audit of practice is performed, the next question becomes how to improve quality. One method is to standardize the procedure, with which some authors have reported success [7]. Sidiropoulous reported improved adequacy following standardization of technique (needle size and number of passes), preparation of samples including both slide prep and liquid preparation (which is quite time consuming), and personnel (difficult in a teaching institution where residents and fellows are involved). There is further evidence that standardizing the number of passes improves adequacy, as Naim 2013 showed inadequacy rates of 33.8 %, 23.4 %, and 13.7 % with 1, 2 and 3 needle passes respectively.

The utilization of on-site cytopathology is the subject of controversy in the literature. Reports with on-site evaluation approach 95 % [20, 21]. Some comparisons report increase in diagnostic rates from 73 % to over 90 % [22] once the process is implemented. Olson showed that both cytopathologists and less expensive technologists are able to achieve similar levels of on-site evaluation of adequacy [23]. The issue of course with implementation is cost. Eedes calculated that in Boston, the cytopathologist would spend 220 min of time for each additional diagnostic case [24]. Zanocco performed a formal cost-effectiveness analysis using a decision model to compare strategies in the U.S. health system. He found that when the adequacy rate without on-site evaluation is less than 85 %, on-site evaluation became cost-effective [25].

This review has several limitations owing to design. Without prospectively collected data, factors such as surgical technique, amount of passes, and recording of nodule characteristics on ultrasound reports will be variable. One of the main challenges faced was the lack of consistent reporting of characteristics, which made analysis difficult. We did not have consistent data regarding the specific indication for biopsy. Future audits will include prospectively collected data using standardized forms. Although complications were not specifically recorded in this database, to the author's knowledge there were no complications.

## Conclusion

Analysis of nodules' characteristics revealed that cystic lesions are more likely to yield non-diagnostic sampling, which can help to explain why we have a less than perfect adequacy rate with UG-FNAB, even after a physician achieves expertise. However, this report ultimately concluded that surgeon performed ultrasound guided FNA of the thyroid is a useful tool that can be implemented in the head and neck surgeon's office with ease.

### Abbreviations
FNA: Fine needle aspirate; UG-FNAB: Surgeon preformed ultrasound-guided fine needle aspirate biopsy; SHSC: Sunnybrook health sciences centre; FNAB: Fine needle aspirates biopsy; OR: Odds ratio; CI: Confidence interval.

### Competing interests
The authors declare that they have no competing interests.

### Authors' contributions
VTF was involved with the acquisition of data and drafting of the manuscript. RJD was involved in completing the statistical analysis and figures for the manuscript. All authors were involved with the conception and design, analysis and interpretation of data, revising the manuscript and have given final approval.

### Acknowledgments
We thank Lindsay Wilson who contributed toward the acquisition of data.

### Author details
[1]Department of Otolaryngology-Head & Neck Surgery, University of Toronto, Toronto, Canada. [2]Sunnybrook Health Sciences Centre, 2075 Bayview Avenue, Suite M1 102, Toronto, ON M4N 3 M5, Canada. [3]Department of Otolaryngology–Head & Neck Surgery, University of Toronto, Sunnybrook Health Sciences Centre, 2075 Bayview Avenue, Suite M1 102, Toronto, ON M4N 3 M5, Canada.

### References
1. Bhatki AM, Brewer B, Robinson-Smith T, Nikiforov Y, Steward DL. Adequacy of surgeon-performed ultrasound-guided thyroid fine-needle aspiration biopsy. Otolaryngol Head Neck Surg. 2008;139:27–31.
2. Bohacek L, Milas M, Mitchell J, Siperstein A, Berber E. Diagnostic accuracy of surgeon-performed ultrasound-guided fine-needle aspiration of thyroid nodules. Ann Surg Oncol. 2012;19:45–51.
3. Carr S, Visvanathan V, Hossain T, Uppal S, Chengot P, Woodhead CJ. How good are we at fine needle aspiration cytology? J Laryngol Otol. 2010;124:765–6.
4. Howlett DC, Harper B, Quante M, Berresford A, Morley M, Grant J, et al. Diagnostic adequacy and accuracy of fine needle aspiration cytology in neck lump assessment: results from a regional cancer network over a one year period. J Laryngol Otol. 2007;121:571–9.
5. Al-azawi D, Mann GB, Judson RT, Miller JA. Endocrine surgeon-performed US guided thyroid FNAC is accurate and efficient. World J Surg. 2012;36:1947–52.
6. Sidiropoulos N, Dumont LJ, Golding AC, Quinlisk FL, Gonzalez JL, Padmanabhan V. Quality improvement by standardization of procurement and processing of thyroid fine-needle aspirates in the absence of on-site cytological evaluation. Thyroid. 2009;19:1049–52.
7. Baier ND, Hahn PF, Gervais DA, Samir A, Halpern EF, Mueller PR, et al. Fine-needle aspiration biopsy of thyroid nodules: experience in a cohort of 944 patients. AJR Am J Roentgenol. 2009;193:1175–9.
8. Cai XJ, Valiyaparambath N, Nixon P, Waghorn A, Giles T, Helliwell T. Ultrasound-guided fine needle aspiration cytology in the diagnosis and management of thyroid nodules. Cytopathology. 2006;17:251–6.
9. Mittendorf EA, Tamarkin SW, McHenry CR. The results of ultrasound-guided fine-needle aspiration biopsy for evaluation of nodular thyroid disease. Surgery. 2002;132:648–53. discussion 653–4.
10. Naïm C, Karam R, Eddé D. Ultrasound-guided fine-needle aspiration biopsy of the thyroid: methods to decrease the rate of unsatisfactory biopsies in the absence of an on-site pathologist. Can Assoc Radiol J. 2013;64:220–5.
11. Isaac A, Jeffery CC, Seikaly H, Al-Marzouki H, Harris JR, Connell DA O. Predictors of non-diagnostic cytology in surgeon-performed ultrasound guided fine needle aspiration of thyroid nodules. J Otolaryngol Head Neck Surg. 2014;43(1):48.
12. Schwartz J, How J, Lega I, Cote J, Gologan O, Rivera JA, et al. Ultrasound-guided fine-needle aspiration thyroid biopsies in the otolaryngology clinic. J Otolaryngol Head Neck Surg. 2010;39(4):356–60.
13. Cibas ES, Ali SZ, NCI Thyroid FNA State of the Science Conference. The Bethesda system for reporting thyroid cytopathology. American Society for Clinical Pathology. 2009;132:658–65.
14. Wright TP. Factors affecting the cost of airplanes. Journal of Aeronautical Science. 1936;3:122–8.
15. Lee YJ, Kim DW, Jung SJ. Comparison of sample adequacy, pain-scale ratings, and complications associated with ultrasound-guided fine-needle aspiration of thyroid nodules between two radiologists with different levels of experience. Endocrine. 2013;44:696–701.
16. Mahony GT, Mahony BS. Low nondiagnostic rate for fine-needle capillary sampling biopsy of thyroid nodules: a singular experience. J Ultrasound Med. 2013;32:2155–61.
17. Lieu D. Cytopathologist-performed ultrasound-guided fine-needle aspiration and core-needle biopsy: a prospective study of 500 consecutive cases. Diagn Cytopathol. 2008;36:317–24.
18. Hopper AN, Jamison MH, Lewis WG. Learning curves in surgical practice. Postgrad Med J. 2007;83:777–9.
19. DelGaudio JM, Dillard DG, Albritton FD, Hudgins P, Wallace VC, Lewis MM. Computed tomography–guided needle biopsy of head and neck lesions. Arch Otolaryngol Head Neck Surg. 2000;126:366–70.

20. Baloch ZW, Tam D, Langer J, Mandel S, LiVolsi VA, Gupta PK. Ultrasound-guided fine-needle aspiration biopsy of the thyroid: role of on-site assessment and multiple cytologic preparations. Diagn Cytopathol. 2000;23:425–9.
21. Ghofrani M, Beckman D, Rimm DL. The value of onsite adequacy assessment of thyroid fine-needle aspirations is a function of operator experience. Cancer. 2006;108:110–3.
22. Moberly AC, Vural E, Nahas B, Bergeson TR, Kokoska MS. Ultrasound-guided needle aspiration: impact of immediate cytologic review. Laryngoscope. 2010;120:1979–84.
23. Olson MT, Tatsas AD, Ali SZ. Cytotechnologist-attended on-site adequacy evaluation of thyroid fine-needle aspiration: comparison with cytopathologists and correlation with the final interpretation. Am J Clin Pathol. 2012;138:90–5.
24. Eedes CR, Wang HH. Cost-effectiveness of immediate specimen adequacy assessment of thyroid fine-needle aspirations. Am J Clin Pathol. 2004;121:64–9.
25. Zanocco K, Pitelka-Zengou L, Dalal S, Elaraj D, Nayar R, Sturgeon C. Routine on-site evaluation of specimen adequacy during initial ultrasound-guided fine needle aspiration of thyroid nodules: a cost-effectiveness analysis. Ann Surg Oncol. 2013;20:2462–7.

# 29

# An outcomes analysis of anterior epistaxis management in the emergency department

E. Newton[1], A. Lasso[3], W. Petrcich[3] and S. J. Kilty[2,3*]

## Abstract

**Background:** Many treatment options exist for the management of anterior epistaxis. However, little is known about treatment outcomes. The objective was to identify the currently utilised methods of management and outcomes for patients with anterior epistaxis presenting to the emergency department (ED) at a Canadian tertiary care center.

**Methods:** A retrospective review of ED visits from January 2012-May 2014 for adult patients with a diagnosis of anterior epistaxis was performed. Patient demographic data, comorbidities, and treatment methods were documented. The effectiveness of different treatment modalities was determined.

**Results:** Three hundred fifty-three primary anterior epistaxis cases were included. Mean patient age was 70 years and 49 % of patients were female. Comorbidities included hypertension (56 %), diabetes (19 %), CAD (28 %), and atrial fibrillation (27 %). A large proportion of the cohort (61 %) was on at least one anticoagulant or antiplatelet therapy. The most common utilised treatment modalities were silver nitrate cauterization, Merocel®, petroleum gauze packing, nasal clip and 15 % were simply observed. Initial treatment success was achieved in 74 % of cases. Of patients receiving specific treatment modalities, silver nitrate cauterization had the highest success rate at 80 %. 26 % of patients returned to the ED for recurrence of epistaxis with highest rates occurring in the nasal clip (59 %), Merocel® (26 %), and petroleum gauze packing (42 %) groups.

**Conclusions:** The differences in recurrence rate among the different treatment modalities observed may be due to true differences in effectiveness or differences in treatment selection by the ED physicians based on severity of epistaxis. Cauterization with silver nitrate, however, offers the added benefit of no need for follow up. Further study is needed to elucidate the most efficacious treatment modality based on epistaxis severity.

**Keywords:** Epistaxis, Treatment, Anterior epistaxis, Tertiary care, Emergency department

## Background

Epistaxis, is an exceedingly common presenting problem to hospitals in North America accounting for approximately 1 in 200 emergency department (ED) visits in the United States [1]. Although difficult to truly assess, it has been estimated that 60 % of the population has at least 1 episode of epistaxis in their lifetime of which 6 % seek medical treatment [2]. The sheer incidence of

epistaxis constitutes it as an important condition in terms of cost, time and resource management. Thus, it is important to identify the most efficacious treatment modality in the realms of treatment success.

There are many treatment modalities and algorithms for epistaxis described in the literature [3–9]. Most approaches describe initiating packing and nasal pressure and escalating to more invasive and time consuming treatments if that fails. For anterior epistaxis there is evidence for the use of chemical cautery [10], anterior packing [5], and other hemostatic matrices [4]. All of these modalities have been shown to have good efficacy in achieving hemostasis. However, there is insufficient

* Correspondence: kiltysj@gmail.com
[2]Department of Otolaryngology - Head and Neck Surgery, University of Ottawa, Ontario, Canada
[3]Ottawa Hospital Research Institute (OHRI), Ottawa, ON, Canada
Full list of author information is available at the end of the article

literature evaluating these modalities and their effectiveness when utilised in the ED. Further, at this time there are no widely accepted treatment guidelines and treatment selection is a matter of individual ED physician preference.

## Importance
Considering that anterior epistaxis is a very common and treatable condition it is important to optimize efficiency and effectiveness when treating this disorder. Although, there is evidence for each individual treatment modality, the literature is deficient as to current ED physician practices and the outcomes for use of the many modalities.

## Goals of this investigation
The purpose of this study was twofold, first to assess the current practices utilised in a Canadian Tertiary Care center for anterior epistaxis management and second, to evaluate the outcomes of these treatments.

## Methods
### Study design and setting
With the approval of the Research Ethics Board at the Ottawa Hospital Research Institute a retrospective review of all patient visits to the ED at The Ottawa Hospital (TOH), a Canadian tertiary care center, with a primary diagnosis of anterior epistaxis during the period of January 2012 to May 2014 was performed.

## Selection of participants
Adult patients with a primary diagnosis of epistaxis in the emergency department were included in this study. Records were identified by the health records department using the ICD-10 code for epistaxis (R04-0). The epistaxis codes do not differentiate between anterior and posterior epistaxis; thus all records were hand searched and patients with a diagnosis of posterior epistaxis or concurrent anterior and posterior epistaxis were excluded. Patients that presented with epistaxis due to a complication of pre-existing conditions such as end stage cancer were excluded. Patients who died during the ED visit for reasons other than epistaxis were also excluded. Patients with an initial visit to the ED for packing removal that had been placed at a different institution and patients who were treated as posterior epistaxis despite having an anterior epistaxis diagnosis were also excluded. Patients who received treatment with a modality that was used in five or fewer cases were also excluded from analysis. See Fig. 1 for study flow chart.

## Methods and measurements
From the identified charts data was abstracted including patient demographics, comorbidities, the treatment modalities used, course in the emergency department, admission, concurrent medical disorders, medications and finally recurrence or ED follow-up information. Treatment modalities identified for data abstraction included conservative (no treatment), nasal clip, petroleum gauze

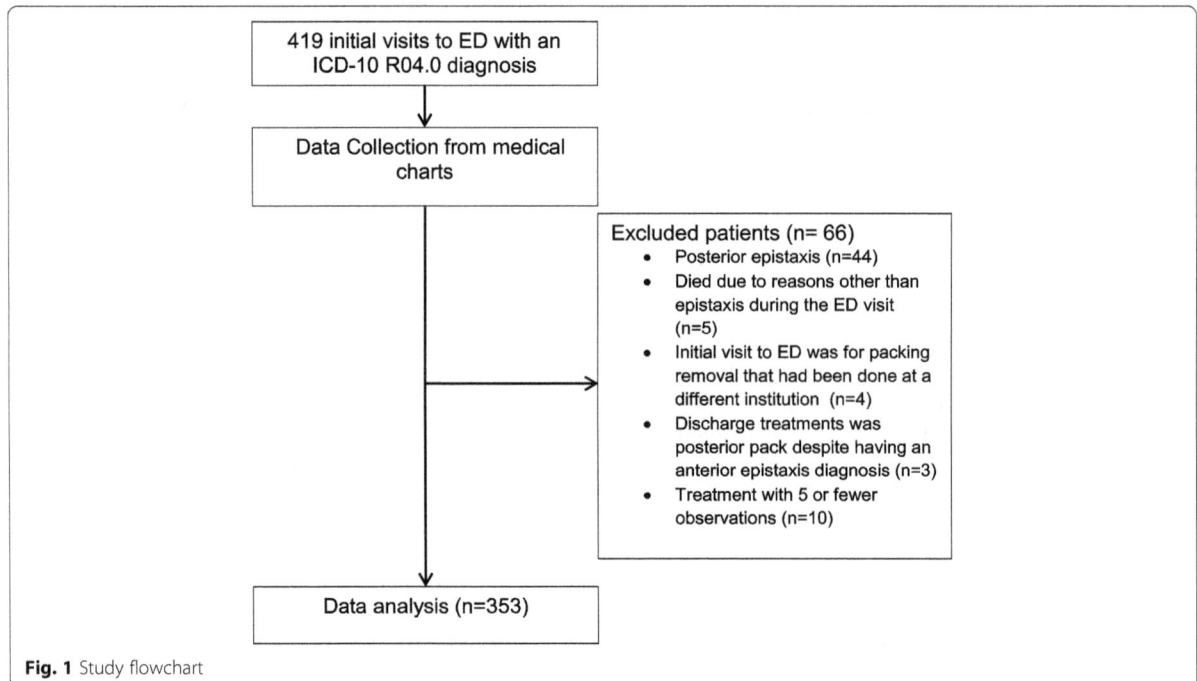

**Fig. 1** Study flowchart

packing, Merocel® packing, Floseal®, Surgicel®, Epistat®, silver nitrate cautery, electrocautery, endoscopic surgery, arterial embolization and other treatments not otherwise specified (NOS). The "other packing" group in this study received anterior petroleum gauze packing or equivalent.

## Outcomes

For each treatment modality, success was defined as patients who were diagnosed with anterior epistaxis, who received treatment and did not present with a recurrence within 14 days of their original date of presentation [11]. Conversely, failure was defined as the patients who had an ipsilateral recurrence of epistaxis within 14 days of initial treatment. The treatment type was recorded based on the treatment modality used to arrest the bleeding that led to the patient's discharge from the ED. Follow-up was defined as patients who were administered a specific treatment and who were subsequently booked and received follow-up care in the ED for either packing removal or to check the site of epistaxis or for any other reason. For patients requiring an inpatient admission, the length and reason for admission were recorded.

## Analysis

All statistical calculations were done using SAS (version 9.3). Categorical variables were summarized using frequency counts and percentages, while continuous variables were summarized using the mean (SD) or median (IQR), as appropriate. Where necessary, initial testing for associations between categorical variables was done using either chi-square or Fisher's Exact tests. Modeling of categorical outcomes was done using logistic regression.

## Results

### Characteristics of study subjects

A total of 419 visits to the ED with a primary diagnosis of epistaxis occurred from January 2012 to May 2014. Sixty-six visits were excluded from this analysis, reasons for exclusion are shown in Fig. 1. Overall, 353 anterior epistaxis cases were included in this study; the demographics and comorbidities are summarized in Table 1. The individuals included in this study had a mean age of 70 and 49 % were women. A large proportion (61 %) of the patients were on some type of anticoagulant or antiplatelet medication. Of the comorbidities recorded, hypertension, diabetes, coronary artery disease, atrial fibrillation, did not have a statistically significant impact on treatment failure ($p > 0.05$).

### Main results

The outcome of each treatment is summarized in Table 2. In all, the overall primary treatment failure rate was 26 % (91 patients) and in total 26.6 % (94 patients)

**Table 1** Patient demographics

| Characteristic | Value |
|---|---|
| Age mean y (range), | 70 (14–97) |
| Sex no. (%) | |
| Male | 180 (51) |
| Female | 173 (49) |
| Comorbidities N (%) | |
| Hypertension | 198 (56) |
| Diabetes | 67 (19) |
| CAD[a] | 97 (28) |
| Afib[b] | 94 (27) |
| HHT[c] | 3 (1) |
| Other blood disorders | 12 (3) |
| AC/AP[d] medication use | 217 (62) |

[a]Coronary artery disease
[b]Atrial fibrillation
[c]Hereditary hemorrhagic telangiectasia
[d]Anticoagulation or antiplatelet

returned to the ED for a scheduled follow-up after discharge from the ED. Of the individuals requiring follow-up, 89 (95 %) returned for packing removal (53 patients had Merocel® packing), in 3 (3.1 %) patients packing was left in situ at the follow up visit and 2 (2.1 %) patients attended the follow up visit even though their packing had fallen out on its own before their appointment. Of the 94 patients requiring follow up, 22 (23 %) required further intervention (10 patients with Merocel® packing) for epistaxis at the time packing removal. There was no difference in bleeding rates post pack removal between the different types of packing.

When silver nitrate was compared to petroleum gauze packing, those in silver nitrate group were less likely to fail (OR 0.335, 95 % CI 0.160–0.703 $p = 0.0038$). When silver nitrate was compared to Merocel® packing, the odds of recurrence were lower with silver nitrate than with Merocel® (OR 0.694, 95 % CI 0.364–1.322, $p = 0.27$), however this was not statistically significant.

When evaluating potential risk factors for the development of epistaxis, anticoagulation was identified

**Table 2** Treatment outcomes for management of anterior epistaxis

| Treatment | N (%) | Failure N (%) |
|---|---|---|
| Silver nitrate | 122 (35) | 24 (20) |
| Merocel | 92 (26) | 24 (26) |
| No treatment | 54 (15) | 11 (20) |
| Other packing[a] | 45 (13) | 19 (42) |
| Other[b] | 23 (6) | 3 (13) |
| Nasal clip | 17 (5) | 10 (59) |

[a]Other packing included non-dissolvable anterior packs the majority being Vaseline gauze packing
[b]Other included surgicel, decongestant with topical anesthetic alone

from the patient characteristics, through logistical regression. The type of anticoagulant or antiplatelet medication individuals in the study were receiving is summarized in Table 3. Given the large variety of anticoagulation and antiplatelet medications, they were grouped into 3 categories for analysis as seen in Table 4. Overall, 61 % of the individuals were on at least one antiplatelet or anticoagulant medication. Of those not on any anticoagulant or antiplatelet agent, the failure rate for anterior epistaxis treatment was 18 %. In contrast, for individuals on any anticoagulant/antiplatelet agent the failure rate was 30 %. There was a statistically significant association between the use of anticoagulant/antiplatelet medication and the recurrence of epistaxis ($p = 0.0119$). 73 % of all patients who failed treatment were on at least one antiplatelet or anticoagulant medication.

## Discussion

Overall there were 353 cases of anterior epistaxis analyzed in this study for outcomes of treatment received in the ED. Silver nitrate cautery was the most popular modality used accounting for 35 % of initial treatment. However, the treatment of anterior epistaxis proved to be quite variable with Merocel®, petroleum gauze packing/other packing or a nasal clip commonly being used.

The group of patients who received no treatment at the ED was not used as a control to compare other treatment modalities given those patients not requiring treatment had stopped bleeding when seen by the ED physician or they did not have a bleeding episode of such a severity that it required any treatment. It would be an unfair comparison due to the inherent clinical difference in epistaxis severity. When the silver nitrate group was compared to the petroleum gauze packing, those in silver nitrate group were less likely to fail ($p = 0.0038$).

**Table 3** Types of anticoagulation (AC)/antiplatelet (AP) medications used by patient population

| Medication | N (%) |
| --- | --- |
| Any AC/AP | 217 (62) |
| ASA | 122 (34) |
| Coumadin | 78 (23) |
| Rivaroxaban | 14 (4) |
| Dabigatran | 4 (1) |
| Apixaban | 4 (1) |
| Clopidogrel | 33 (9) |
| Ticagrelor | 2 (1) |
| Other anticoagulant | 7 (2) |

**Table 4** Outcomes of treatment success and failure based on anticoagulation/antiplatelet use profile

| Anticoagulant/Antiplatelet | N | Failure N (%) |
| --- | --- | --- |
| None | 136 | 25 (18) |
| Any anticoagulant/antiplatelet | 217 | 66 (30) |
| ASA only | 85 | 28 (33) |
| Other regimen | 132 | 38 (29) |

In this cohort, silver nitrate treatment had the lowest rate of treatment failure (20 %) of the most utilised treatment modalities and it also had the added benefit of not requiring an additional routine ED visit, as non-dissolvable packing did. Selection bias may have affected this observation as silver nitrate may have been used by ED physicians only in less severe cases. Other literature has described good success rates for anterior dissolvable packing [3, 4, 11, 12] and surgical techniques [3], however the number of individuals receiving these treatments in our cohort were too small for analysis.

Epistaxis management, as with any medical condition, should be tailored to the patient and the clinical situation [8]. In this study most patients with anterior epistaxis received successful management with silver nitrate cautery or Merocel® packing being the most commonly used modalities. Silver nitrate was particularly advantageous as it showed promising results insofar as treatment success without a need for follow-up. However, in these cases the site of bleeding was identifiable on anterior rhinoscopy examination and amenable to cautery with silver nitrate. This is in keeping with other studies which have shown that when the source of bleeding in epistaxis is identifiable chemical cautery has excellent success in the treatment of anterior epistaxis [2, 8–10].

Exploring the reasons for treatment failure, the use of blood thinners is largely believed to have an effect. In our study it was found that being on any anticoagulant or antiplatelet agent, including ASA, significantly increased the odds of recurrence after discharge from the ED ($p = 0.0106$). The rate of treatment failure in patients on any anticoagulant/antiplatelet agent was 30 %, in ASA alone was 33 % and in another regimen was 29 %, these were significantly greater than the failure rate of 18 % seen in the individuals not on any such therapy ($p < 0.0119$).

As with any study, this study has some limitations. The population size studied was not large enough to accurately comment on less commonly used forms of management for anterior epistaxis. Similarly, there was no data or rating on the severity of epistaxis on arrival to the ED that, in the end, may have affected physician treatment selection and also affected recurrence. This may confound the relationship between the treatment modality used and outcomes. At the institution of this study, patients presenting acutely with anterior epistaxis are seen first by an emergency physician, who may or may not utilise nasal endoscopy if the bleeding site is not readily identified on anterior rhinoscopy. Similarly, a standardized approach to patient evaluation prior to treatment selection was not utilised for the patients in this series. A standard approach to patient evaluation for anterior epistaxis such as the application of a topical decongestant/vasoconstrictor and analgesia prior to assessment for a bleeding site is needed. Given that the decision to use cautery requires visualization of the bleeding site the choice between packing and cautery for an ED physician may then have been affected. Further, there may also have been patients who were lost to follow up due to ED visits at other locations in the case of re-bleeding. Despite the limitations in this study, the large patient population allowed for informative evaluation of the treatment data.

## Conclusions

In summary, the current practices for the treatment of anterior epistaxis in the ED are quite variable. There are many modalities currently in use and there is not yet an accepted evidence-based recommendation to help guide treatment decisions. Looking at the four most common modalities used to treat anterior epistaxis in the ED from this study, the use of silver nitrate appears to be an effective management option taking into account the time and resources used for any other modality necessitating a patient to return to the ED. This suggests that if the anterior site of bleeding is identifiable, it is likely amenable to chemical cautery, silver nitrate be the first line treatment. However, due to limitations of the study, and that there was no grading system to identify epistaxis severity, a recommendation of silver nitrate cautery for all occurrences of anterior epistaxis cannot be given at this time. Further study is needed to determine the most efficacious treatment modality based on epistaxis severity.

### Competing interests
The authors declare that they have no competing interests.

### Authors' contributions
SK conceived the study, and obtained ethics approval. SK supervised the conduct of the trial and data collection. EN and AL undertook collecting patient data, and management of the. EN, AL and WP provided statistical advice on study design and helped analyze the data. EN drafted the manuscript, and all authors contributed substantially to its revision. SK takes responsibility for the paper as a whole. All authors read and approved the final manuscript.

### Author details
[1]University of Ottawa, Ottawa, ON, Canada. [2]Department of Otolaryngology - Head and Neck Surgery, University of Ottawa, Ontario, Canada. [3]Ottawa Hospital Research Institute (OHRI), Ottawa, ON, Canada.

### References
1. Pallin DJ, Chng YM, McKay MP, Emond JA, Pelletier AJ, Camargo Jr CA. Epidemiology of epistaxis in US emergency departments, 1992 to 2001. Ann Emerg Med. 2005;46:77–81.
2. Viehweg TL, Roberson JB, Hudson JW. Epistaxis: diagnosis and treatment. J Oral Maxillofac Surg. 2006;64:511–8.
3. Abdelkader M, Leong SC, White PS. Endoscopic control of the sphenopalatine artery for epistaxis: long-term results. J Laryngol Otol. 2007;121:759–62.
4. Bachelet JT, Bourlet J, Gleizal A. Hemostatic absorbable gel matrix for severe post-traumatic epistaxis. Rev stomatol Chir Maxillofac Chir Orale. 2013;114: 310–4.
5. Badran K, Malik TH, Belloso A, Timms MS. Randomized controlled trial comparing Merocel and RapidRhino packing in the management of anterior epistaxis. Clin Otolaryngol. 2005;30:333–7.
6. Biggs TC, Baruah P, Mainwaring J, Harries PG, Salib RJ. Treatment algorithm for oral anticoagulant and antiplatelet therapy in epistaxis patients. J Laryngol Otol. 2013;127:483–8.
7. Killick N, Malik V, Nirmal Kumar B. Nasal packing for epistaxis: an evidence-based review. Br J Hosp Med (London, England: 2005). 2014;75:143–4.
8. Kucik CJ, Clenney T. Management of epistaxis. Am Fam Physician. 2005; 71:305–11.
9. Morgan DJ, Kellerman R. Epistaxis: evaluation and treatment. Prim Care. 2014;41:63–73.
10. Toner JG, Walby AP. Comparison of electro and chemical cautery in the treatment of anterior epistaxis. J Laryngol Otol. 1990;104:617–8.
11. Kilty SJ, Al-Hajry M, Al-Mutairi D, et al. Prospective clinical trial of gelatin-thrombin matrix as first line treatment of posterior epistaxis. Laryngoscope. 2014;124:38–42.
12. Mathiasen RA, Cruz RM. Prospective, randomized, controlled clinical trial of a novel matrix hemostatic sealant in patients with acute anterior epistaxis. Laryngoscope. 2005;115:899–902.

# 30

# Avoiding allogenic blood transfusions in endoscopic angiofibroma surgery

Hisham Wasl[*], Jessica McGuire and Darlene Lubbe

## Abstract

**Background:** Surgical approaches for many tumours are often limited by blood loss, exposure and risk to vital anatomical structures. Therefore, the standard of care for certain skull base tumours has become endoscopic transnasal resection. Other surgical disciplines often use cell salvage techniques, but review of the otolaryngology literature revealed very few case reports. This study investigated the value and safety of salvage-type autologous blood transfusion during the endoscopic resection of juvenile nasopharyngeal angiofibromas (JNA).

**Methods:** JNA is a rare vascular nasal tumour and the study extended over a 3-year period to obtain adequate patient numbers. All patients undergoing endoscopic resection during this period were included in the population sample. Ten patients with JNA were identified and underwent embolization prior to the endoscopic resection. In all cases the intraoperative blood salvage apparatus was used. Close post-operative monitoring was performed.

**Results:** Homologous blood transfusion could be avoided in all cases. Postoperative monitoring revealed transient bacteraemia in two cases where the leukocyte filter was not used, but no evidence of septicaemia.

**Conclusions:** Perioperative cell saver and autologous blood transfusion in endonasal JNA surgery is safe. Homologous blood transfusion can be avoided by using this technique. The use of cell salvage allows for single stage surgery without the need to abandon surgery due to excessive blood loss and its future use is promising.

## Background

For more than 25 years, trauma, orthopaedic, urological, liver transplant and cardiac surgery have used intraoperative cell salvage (ICS) techniques [1]. However, in contaminated surgical fields the role of cell salvage techniques has been contentious. Contaminated surgical fields have been previously considered as a relative or absolute contraindication for intraoperative cell salvage. However, it is increasingly being used during trauma surgery even though the surgical field is often deemed contaminated and has been found to be a safe technique. A review of the literature reveals no research about the utilisation of cell salvage techniques in endonasal surgery.

Haemorrhage during tumour surgery often results in the need for intraoperative allogeneic blood transfusion. Many reports have focused on allogenic transfusion risks, such as immunomodulation, transfusion related immune-mediated reactions and infection. It may be associated with increased mortality, myocardial infarction and increased risk of tumour recurrence [2]. ICS autologous blood transfusions reduce the need for allogenic blood transfusions.

Other advantages of ICS autologous blood transfusions are reduced burden on blood donation systems, the blood available is proportional to the blood lost during surgery, there is no haemodilution; and it can be used when significant blood loss is anticipated [3]. Salvaged red cells also have a better oxygen delivery profile, and the system is cost-effective.

Pre-operative embolization is associated with less blood loss. A meta-analysis of the clinical features and treatment outcomes were unable to draw definitive conclusions regarding expected blood loss because most studies do not stratify blood loss according to stage and most studies on JNA are non-comparative case series [4]. At our institute almost all patients with Fisch stage 2c and 3 would require a transfusion, even with pre-operative embolization.

* Correspondence: hisham7070@yahoo.com
Division of Otolaryngology, University of Cape Town, Cape Town, South Africa

The autologous red cell recovery system, also known as the "cell saver", has a double lumen tube that mixes the aspirated blood with a heparin solution and collects it in a reservoir (Fig. 1). A centrifuge is then used to separate erythrocytes from the blood and cell stroma, free haemoglobin and plasma flow to the waste bag. The leukocyte filter is used to provide further protection, and blood is then re-infused into the patient (Fig. 1). The mechanisms of leukocyte reduction by leukocyte depletion filter (LDF) are insufficiently understood. It is widely accepted that centrifugal effects are used to eliminate bacteria with cell saver methods. Bacterial removal mechanisms of the leukocyte depletion filter (LDF) cannot depend on the size of bacteria alone and may be more dependent on adhesive characteristics of the filter, such as the surface structure of the material used in the filter, wettability, surface charge, the disintegration of cells, and deformability of infected cells in the filter [5, 6]. Reports indicate that 97.6 to 100 % of bacterial colony-forming units may be cleared when blood is subjected to a leukocyte filtration system and is washed.

According to our reading, there has been no research done with regards to the role of red cell salvage in endoscopic JNA surgery. This research forms a preliminary study into the role of cell salvage during JNA surgery.

## Methods

We conducted a prospective study over a 3 year period of all patients undergoing endoscopic resection of JNA at 2 centres, by a single surgeon. Ten patients were enrolled, they all had Fisch stage 3 or 4 tumours and all underwent pre-operative embolization, had intra-operative cell salvage and close postoperative monitoring. We received ethics approval from the *Human Research Ethics Committee* of the *University of Cape Town*. Inclusion criteria were an estimated blood loss of more than 500 ml and a patient that may qualify for an intraoperative blood transfusion. No JNA patients were excluded.

Patients were all male and aged between 12 and 20 years. The first patient was a Jehovah's Witness and refused allogeneic blood transfusion; however the church found autologous blood transfusion via a salvage system acceptable if transfusion was required. No leucocyte filter was available in the government sector hospital and the surgeons advised against surgery since the transfusion likelihood was 100 % for a stage 2c tumour at our institution. However, due to state policy the surgeons were obligated to perform surgery.

The Fisch staging system for JNA grades tumours invading pterygomaxillary fossa and paranasal sinuses with bony destruction as stage 2. Stage 3 tumours invade the infratemporal fossa, orbit and/or parasellar region, remaining lateral to cavernous sinus (Fig. 2).

Based on the Fisch staging system for JNA, 6 patients had stage 2 tumours and 4 had stage 3 tumours (Table 1). Two patients with stage 3 disease had staged procedures with initial incomplete resection and the rest of the patient had successful complete resection of the tumour at the first surgery. Of the 2 patients requiring a second stage procedure, 1 had unsuccessful preoperative embolization and the first surgery was terminated as a result of bleeding and the other patient had extensive disease and residual tumour which required a second look procedure.

An intra-operative nasal swab was taken to determine the presence of bacteria in the surgical field and to obtain sensitivities in the event that antibiotics were required postoperatively. The cell saver system was used to salvage autologous blood. A second specimen for microscopy, culture and sensitivity (MCS) was taken from the cell saver system to detect the presence of organisms in the autologous blood that was to be transfused back to the patient.

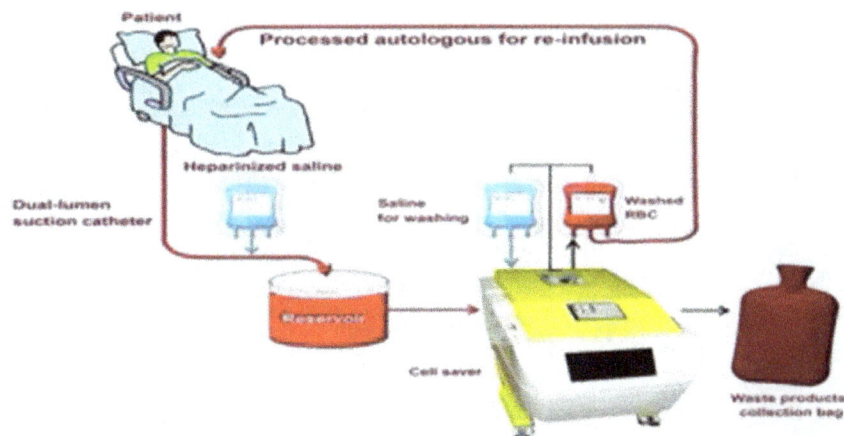

**Fig. 1** Cell salvage techniques

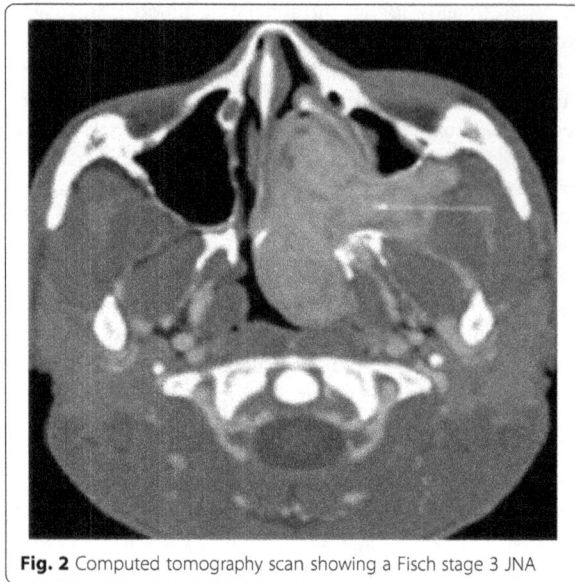

**Fig. 2** Computed tomography scan showing a Fisch stage 3 JNA

The anaesthetist and surgeon based decisions to transfuse each patient on their haemoglobin and clinical stability. The transfusion trigger was a haemoglobin of 7.0 g/dL or a falling pH level or an increasing anion gap. Blood was collected from the cell saver unit by a technician. Heparin was added to the collected blood, and only processed if a sufficient volume was recovered, or if the patient required a blood transfusion based on the above parameters. The disposables and the leukocyte filter need only be set up when a decision to process the blood is made. We found that using this standby technique could reduce the costs of cell salvage by 90 % if no blood was processed. This is important in resource-restricted hospitals.

The leukocyte filter was not used in two cases, as it was not available in the state hospital at that time. The rationale for proceeding with the autologous blood transfusion was that the patients were covered with broad spectrum antibiotics and the surgical site, although colonised by bacteria, was not infected. United Kingdom guidelines for autologous intraoperative blood transfusion recommend the use of a LDF in surgery for malignant disease, although they state that extensive clinical experience suggests the risk of seeding is not significant. JNA are benign tumours with no risk of distant metastases [7].

Our decision to use the LDF was based on knowledge that the nasal cavity is colonised by bacteria. There are no specific guidelines for the use of LDF in uncontaminated, colonised surgical fields [7].

All patients received prophylactic intraoperative antibiotics and a post-operative course of broad spectrum antibiotics for 48 h. Patients were monitored for signs of infection/ septicaemia by routine methods of temperature and pulse rate. A blood culture was performed 1 day following surgery to exclude a bacteraemia or septicaemia.

Postoperatively, all patients were admitted to the intensive care unit (ICU) for one day for monitoring. Laboratory coagulation tests were taken on admission to ICU, and the international normalised ratio (INR) in the laboratory control group was 1.1.

The mean hospital stay for all patients was 3 days. Nasal packs were removed on the second day after surgery and no patients needed a relook procedure for haemostasis. All patients were seen in the clinic 7 days after surgery for routine endoscopic examination and nasal debridement. They had post-operative magnetic resonance imaging 3 months post-surgery and after 6 months; yearly follow up was planned for all patients.

**Table 1** Summary of results

| Patient | Age | Tumour stage Fisch | Intraoperative blood loss (ml) | Cell saver blood transfusion | Nasal swab | Cell saver blood culture | Postoperative blood culture |
|---|---|---|---|---|---|---|---|
| Patient 1 | 12 | 2 | 500 ml | 200 ml | Staphylococcus Aureus | No growth | No growth |
| Patient 2 | 19 | 2 | 500 ml | 300 ml | Staphylococcus Aureus | No growth | No growth |
| Patient 3 | 18 | 3 | 1700 ml | 700 ml | Staphylococcus Aureus | No growth | No growth |
| Patient 4 No LDF | 13 | 3 | 2000 ml | 1500 ml | Staphylococcus Aureus | Staphylococcus Aureus | Staphylococcus Aureus |
| Patient 5 Johavah's Witness | 16 | 3 | 4000 ml | 2500 ml | Streptococcus Viridans | No growth | No growth |
| Patient 6 | 14 | 3 | 3000 ml | 1700 ml | Methicillinresistant Staphylococcus Aureus (MRSA) | No growth | No growth |
| Patient 7 | 15 | 2 | 1000 ml | 600 ml | Staphylococcus Epidermidis | No growth | No growth |
| Patient 8 | 13 | 2 | 900 ml | 400 ml | Streptococcus Viridans | No growth | No growth |
| Patient 9 | 16 | 2 | 1000 ml | 600 ml | Moraxella Catarrhalis | No growth | No growth |
| Patient 10 No LDF | 14 | 2 | 700 ml | 250 ml | Staphylococcus Aureus | Staphylococcus Aureus | Staphylococcus Aureus |

## Results

The mean volume of blood lost from the 10 patients was 1530 mL (500–4000 mL). The mean volume of re-infused blood was 875 mL (200–2600 mL) (Table 1).

Bacterial growth was detected on all nasal swabs. Organisms that were cultured included: *Staphylococcus aureus*, *Staphylococcus epidermidis*, *Streptococcus viridans*, and *Moreaxella catarrhalis* (Table 1).

In both cases in which a LDF was not available, the same organism that was isolated from the nasal cavity was also cultured from the cell saver washed blood. Postoperatively the 2 patients developed a transient bacteraemia with a raised temperature and pulse rate and a positive blood culture, in which the same organism was grown (Table 1). Both were treated with the appropriate intravenous antibiotics according to sensitivities and both recovered completely.

Routine postoperative monitoring revealed that haemoglobin and coagulation levels were within the normal range for all patients, with no evidence of major complications such as haemoglobinuria, coagulopathy, cardiopulmonary issues or sepsis. None of the patients had postoperative epistaxis. None of the patients required any allogeneic blood products. Regular follow up after discharge showed no adverse events (minimum follow-up time was 18 months).

## Discussion and conclusions

The most common benign vascular neoplasm of the nasopharynx is juvenile angiofibroma (JNA) [5]. It is locally destructive and causes bony erosion despite its benign histology. JNA can extend intracranially and cause complications that are potentially life threatening, such as massive blood loss and fatal epistaxis [5]. There are both fibrotic and vascular elements within the tumours, but the vessels lack an elastic lamina and this precludes constriction and is partially responsible for their propensity to bleed [6, 8]. The management of JNA can be challenging because of its aggressive growth pattern, vital adjacent anatomical structures and rich blood supply.

Our institute uses two methods to control blood loss during JNA surgery: the first method is preoperative embolization which was performed in all our patients. The second method is intraoperative cell salvage technique.

Our greatest concern was that we were re-infusing blood from a bacterially colonised surgical field. This has been done previously in gastrointestinal surgery for perforated peptic ulcers. They covered the patients with broad spectrum antibiotics perioperatively and the only post-operative complication they had were wound infections in 3 out of 11 patients, which may have been unrelated to the transfusion [9]. This was reinforced by a study of patients undergoing liver transplantation who received ICS blood transfusion and despite there being positive bacterial cultures in 8 out of 28 re-transfusion bags, no post-operative infections were observed. The patients' blood cultures remained negative 1 week post-surgery [10]. Other surgical disciplines have also demonstrated the successful use of culture-positive cell saver blood with no reported adverse clinical consequences [11-13]. Another concern associated with cell salvage blood is the promotion of coagulopathy, but no evidence of coagulopathy was revealed in any of our patients, and all laboratory parameters were normal.

The use of cell salvage autologous blood transfusion is cost effective and reduces the need for allogenic transfusions. This is associated with shorter hospital stays, reduced blood transfusion reactions and reduced postoperative infection rates. The cost of leukocyte filters should be a consideration, especially in resource limited settings. Although these filters are not expensive; additional savings may be instituted by employing a standby technique in JNA surgery, which includes collecting blood from the operative field but only using it if necessary.

The combination of washing blood cells and using a leucocyte filter significantly reduced the bacterial load in processed blood that could then be safely re-transfused to the patient. Leukocyte depletion filters have been widely used during the processing of donated blood to remove white blood cells and their use is now acknowledged to improve cell salvage safety and to reduce the incidence of any cell salvage adverse effects [14]. Various findings have revealed that leukocyte depletion filters are effective in removing white blood cells, tumour cells [15–17], amniotic fluid [18], and bacteria [3].

Our study has shown that cell saver techniques are beneficial in JNA surgery, as the surgery can be completed in a single stage, there is a decreased need for allogenic blood transfusion, and it is often acceptable to Jehovah's Witness patients. This study has also demonstrated that intraoperative cell salvage is a safe technique in endoscopic JNA surgery. We recommend the use of leucocyte depletion filters and perioperative broad-spectrum antibiotics. Our findings indicate that the commensal bacteria that are introduced with the re-transfused blood are successfully eliminated by an intact immunological system. This explains the good tolerance to the iatrogenic bacteraemia that was caused.

In conclusion, cell salvage autologous blood transfusion is safe and effective in reducing allogenic blood transfusion requirements in endoscopic JNA surgery. Cell salvage should be considered in all cases of JNA surgery as significant blood loss is usually anticipated. This can also be used in situations when patients refuse allogenic blood products. The standby technique allows cell salvage to be used in cases where blood transfusion is not required, but significant bleeding is a possibility, which contributes to relieving the stress on blood donation services.

Leukocyte depletion filters are recommended to provide an additional element of safety, and should be used
in all cell salvage autologous blood transfusions. In addition,
a contaminated surgical field is not a contraindication for
the use of cell salvage blood as long as adequate pre-
cautions are taken. Recent evidence has shown that cell
salvage may be used in malignancy surgery, and that the
only contraindication to using cell salvage blood, is the
patient's refusal to accept autologous blood.

A limitation of our study is the small number of patients
due to the rarity of the disease. Further research is needed
with a larger population sample to define the efficacy of
this technique in avoiding allogeneic blood transfusions
and its impact on several outcome variables.

## Consent
Written informed consent was obtained from the patients
and their parents for publication of this case report and
accompanying images. A copy of the written consent is
available for review by the Editor-in-Chief of this journal.

### Competing interests
The authors declare that they have no competing interests.

### Authors' contributions
HW carried out the Conception, drafting, data analysis, and major revisions.
JM participated in the sequence alignment, drafted the manuscript, and major
revisions. DL participated in the sequence alignment, drafted the manuscript,
and major revisions. DL was also the supervisor and surgeon for all the cases.
All authors read and approved the final manuscript.

### Acknowledgements
We thank Professor Fagan for sharing his pearl of wisdom with us during the
course of this research.

## References
1.  Anderson S. Are cell salvage and autologous blood transfusion safe in
    endonasal surgery? Otolaryngol Head Neck Surg. 2010;142:S3–6.
2.  Leal-Noval SR, Rincon-Ferrari MD, Garcıa-Curiel A, Herruzo-Aviles A,
    Camacho-Larana P, Garnacho-Montero J, et al. Transfusion of blood
    components and postoperative infection in patients undergoing cardiac
    surgery. Chest. 2001;119:1461–8.
3.  Waters J, Tuohy M, Hobson D, et al. Bacterial reduction by cell salvage
    washing and leukocyte depletion filtration. Anaesthesiology. 2003;99:652–5.
4.  Khoueir N, Nicolas N, Rohayem Z, Haddad A, Abou Hamad W. Exclusive
    endoscopic resection of juvenile nasopharyngeal angiofibroma: a systematic
    review of the literature. Otolaryngol Head Neck Surg. 2014;150(3):350–8. doi:
    10.1177/0194599813516605. Epub 2013 Dec 31.
5.  Renkonen S, Hagström J, Vuola J, et al. The changing surgical management
    of juvenile nasopharyngeal angiofibroma. Eur Arch Otorhinolaryngol. 2011;
    268(4):599–607.
6.  Blount A, Riley KO, Woodworth BA. Juvenile nasopharyngeal angiofibroma.
    Otolaryngol Clin N Am. 2011;44(4):989–1004.
7.  Joint United Kingdom Blood Transfusion and Tissue Transplantation
    Services Professional Advisory Committee. 6.1: Autologous blood
    transfusion: 6.1.2: Intraoperative cell salvage. http://www.transfusionguidelines.
    org/transfusion-handbook/6-alternatives-and-adjuncts-to-blood-transfusion/6-
    1-autologous-blood-transfusion-collection-and-reinfusion-of-the-patient-s-own-
    red-blood-cells. [5 January 2016].
8.  Fyrmpas G, Konstantinidis I, Constantinidis J. Endoscopic treatment of
    juvenile nasopharyngeal angiofibromas: our experience and review of the
    literature. Eur Arch Otorhinolaryngol. 2012;269(2):523–39.
9.  Timberlake GA, MeSwain NE. Autotransfusion of blood contaminated by
    enteric contents: a potentially life-saving measure in the massively
    haemorrhaging trauma patient? J Trauma. 1988;28:855.
10. Kang Y, Aggarwal S, Virji M, Pasculle AW, Lewis JH, Freeman JA, Martin LK.
    Clinical evaluation of autotransfusion during liver transplantation. Anesth
    Analg. 1991;72:94.
11. Sugai Y, Sugai K, Fuse A. Current status of bacterial contamination of
    autologous blood for transfusion. Transfus Apher Sci. 2001;24(3):255–9.
12. Ezzedine H, Baele P, Robert A. Bacteriologic quality of intraoperative
    autotransfusion. Surgery. 1991;109(3Pt1):259–64.
13. Locher MC, Sailer HF. The use of the Cell Saver in transoral maxillofacial
    surgery: a preliminary report. J Craniomaxillofac Surg. 1992;20(1):14–7.
14. Duffy G, Neal KR. Differences in post-operative infection rates between
    patients receiving autologous and allogeneic blood transfusion: a meta-
    analysis of published randomised and nonrandomised studies. Transfus
    Med. 1996;6:325–8.
15. Innerhofer P, Klingler A, Klimmer C, Fries D, Nussbaumer W. Risk of
    postoperative infection after transfusion of white blood cell-filtered
    allogeneic or autologous blood components in orthopaedic patients
    undergoing primary arthoplasty. Transfusion. 2005;45:103–10.
16. Catling S, Williams S, Freites O, Rees M, Davis C, Hopkins L. Use of a
    leucocyte filter to remove tumour cells from intra-operative cell salvage
    blood. Anaesthesia. 2008;63:1332–8.
17. Laing TB, Li DL, Laing L, Zhang JM. Intraoperative blood salvage during liver
    transplantation in patients with hepatocellular carcinoma: efficiency of
    leukocyte depletion filters in the removal of tumour cells. Transplantation.
    2008;85:863–9.
18. Sullivan I, Faulds J, Ralph C. Contamination of salvaged maternal blood by
    amniotic fluid and foetal red cells during elective caesarean section. Br J
    Anaesth. 2008;101:225–9.

# 31

# Monoscopic photogrammetry to obtain 3D models by a mobile device: a method for making facial prostheses

Rodrigo Salazar-Gamarra[1*], Rosemary Seelaus[2], Jorge Vicente Lopes da Silva[3], Airton Moreira da Silva[4] and Luciano Lauria Dib[1,5]

## Abstract

**Purpose:** The aim of this study is to present the development of a new technique to obtain 3D models using photogrammetry by a mobile device and free software, as a method for making digital facial impressions of patients with maxillofacial defects for the final purpose of 3D printing of facial prostheses.

**Methods:** With the use of a mobile device, free software and a photo capture protocol, 2D captures of the anatomy of a patient with a facial defect were transformed into a 3D model. The resultant digital models were evaluated for visual and technical integrity. The technical process and resultant models were described and analyzed for technical and clinical usability.

**Results:** Generating 3D models to make digital face impressions was possible by the use of photogrammetry with photos taken by a mobile device. The facial anatomy of the patient was reproduced by a *.3dp* and a *.stl* file with no major irregularities. 3D printing was possible.

**Conclusions:** An alternative method for capturing facial anatomy is possible using a mobile device for the purpose of obtaining and designing 3D models for facial rehabilitation. Further studies must be realized to compare 3D modeling among different techniques and systems.

**Clinical implication:** Free software and low cost equipment could be a feasible solution to obtain 3D models for making digital face impressions for maxillofacial prostheses, improving access for clinical centers that do not have high cost technology considered as a prior acquisition.

**Keywords:** 123D Catch, 3D photography, Maxillofacial rehabilitation, Facial prosthetics, Photogrammetry, Oral rehabilitation

## Background

Facial mutilation and defects could derive from cancer, tumors, trauma, infections, congenital or acquired deformation and affect quality of life due to the impact on essential functions such as communication, breathing, feeding and aesthetics [1–5]. Rehabilitation of these patients is possible with adhesive-retained facial prosthetics, implant supported facial prosthetics and plastic surgery [2, 6–12]. Although some aesthetic results can be achieved by plastic surgery [13, 14], frequently this requires multiple attempts which

are time consuming and costly [15]. In most cases worldwide, defects of external facial anatomy are primarily treated by prostheses [16, 17]. Still, for the realization of a prosthesis, a highly trained and skilled specialist is required to sculpt a form mimicking the lost anatomy, and to handle the time-consuming technical fabrication process.

To make a facial prosthesis, an impression is required to record the anatomic area of the defect. Some impression materials have demonstrated high and accurate precision registering details of defects and the surrounding anatomy [18–21], but present other difficulties and limitations [22, 23]. Some challenges are related to the technical sensitivity of the material, working time and setting time. Training and experience is needed to handle the materials, especially

* Correspondence: rodrigo_eb@hotmail.com
[1]UNIP Postgraduate Dental School, Universidade Paulista, Rua Afonso Braz, 525 - Cj. 81 Vila Nova Conceição, São Paulo CEP 04511-011, SP, Brazil
Full list of author information is available at the end of the article

when working near the airway, and frequently require the assistance of a second professional to help in the procedure. In cases of large facial defects, there is a need to cover all the face which can be claustrophobic for the patient. Also the weight of the materials and the use of cannulas, to allow free airway during the procedure with the mouth opening, can deform the residual facial tissues, causing distortion in the impression [22]. The economic cost of large usage of impression materials is also a topic of concern. A limitation of conventional facial impressions is that they cannot predict information about results of the final rehabilitation because they only register detail of the defect and surrounding tissues.

To address these difficulties of conventional facial impressions, some authors reported [24, 25] clinical cases using Computerized Tomography (CT-Scan) [26, 27], Magnetic Resonance Imaging (MRI) [27, 28], Laser impressions [27, 29–32] and 3D photography [33, 34] to record extra-oral digital impressions. Digital impressions are also used to print working models [34], design prostheses digitally by mirroring from a healthy side [36], digitally capturing structures from a healthy donor patient [37]' for designing templates of the final prostheses and prototyping it, or to design a prototype model of the flask where the silicone is directly packaged [31, 38]. These reports represent a viable way to rehabilitate patients in less time, with more effectiveness, improved accuracy and less effort by the patient and the professional. However the use of such technologies can produce even higher costs in software, hardware or other equipment. Different authors have sought alternatives to transform these impressions with low cost solutions [38], but there is still no consensus nor a concept widely accepted.

Among all the possible methods for 3D surface imaging and data acquisition, 3D photogrammetry is attractive for its capacity to obtain 3D models from 2D pictures, the capture and process speed, absence of radiation for patient, good results and non-complex training [39–41]. 3D photography is performed by a method called photogrammetry, that emerged from radiolocation, multilateration and radiometry and it has been used since the mid-19th century in industries of space, aeronautics, geology, meteorology, geography, tourism, and entertainment. More recently, applications in general medicine have been reported. Photogrammetry allows "Structure from Motion" (SFM) where the software examines common features in each image and is able to construct a 3D form from overlapping features, by a complex algorithm that minimizes the sum of errors over the coordinates and relative displacements of the reference points. This minimization is known as "bundle adjustment" and is often performed using the Levenberg-Marquardt algorithm. Photogrammetry can be used in a stereophotogrammetry technique, where all captures are made simultaneously by different cameras at different heights and angles relative to the object/subject; or, by a monoscopic technique, where only one camera is used to do sequential captures at different heights and angles from to the object/subject [39–41]. This industry has developed different products and systems for simplifying the clinical application obtaining increasingly better results. On the other hand, this technology demands high costs for hardware, software and infrastructure and may not be possible for many centers worldwide.

Alternatives for expensive photogrammetry are free software that can be used by computers, tablets and other mobile devices to generate 3D models from 2D pictures by similar methods (Autodesk 123D Catch®, California, US) [42, 43]. Initially, the target of these software was entertainment and other non-medical use. Recently Mahmoud [42] used this free software for medical educational reasons and Koban [43] for making an evaluation and analysis for plastic surgery planning on a plastic mannequin. To the authors best knowledge, monoscopic photogrammetry has not been published for facilitating the process of fabrication of facial prostheses in humans, by adapting this low cost technology into a clinical solution. The possibility to decrease the cost of fabrication of facial prostheses with the use of mobile devices and free software would warrant investigation for the benefit of most parts of the world.

The incorporation of technology into the fabrication process of facial prostheses has the potential to transform the rehabilitation, from a time-consuming artistically driven process to a reconstructive biotechnology procedure [24]. One of the methods for surface data acquisition and 3D modeling is 3D photography (photogrammetry) that has been used in medical sciences since 1951[44–46]. In recent years, techniques and methods have been improving to the benefit of the surgical and prosthetic team [47, 48]. Technical validation and evaluation of sophisticated photogrammetry systems have reported beneficial applications in facial prosthetic treatment [49–57]. 3D photography has been a practical solution in clinical practice compared with other 3D model obtaining methods (MRI, CT-Scan & Laser) [26–37, 58–64]. Still this technology requires substantial investment in infrastructure, hardware and software for clinical practice [65, 66]. For this reason, some authors have pursued low cost processes for fabrication of facial prosthetics [38], with the use of free software and the monoscopic photogrammetry technique with mobile devices [42, 43].

## Methods
### Patient selection
One subject, who attended the Maxillofacial Prosthetic Clinic of the *Universidade Paulista* in *São Paulo* for prosthetic rehabilitation, was selected after being advised about ethical aspects of the research and freely accepted

to participate. Informed consent was obtained from the patient.

## Data acquisition

### Subject and operator positioning

The subject was positioned in a 45 cm-high chair in an upright seated position, with 1 meter of floor space between the chair and the position of the operator with 0° − 180° of clearance laterally, where 90° was the primary area of interest to capture. Floor clearance allowed sufficient room for the operator to move around the subject during the capture process. An adjustable-height (30 cm to 50 cm) chair with wheels for mobility was used by the operator. Earrings, hats, glasses or other accessories that could interfere with the area of capture were removed from the subject prior to photo capture. The subject was instructed to remain still in order to eliminate balance movement and maintain the head in an orthostatic position with the Frankfurt plane parallel to the floor. If balance of the head was detected after giving the instruction of not moving, a head support was used between the head and a wall. The subject was also instructed to: maintain a neutral facial expression, with jaw and lips closed without force (maximal intercuspal occlusion); to wear his intraoral removable prostheses for giving support to the facial tissues; and, to blink between photographs repeating the same eye position. Visual color contrast between the background and the colors of the skin and hair of the subject was established. A clinical measurement of the inter-alar nasal distance was registered for further scale verification.

### Lighting

Sufficient lighting in the room was ensured such that the ambient light enabled taking clear images without flash and without underexposing or overexposing images. Lights of the room, blinds and curtains of the windows were opened and orientation of the ambient light was considered to avoid getting shadows on the area of interest through the process of capture. Irregular lighting was avoided, like strong back-lighting and direct, intense light to the subject. Objects with strong reflective or shiny surfaces were eliminated from the camera's field of view during the photo capture process.

### Mobile device and application

An internet Wi-Fi 5Ghz network connection was used. A free photogrammetry application (Autodesk 123D Catch®, California, US) was downloaded by a mobile device (Samsung Galaxy Note 4® - Seoul, South Korea) through the Android® Google Playstore® (California, US). A 123D Catch® and a free account was created. All automatic features of the mobile device were enabled as needed by the application for the data acquisition process. Features of the mobile device are outlined in (Table 1). 123D Catch® PC version

**Table 1** Mobile Device technical features

| Samsung galaxy note 4 - Brasilian standard version, software actualized at 10/03/2015 |
| --- |
| Hardware & Software |
| 1. Model: SM-N910C |
| 2. Android version 4.4.4 |
| 3. Kernel version 3.10.9-3317155 (Fundamental software of the operating system) |
| 4. KNOX version 2.2 (Informatic security) |
| 5. 2.7GHz Quad Core Process, 1.9GHz Octa Core (1.9GHz Quad + 1.3GHz Quad Core) Process |
| 6. MEMORY 3GB RAM + 32GB Internal memory |
| 7. NETWORK 2.5G (GSM/GPRS/EDGE) : 850/900/1800/1900 MHz. 3G (HSPA+ 42Mbps): 850/900/1900/2100 MHz, 4G (LTE Cat.4 150/50Mbps) or 4G (LTE Cat.6 300/50Mbps) |
| 8. CONNECTIVITY Wi-Fi 802.11 a/b/g/n/ac (2X2 MIMO) |
| 9. Camera F1.9 lens camera and 16MP Smart OIS, 31 mm focal length |
| 10. Accelerometer sensor (identify the position and movement of the cellphone and registers data in axis X, Y & Z) |
| 11. Gyroscope sensor (Identify the status of rotation of the telephone in axis X and Y) |

was also downloaded in a Windows PC (Dell Inspiron 1525 Dual Core).

### Photo capture

The photogrammetry application was opened from the mobile device and new capture was selected by pressing the "+" button in the upper right corner. A planned sequence of 15 conventional 2D photos were taken, always with the area of interest for capturing as the center of the picture and with the operator maintaining a 30 cm distance between his eyes and the mobile device, raising it up to his same eye-height position. Photo captures were taken at three different heights. The first height (H1) was the standup-height of the operator (1.75 m) with the mobile device at 1.50 m of height from the floor. (Figure 1a) The second height (H2) was with the operator seated on the moveable chair at its maximum adjustable height (50 cm) and maintaining the mobile device at 1.25 m from the floor. (Figure 1b) The third height (H3) was with the operator seated on the same chair at its lowest adjustable height (30 cm) with the mobile device at 1 m of height above the floor. (Figure 1c) Each height repeated the same positions for taking the photo captures and was taken at the 0°, 45°, 90°, 135° and 180°, considering 0° as subject's right side, 90° as the midline of the face and 180° as the subject's left side (Fig. 2). All photo captures were perpendicular to the primary area of interest. The operator took the first picture starting from H1-0° at a one meter distance from the subject. The complete sequence was H1-0°, H1-45°, H1-90°, H1-135° H1-180°, H2-

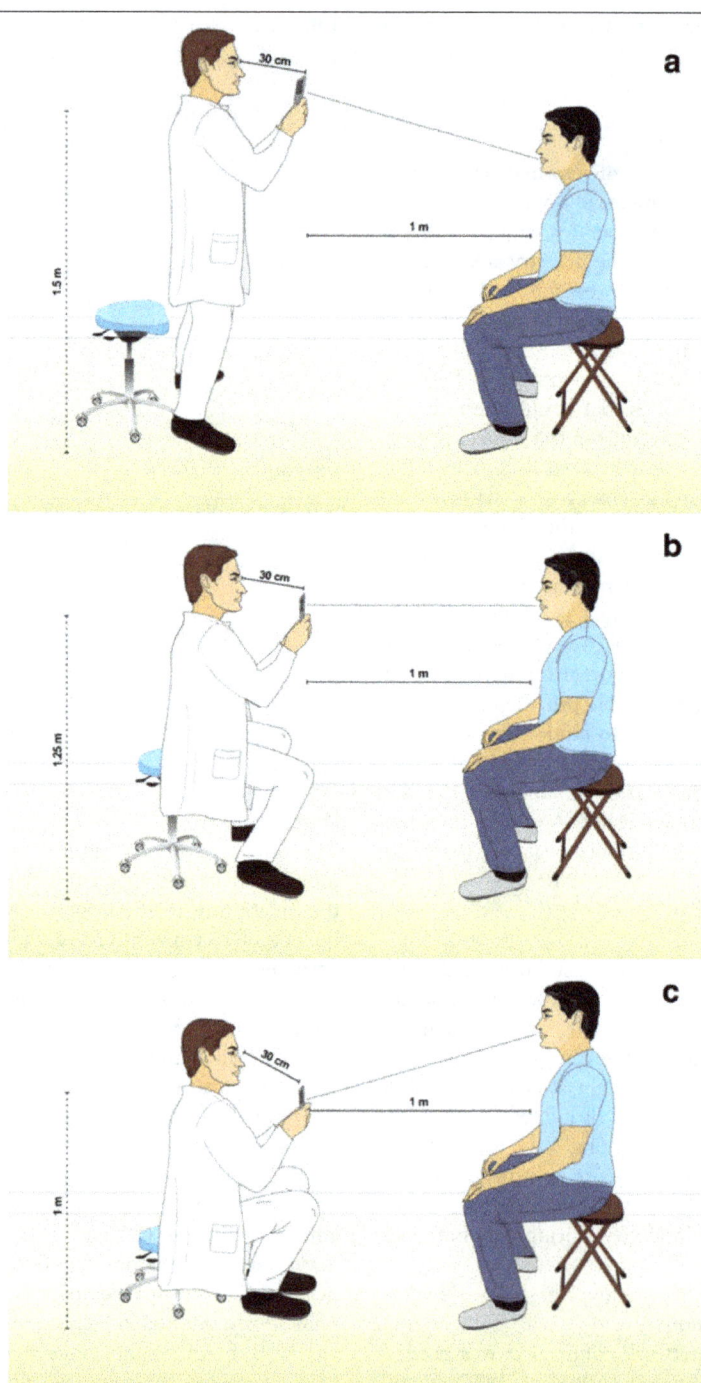

**Fig. 1 a**. Simulation of the Height 1, where the operator is at a stand up height and maintain the mobile device 30 cm from his head, 1.5 m from the floor and 1 meter from the patient. **b**. Simulation of the Height 2, where the operator sits on the higher height of the chair with wheels and maintain the mobile device 30 cm from his head, 1.25 m from the floor and 1 meter from the patient. **c**. Simulation of the Height 3, where the operator sits on the lower height of the chair with wheels and maintain the mobile device 30 cm from his head, 1 m from the floor and 1 meter from the patient

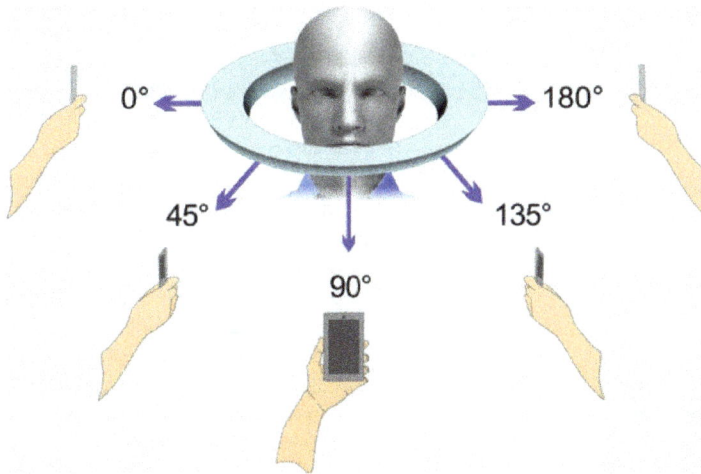

**Fig. 2** Simulation of angles of photo captures per each height

180°, H2-135°, H2-90°, H2-45°, H2-0°, H3-0°, H3-45°, H3-90°, H3-135° and H3-180°, completing the 15 photo captures (Fig. 3). For photo capture, the "autofocus" was used at the center of the area of interest, avoiding blurry photographs. The "position-in-space-recognition gadget" of the application was used to guide the position of photo captures and to register total numbers of photos recorded in the process (Fig. 4). Following the photo capture, the operator reviewed the integrity of each picture, verifying that there were no illumination irregularities, blurry images, incomplete parts of the face of the subject or any other evident errors in the picture that would compromise data processing. After ensuring the good quality of the photo captures, the subject was released from his static position and the "check" button was pressed for uploading the pictures for processing.

### Photo capture review and 3D processing

When all 15 photo captures were taken, the "check" button in the upper right corner of the application was pressed and captures were shown in the visor to be reviewed and approved with another pressing of the "Check" button. The application started automatically to upload and process the captures into the 123D Catch® servers. Once finished, the digital model was reviewed through the mobile device to verify its integrity.

All photo captures taken by the mobile device were downloaded from 123D Catch® website and meshed through the 123D Catch® PC version with the maximum quality of meshing. A *.3Dp and *.stl files were obtained. The *.3Dp file was opened and reviewed from 123D Catch® PC version for primary analyzing and the *.stl file was opened and edited from Autodesk Meshmixer (California,

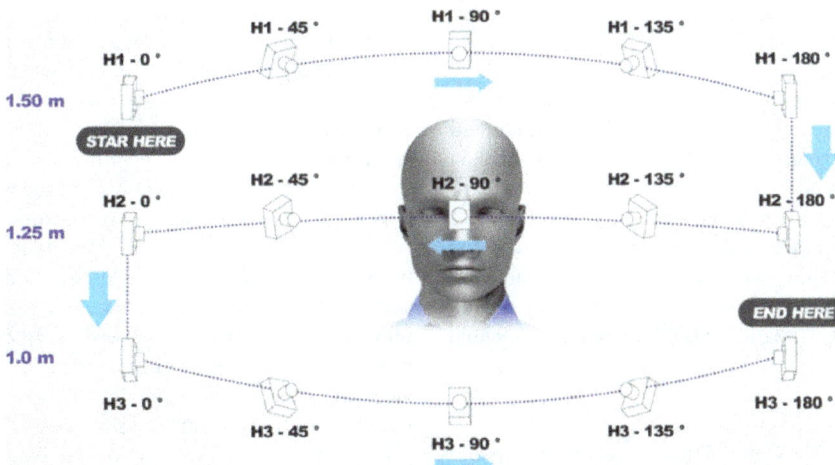

**Fig. 3** Simulation of the complete sequence of photo capture protocol around the area of interest for capture

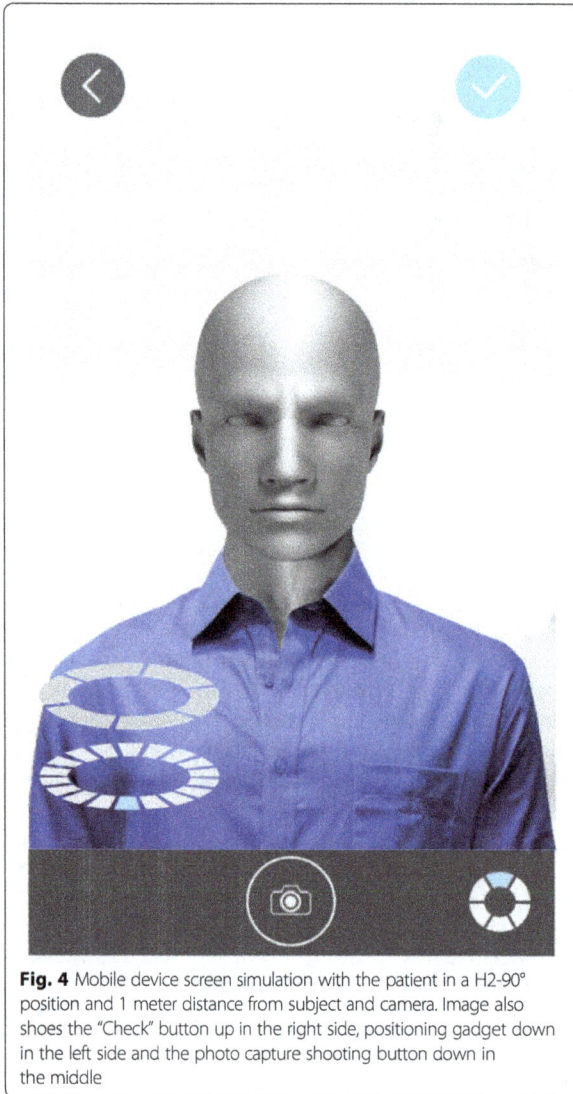

**Fig. 4** Mobile device screen simulation with the patient in a H2-90° position and 1 meter distance from subject and camera. Image also shoes the "Check" button up in the right side, positioning gadget down in the left side and the photo capture shooting button down in the middle

file format. Automatically, according to the mobile device camera features, sizes of photo captures varied from 4710 kb to 5931 kb with an average size of 5118 kb. Revision of the captured photos before processing detected that all captures were compatible with the protocol (Fig. 5). The revision of the created digital model through the mobile device before downloading found no major irregularities which could interrupt the process (Fig. 6).

Digital model and photo captures were downloaded from the Autodesk webpage. Photo captures were re-processed in high quality through the 123D Catch® PC version (Fig. 7). The combined use of 123D Catch® mobile device application and pc version created high quality *.3Dp and *.stl files from the 15 individual 2D photographs, with file sizes of *.3Dp and *.stl of 5 kb and 39,918 kb respectively (Fig. 8a, b).

By the use of Meshmixer®, it was possible to manually eliminate the triangles beyond the head, to reposition in space and to scale the digital model. This final manipulated digital model obtained appropriately represented the shape and proportions of the original face of the patient, leading to a printed polyamide model which also showed similarity of representation; although, some minor irregularities were detectable in the surface of eyebrows, hair and lateral sides of the patient (Figs. 8b and 9).

## Discussion

This study aimed to develop a technique to obtain 3D models by mobile device photogrammetry and the use of free software as a method for making facial impressions of patients with facial defects for the final purpose of 3D printing of facial prostheses. For this purpose a patient that voluntarily accepted to participate in the study was submitted to the proposed protocol and methods. Captures were taken by the use of 123D Catch through a mobile device by a controlled sequence, illumination and position of the operator and patient.

The rational for using a cellphone for making photo captures through the 123D Catch® application was that all modern mobile devices have an integrated accelerometer and a gyroscope sensor, which are automatically run by the application to guide the operator in a 3D position during the photo capture sequence. Also in today's market, mobile devices are equipt with faster processors, fast network and connection qualities, high quality cameras and added features, (Table 1), at a reasonable cost to the consumer as a personal tool, and not as a clinical equipment. Monoscopic photogrammetry has been used with different kinds of cameras like SLR, prosumer, point and shoot, mobile devices and others, principally for non-medical reasons [67], but also recently, for medical purposes [42, 43].

Developers of 123D Catch® published through their web tutorials some general indications for the photo capture process, and for that reason, in the present study, a

US). Editing in Meshmixer® only considered model repositioning in space (x-y-z axis transform tool) into a straight position, deleting triangles beyond the face and re-scaling model into the inter-alar nasal distance that had been clinically registered. 360° degrees observation and in all x-y-z axis angles for descriptive analysis was performed and the model of the face of the patient was printed in Duraform Polyamide C15 degraded material by a Sinterstation HiQ by Selective Laser Sinterization (SLS) (3D Systems, Rockhill SC, USA).

## Results

With the use of 123D Catch® mobile device application using the described photo capture protocol, fifteen two-dimensional colored photo captures were obtained in *.jpeg

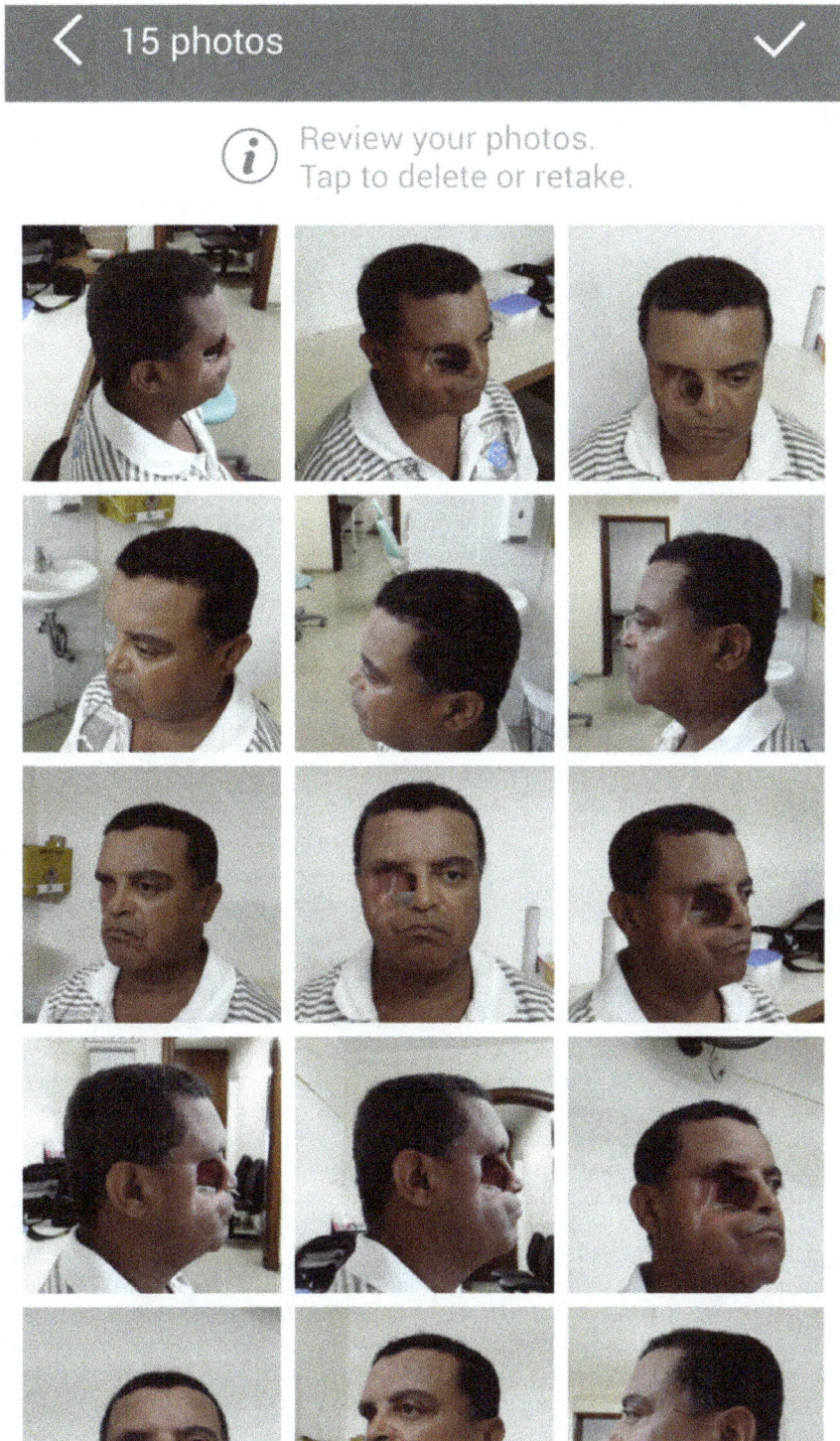

**Fig. 5** Mobile device screen with the 15 photo captures of the patient in the sequence of our protocol

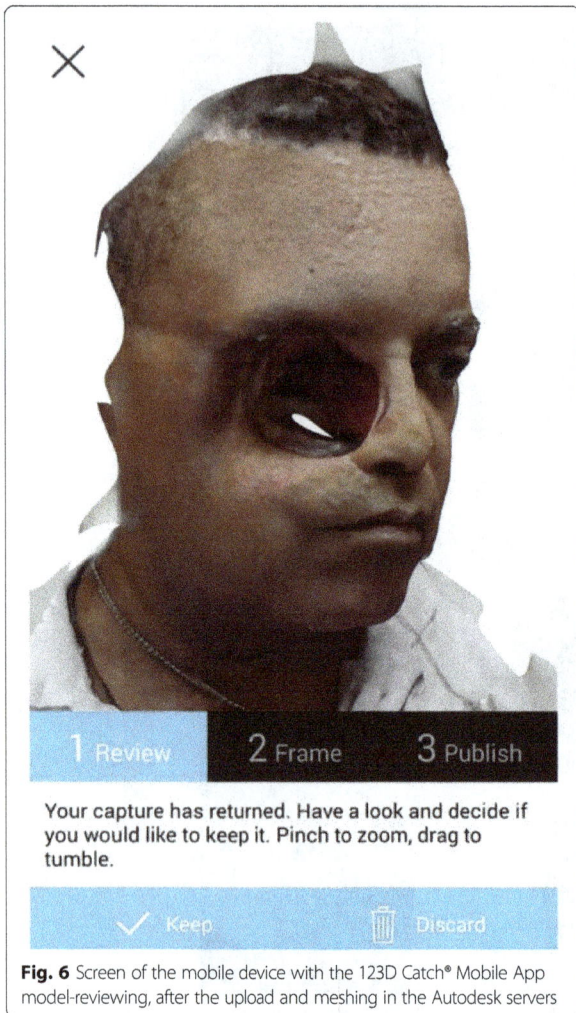

**Fig. 6** Screen of the mobile device with the 123D Catch® Mobile App model-reviewing, after the upload and meshing in the Autodesk servers

standardized sequence protocol of photo capturing was designed into a user-friendly sequence, which satisfies both the requirements of 123D Catch® and the clinical needs for maxillofacial rehabilitation. The most important considerations are sequence and orientation of capture, illumination, subject and operator positioning and clinical measurement of a stable reference of the subject. This free photogrammetry application recognizes patterns between captures that have more than 50 % of overlap between each capture [67]. For this reason, it was decided to make a sequence with 45° degree intervals between captures at each height, demonstrating acceptable results in the meshing process. If the illumination pattern is different between each capture, or the subject does not keep still during captures, or if photos are taken randomly or arbitrarily, the photo capture overlapping by the algorithm may not be possible, and will show defects, affecting the viability of using the model. It is for this reason that the

flash is not used, and rotating the patient on his own axis is not recommended. Flash will generate its own pattern between each capture, and if the patient is rotated on his own axis during capture, the illumination pattern over the patient and background will differ among captures and will be unreadable by the software [67]. The ideal is to complete multiple captures, as stereophotogrammetry does, while maintaining the position of the patient during the complete sequence of photo captures, one by one, with consistent conditions of ample indirect ambient light. The position of the operator is equally important to allow capture of the entire area of interest without losing detail from too great a distance, or producing shadows by being too close to the patient. One meter of distance between the subject and the camera is compatible with aforementioned technical requirements. Distance and position are important in the capture protocol, but absolute exactness is not critical since the application still recognizes patterns with consistent light reflection [67]. Currently, no information is available about a tolerance of acceptable variance in photo capture, and how this might impact the meshing process. While there are not objective protocols for evaluating the model, the clinician must subjectively evaluate the model to see if it is below a threshold of being usable. The time-consuming process of photo capture is prone to have some irregularities [43]. In this workflow, the 3D position of the reproduced anatomy is a very well startup for sculpture. All possible errors and small texture details may not have much importance because the digital model of the prostheses will serve to produce a prototype that will be duplicated in a wax for final handwork to obtain a sculpture with finishing details, texture, and adaptation into the patient. That's why small digital discrepancies on surface will not affect the final result of the definitive prosthesis. Actual technology, neither the expensive stereophotogrammetry systems, have not the enough imaging detail to reproduce skin texture, expression lines of the patient or others, resulting in a mandatory handwork finishing sculpture. A clinical measurement is needed for registration because 123D Catch® generates a reduced model and this is not unexpected since the application was meant for entertainment and desktop 3D printing objectives. Subsequently, scaling is required and a reliable, stable distance must be used. In our subject, the inter-alar distance of the nose was used. In other patients that have both eyes, the intercanthal or inter-pupilar distance could be to ensure stable measurement. Small ruler or fiducial markers fixed on the patient could be used for registration and scaling purposes.

Once the models were obtained (*.3Dp & *.stl), *.3Dp models showed good appearance in color and proportions of the subject through the 123D Catch® mobile device app and PC version. The *.3Dp file was useful only by this application but can be exported as other file types like *.obj or *.stl. Alternatively, multiple file types

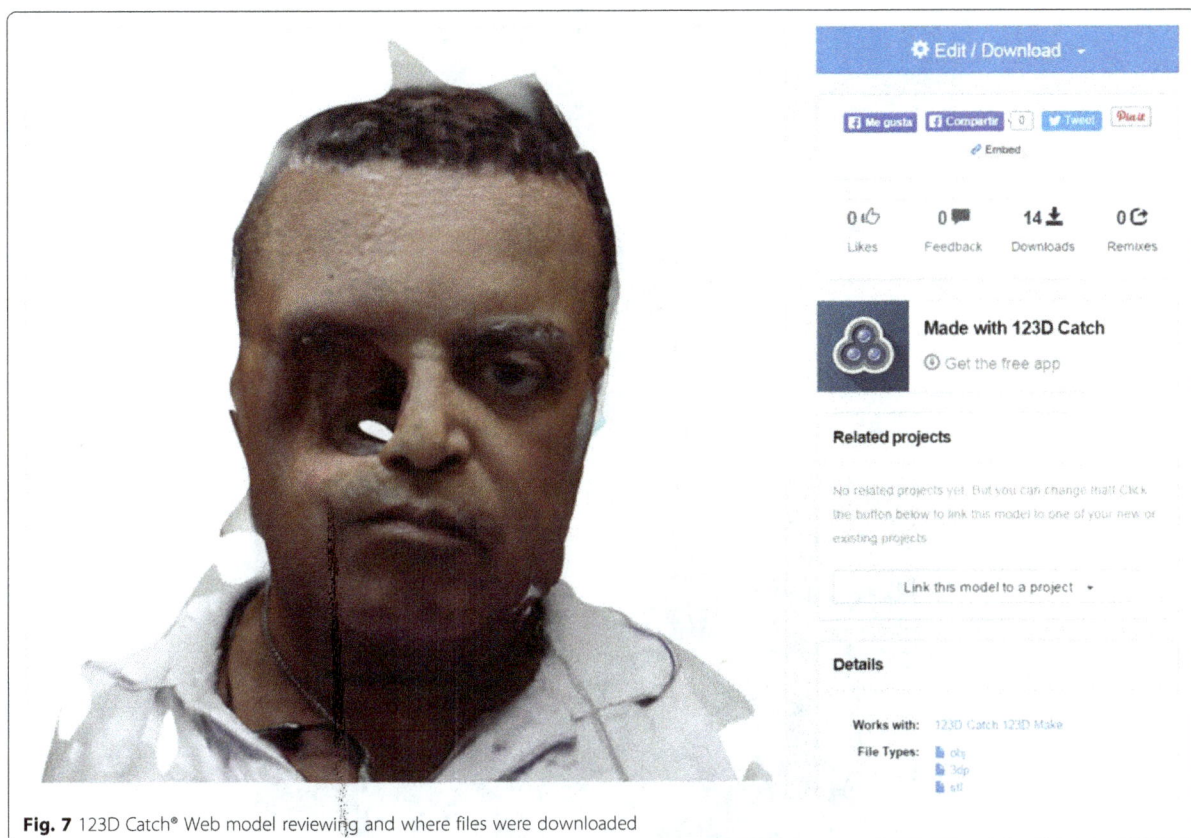

**Fig. 7** 123D Catch® Web model reviewing and where files were downloaded

can be directly downloaded from the web, as was done in this study. Reviewing this file on the PC version provides the colored model, which can be helpful to show to the patient, and for explanation and education of the anatomy and planning. It also provides an indication of the quality of the meshing. If substantial errors were found in this step, they were more evident in the *.stl version. Through the PC version of 123D Catch, it is possible to press the "print" button and that will take you to the *.stl in Meshmixer®, or it is possible to open the *.stl file directly from Meshmixer® as was done in the present study. Once opened the model needed to be up righted, repositioned, and rescaled according to the clinical measurement previously recorded. It was then edited to eliminate all the background and body parts of the model, which are beyond the area of interest for capture.

In the present study the models generated by the mobile device were not used directly for 3D printing. Instead, the captures made by the mobile device were meshed through the PC version of 123D Catch®. They showed better results in the surface of the models virtually and were therefore selected for printing purposes. Further studies should be conducted to better evaluate the accuracy of the respective virtual models. The PC version of 123D Catch® has an option to re-mesh the model with higher quality than the originally configured application for mobile devices. The application was not originally created for medical purposes, but rather, for more simplified CAD designs; complex organic shapes of anatomical models represent a heavier burden for mobile applications, and would run more slowly on smartphones [67].

This *.stl file showed a very acceptable replica of the anatomy of the patient. Once it was re-scaled and printed it showed that it subjectively met the needs for facial prosthetic fabrication, but further studies are needed to evaluate the precision and accuracy of this process.

While not a part of the objective of this study, once an *.stl of the patient is acquired through this process, that sufficiently recreates the anatomy, a digital prostheses design is possible. This is possible through the manipulation of the healthy side of the patient by selecting, isolating, duplicating, mirroring, transforming, editing and sculpting up to have an adequate adaptation of the prostheses model using Meshmixer®. The virtually designed prosthesis model would need to be extruded to provide a volume from the surface data, to produce the final prosthesis design for printing.

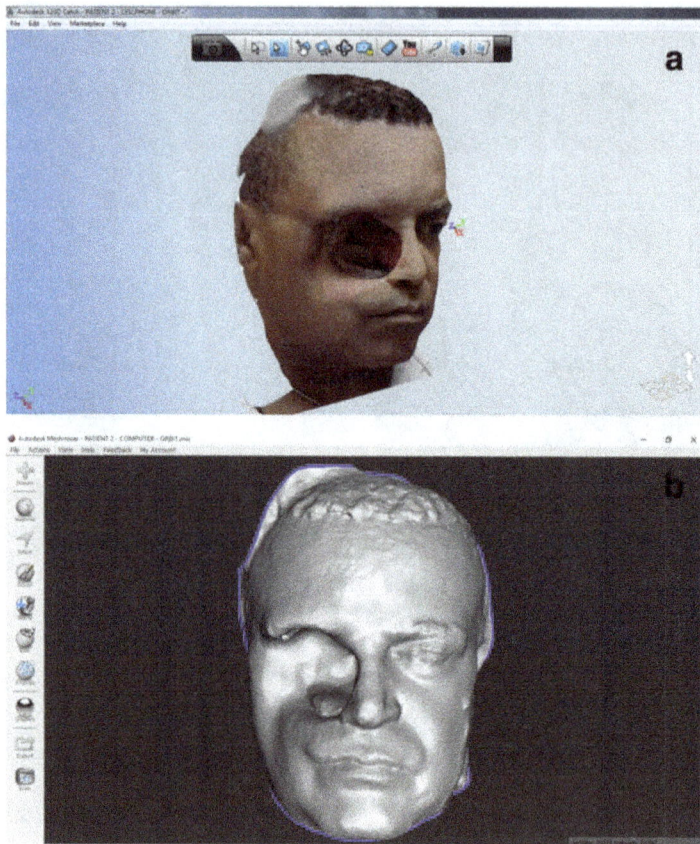

**Fig. 8 a**. 123D Catch® PC version review of the *.3Dp model. **b**. Screen capture of Meshmixer® reviewing the *.stl model after setting up-right position, rescaling and deleting triangles beyond the face

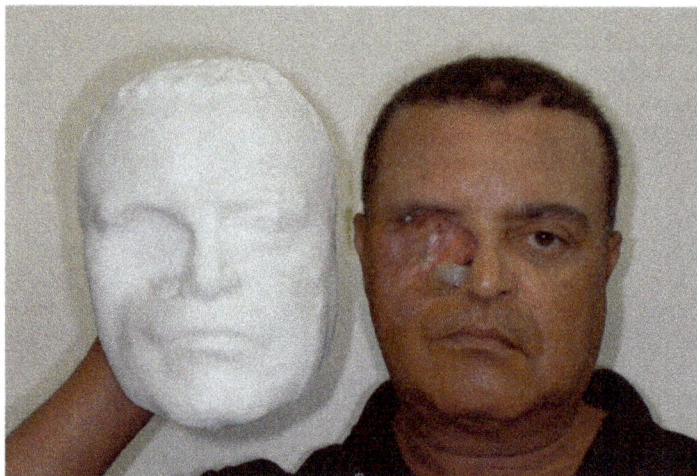

**Fig. 9** Shows the Duraform Polyamide C15 degraded material, for the impression of the model of the patient, with the patient holding it

Mahmoud, et al., demonstrated that three-dimensional printing of human anatomic pathology specimens is achievable by the use of 123D Catch® and recognize that advances in 3D printing technology may further improve [42]. Koban et al. founded in a comparison between Vectra® and 123D Catch® on a labeled plastic mannequin head with landmarks, that no significant ($p > 0.05$) difference was found between manual tape measurement and digital distances from 123D Catch® and Vectra®. Also they describe that sufficient results for the 3D reconstruction with 123D Catch® is possible with 16, 12 and 9 photo captures, but with higher deviations on lateral units than in central units. Also they found that 123D Catch® needed 10 minutes on average to capture and compute 3D models (5 times more than Vectra) [43]. The present study obtained similar results in the lateral views of our models, with more irregularities compared to the primary area of interest to be captured (center of the face). This phenomenon could be associated with less intersection of overlapping triangles in those areas which are not the primary area of interest to be captured. Time was not measured as a variable of our study, but we experienced that during the automatic software uploading, meshing and downloading process, the operator's attention could be dedicated to other tasks.

While the technology process does not print the final adapted prosthesis, some small errors in the surface of the model are acceptable, because a finishing work by hand on the wax replica of the prototyped prosthesis will be done chairside which will eliminate any "stair-stepping" from printing, ensuring appropriate adaptation to the skin surface and applying naturalistic surface texture. While finishing work in the clinic and laboratory is still required, this protocol provides a very helpful advancement in the macro-sculpture of the prosthesis, which can be tested and adapted as needed directly on the patient.

Prolonged capture time with multiple pictures is prone to errors [43] and it is for this reason that standardizing a photo capture protocol for data capture and processing is essential. A standardized photo capture protocol will simplify the process of capture-to-print-prototyping (CPP). 123D Catch® computed models suggest good accuracy of the 3D reconstruction for a standard mannequin model [43] and so is demonstrated in this study for a maxillofacial prosthetic patient.

## Conclusion

It was possible to generate 3D models as digital face impressions with the use of monoscopic photogrammetry and photos taken by a mobile device. Free software and low-cost equipment are a feasible alternative for capturing patient facial anatomy for the purpose of generating physical working models, designing templates for facial prostheses, improving communication with patients before and during treatment and improving access to digital clinical solutions for clinical centers that do not have high cost technology allowances in their budget. Further studies are needed to evaluate quality variables of these models. Clinical data capture protocols like the one described in this report must be validated clinically to optimize the process of data acquisition.

### Acknowledgements
The authors acknowledge the close collaboration of all the professionals of the "Centro Tecnológico Da Informação Renato Archer" which have collaborated in the design and printing for this project: Amanda Amorin, Paulo Inforçatti, Marcelo Oliveira, Dr. Augusto Oliveira, Ana Cláudia Matzenbacher, and the large team. Also to Dra. Crystianne Signiemartin and Dr. Joaquim Piras De Oliveira who guide the maxillofacial rehabilitation needs of our patient.

### Funding
No grant was required for this work. It was supported by own resources of the authors and the printing model was donated by the Centro Tecnológico Renato Archer as partnership in research.

### Ethical approval
This article does not contain clinical procedures on a human, but contain the image of a human participant. Only photo captures were taken from him, after he was fully informed about the clinical implication of our study. He voluntarily accepted to participate.

### Informed consent
Formal consent was obtained from the patient to use his image and to submit and publicate this article.

### Competing interests
The authors are not part of Autodesk. Author Rodrigo Salazar-Gamarra declares that he has no conflict of interest, Rosemary Seelaus declares that he has no conflict of interest, Jorge Vicente Lopes da Silva declares that he has no conflict of interest, Airton Moreira da Silva declares that he has no conflict of interest, Luciano Lauria Dib declares that he has no conflict of interest.

### Author details
[1]UNIP Postgraduate Dental School, Universidade Paulista, Rua Afonso Braz, 525 - Cj. 81 Vila Nova Conceição, São Paulo CEP 04511-011, SP, Brazil. [2]The Craniofacial Center, University of Illinois at Chicago, 811 S Paulina St, Chicago, IL 60612, USA. [3]Division of the Centro Tecnológico da Informação Renato Archer, Rodovia Dom Pedro I, Km 143, 6 - Amarais, Campinas, SP 13069-901, Brazil. [4]Centro Tecnológico da Informação Renato Archer Campinas, Rodovia Dom Pedro I, Km 143, 6 - Amarais, Campinas, SP 13069-901, Brazil. [5]Oncology Center, Hospital Alemão Oswaldo Cruz, Rua Afonso Braz, 525 - Cj. 81 Vila Nova Conceição, São Paulo CEP 04511-011, SP, Brazil.

### References
1. Jankielewicz I et al. Prótesis Buco-maxilo-facial. Quintessence: Barcelona; 2003.
2. Alvarez A et al. Procederes básicos de laboratorio en prótesis bucomaxilofacial 2da ed. La Habana: Editorial CIMEQ; 2008.
3. Mello M, Piras J, Takimoto R, Cervantes O, Abraão M, Dib L. Facial reconstruction with a bone-anchored prosthesis following destructive cancer surgery. Oncol Lett. 2012;4(4):682–4.
4. Karakoca S, et al. Quality of life of patients with implantretained maxillofacial prostheses: A prospective and retrospective study. J Prosthet Dent. 2013; 109:44-52
5. Pekkan G, Tuna SH, Oghan F. Extraoral prostheses using extraoral implants. Int J Oral Maxillofac Surg. 2011;40:378–83.
6. Machado L et al. Intra and Extraoral Prostheses Retained by Zygoma Implants Following Resection of the Upper Lip and Nose. J Prosthodont. 2015;24:172–7.
7. Ashab Yamin MR, Mozafari N, Mozafari M, Razi Z. Reconstructive Surgery of Extensive Face and Neck Burn Scars Using Tissue Expanders. World J Plast Surg. 2015;4(1):40–9.

8.  Zhang R. Ear reconstruction: from reconstructive to cosmetic. Zhonghua Er Bi Yan Hou Tou Jing Wai Ke Za Zhi. 2015;50(3):187–91.

9.  Kang SS et al. Rib Cartilage Assessment Relative to the Healthy Ear in Young Children with Microtia Guiding Operative Timing. Chin Med J. 2015;128(16):2209–14.

10. Liu T, Hu J, Zhou X, Zhang Q. Expansion method in secondary total ear reconstruction for undesirable reconstructed ear. Ann Plast Surg. 2014; 73(S1):S49–52.

11. Thiele OC et al. The current state of facial prosthetics - A multicenter analysis. J Craniomaxillofac Surg. 2015;15:130–4.

12. Ariani N et al. Current state of craniofacial prosthetic rehabilitation. Int J Prosthodont. 2013;26(1):57. retrospective study. J Prosthet Dent. 2013;109:44–52.

13. Hickey A, Salter M. Prosthodontic and psychological factors in treating patients with congenital and craniofacial defects. J Prosthet Dent. 2006;95:392–6.

14. Vidyasankari N, Dinesh R, Sharma N, Yogesh S. Rehabilitation of a Total Maxillectomy Patient by Three Different Methods. J Clin Diagn Res. 2014; 8(10):12–4.

15. Negahdari R et al. Rehabilitation of a Partial Nasal Defect with Facial Prosthesis: A Case Report. J Dent Res Dent Clin Dent Prospects. 2014;8(4):256–9.

16. Granström G. Craniofacial osseointegration. Oral Dis. 2007;13:261–9.

17. Martins M et al. Extraoral Implants in the Rehabilitation of Craniofacial Defects: Implant and Prosthesis Survival Rates and Peri-Implant Soft Tissue Evaluation. J Oral Maxillofac Surg. 2012;70:1551–7.

18. Kusum CK et al. A Simple Technique to Fabricate a Facial Moulage with a Prefabricated Acrylic Stock Tray: A Clinical Innovation. J Indian Prosthodont Soc. 2014;14(S1):341–4.

19. Alsiyabi AS, Minsley GE. Facial moulage fabrication using a two-stage poly (vinyl siloxane) impression. Prosthodont. 2006;15(3):195–7.

20. Moergeli Jr JR. A technique for making a facial moulage. J Prosthet Dent. 1987;57(2):253.

21. Taicher S, Sela M, Tubiana I, Peled I. A technique for making a facial moulage under general anesthesia. J Prosthet Dent. 1983;50(5):677–80.

22. Lemon JC, Okay DJ, Powers JM, Martin JW, Chambers MS. Facial moulage: the effect of a retarder on compressive strength and working and setting times of irreversible hydrocolloid impression material. J Prosthet Dent. 2003;90(3):276–81.

23. Pattanaik S, Wadkar A. Rehabilitation of a Patient with an Intra Oral Prosthesis and an Extra Oral Orbital Prosthesis Retained with Magnets. J Indian Prosthodont Soc. 2012;12(1):45–50.

24. Davis BK. The role of technology in facial prosthetics. Curr Opin Otolaryngol Head Neck Surg. 2010;18(4):332–40.

25. Grant GT. Digital capture, design, and manufacturing of a facial prosthesis: Clinical report on a pediatric patient. J Prosthet Dent. 2015;114(1):138–41.

26. Ting Jiao T et al. Design and Fabrication of Auricular Prostheses by CAD/ CAM System. Int J Prosthodont. 2004;17:460–3.

27. Coward T et al. A Comparison of Prosthetic Ear Models Created from Data Captured by Computerized Tomography, Magnetic Resonance Imaging, and Laser Scanning. Int J Prosthodont. 2007;20:275–85.

28. Coward T et al. Fabrication of a Wax Ear by Rapid-Process Modeling Using Stereolithography. Int J Prosthodont. 1999;12:20–7.

29. Yoshiok F et al. Fabrication of an Orbital Prosthesis Using a Non-contact Three-Dimensional Digitizer and Rapid-Prototyping System. J Prosthodont. 2010;19:598–600.

30. Cheah CM et al. Integration of Laser Surface Digitizing with CAD/CAM Techniques for Developing FacialProstheses. Part 1: Design and Fabrication of Prosthesis Replicas. Int J Prosthodont. 2003;16:435–41.

31. Cheah CM et al. Integration of Laser Surface Digitizing with CAD/CAM Techniques for Developing Facial Prostheses. Part 2: Development of Molding Techniques for Casting Prosthetic Parts. Int J Prosthodont. 2003;16:543–8.

32. Tsuji M et al. Fabrication of a Maxillofacial Prosthesis Using a Computer-Aided Design andManufacturing System. J Prosthodont. 2004;13:179–83.

33. Sabol J et al. Digital Image Capture and Rapid Prototyping. J Prosthodont. 2011;20:310–4.

34. Kimoto K, Garrett NR. Evaluation of a 3D digital photographic imaging system of the human face. J Oral Rehabil. 2007;34:201–5.

35. Chen LH et al. A CAD/CAM Technique for Fabricating Facial Prostheses: A Preliminary Report. IntJ Prosthodont. 1997;10:467–72.

36. Feng Z et al. Computer-assisted technique for the design and manufacture of realistic facial prostheses. Br J Oral Maxillofac Surg. 2010;48:105–9.

37. Ciocca L et al. Rehabilitation of the Nose Using CAD/CAM and Rapid Prototyping Technology After Ablative Surgery of Squamous Cell Carcinoma: A Pilot Clinical Report. Int J Oral Maxillofac Implants. 2010;25:808–12.

38. He Y, Xue GH, Fu JZ. Fabrication of low cost soft tissue prostheses with the desktop 3D printer. Sci Rep. 2014;27:1–4.

39. Feng ZH et al. Virtual Transplantation in Designing a Facial Prosthesis for Extensive Maxillofacial Defects that Cross the Facial Midline Using Computer-Assisted Technology. Int J Prosthodont. 2010;23:513–20.

40. Heike CL et al. 3D digital stereophotogrammetry: a practical guide to facial image acquisition. Head Face Med. 2010;6:18.

41. Runte C et al. Optical Data Acquisition for Computer-Assisted Design of Facial Prostheses. Int J Prosthodont. 2002;15:129–32.

42. Mahmoud A, Bennett M. Introducing 3-Dimensional Printing of a Human Anatomic Pathology Specimen: Potential Benefits for Undergraduate and Postgraduate Education and Anatomic Pathology Practice. Arch Pathol Lab Med. 2015;139(8):1048–51.

43. Koban KC et al. 3D-imaging and analysis for plastic surgery by smartphone and tablet: an alternative to professional systems? Handchir Mikrochir Plast Chir. 2014;46(2):97–104.

44. Nyquist V, Tham P. Method of measuring volume movements of impressions, model and prosthetic base materials in a photogrammetric way. Acta Odontol Scand. 1951;9:111.

45. Savora BS. Application of photogrammetry for quantitative study of tooth and face morphology. Am J Phys Anthropol. 1965;23:427.

46. Adams LP, Wilding JC. A photogrammetric method for monitoring changes in the residual alveolar ridge form. J Oral Rehabil. 1985;12:443–50.

47. Fernández-Riveiro P et al. Angular photogrammetric analysis of the soft tissue facial profile. Eur J Orthod. 2003;25:393–9.

48. Charles W et al. Imaging of maxillofacial trauma: Evolutions and emerging revolutions. Oral Surg Oral Med Oral Pathol Oral Radiol Endod. 2005;100:S75–96.

49. Artopoulos A, Buytaert J, Dirckx J, Coward T. Comparison of the accuracy of digital stereophotogrammetry and projection moire profilometry for three-dimensional imaging of the face. Int J Oral Maxillofac Surg. 2014;43:654–62.

50. Winder RJ. Technical validation of the Di3D stereophotogrammetry surface imaging system. Br J Oral Maxillofac Surg. 2008;46:33–7.

51. Wong JY et al. Validity and reliability of 3D craniofacial anthropometric measurements. Cleft Palate Craniofac J. 2008;45(3):233.

52. Plooij JM et al. Evaluation of reproducibilit y and reliability of 3D soft tissue analysis using 3D stereophotogrammetry. Int J Oral Maxillofac Surg. 2009;38:267–73.

53. Kochel J et al. 3D Soft Tissue Analysis – Part 1: Sagittal Parameters. J Orofac Orthop. 2010;71:40–52.

54. Kochel J et al. 3D Soft Tissue Analysis – Part 2: Vertical Parameters. J Orofac Orthop. 2010;71:207–20.

55. Menezes M et al. Accuracy and Reproducibility of a 3-Dimensional Stereophotogrammetric Imaging System. J Oral Maxillofac Surg. 2010;68: 2129–35.

56. Verhoeven TJ, et al. Three dimensional evaluation of facial asymmetry after mandibular reconstruction: validation of a new method using stereophotogrammetry. Int J Oral Maxillofac Surg. 2013;42(1):19-25.

57. Dindaroğlu F, Kutlu P, Duran GS, Görgülü S, Aslan E. Accuracy and reliability of 3D stereophotogrammetry: A comparison to direct anthropometry and 2Dphotogrammetry. Angle Orthod. 2015;12 [Epub ahead of print].

58. Wu G, Bi Y, Zhou B, et al. Computer-aided design and rapid manufacture of an orbital prosthesis. Int J Prosthodont. 2009;22:293.

59. Ciocca L, Fantini M, Marchetti C, et al. Immediate facial rehabilitation in cancer patients using CAD/CAM and rapid prototyping technology: a pilot study. Support Care Cancer. 2009. doi:10.1007/s000520-009-0676-5 [Epub ahead of print].

60. Ciocca L, Scotti R. CAD–CAM generated ear cast by means of a laser scanner and rapid prototyping machine. J Prosthet Dent. 2004;92:591–5.

61. Rudman K, Hoekzema C, Rhee J. Computer-assisted innovations in craniofacial surgery. Facial Plast Surg. 2011;27(4):358-65.

62. Turgut G, Sacak B, Kiran K, Bas L. Use of rapid prototyping in prosthet auricular restoration. J Craniofac Surg. 2009;20:321–5.

63. Ciocca L. CAD–CAM construction of a provisional nasal prosthesis after ablative tumor surgery of the nose: a pilot case report. Eur J Cancer Care (Engl). 2009;18:97–101.

64. Guofeng W et al. Computer-Aided Design and Rapid Manufacture of an Orbital Prosthesis. Int J Prosthodont. 2009;22:293–5.

65. Tzou CH et al. Comparison of three-dimensional surface-imaging systems. Reconstructive & Aesthetic Surgery: Journal of Plastic; 2014. http://dx.doi.org/10.1016/j.bjps.2014.01.003.

66. Menezes M, Sforza C. Three-dimensional face morphometry. Dental Press. 2010;15(1):13–5.

67. Autodesk. 123D Catch Tutorials [Internet]. USA: 123D Catch Tutorials; 2015. Available from: http://www.123Dapp.com/howto/catch.

# Permissions

All chapters in this book were first published in JOHNS, by BioMed Central; hereby published with permission under the Creative Commons Attribution License or equivalent. Every chapter published in this book has been scrutinized by our experts. Their significance has been extensively debated. The topics covered herein carry significant findings which will fuel the growth of the discipline. They may even be implemented as practical applications or may be referred to as a beginning point for another development.

The contributors of this book come from diverse backgrounds, making this book a truly international effort. This book will bring forth new frontiers with its revolutionizing research information and detailed analysis of the nascent developments around the world.

We would like to thank all the contributing authors for lending their expertise to make the book truly unique. They have played a crucial role in the development of this book. Without their invaluable contributions this book wouldn't have been possible. They have made vital efforts to compile up to date information on the varied aspects of this subject to make this book a valuable addition to the collection of many professionals and students.

This book was conceptualized with the vision of imparting up-to-date information and advanced data in this field. To ensure the same, a matchless editorial board was set up. Every individual on the board went through rigorous rounds of assessment to prove their worth. After which they invested a large part of their time researching and compiling the most relevant data for our readers.

The editorial board has been involved in producing this book since its inception. They have spent rigorous hours researching and exploring the diverse topics which have resulted in the successful publishing of this book. They have passed on their knowledge of decades through this book. To expedite this challenging task, the publisher supported the team at every step. A small team of assistant editors was also appointed to further simplify the editing procedure and attain best results for the readers.

Apart from the editorial board, the designing team has also invested a significant amount of their time in understanding the subject and creating the most relevant covers. They scrutinized every image to scout for the most suitable representation of the subject and create an appropriate cover for the book.

The publishing team has been an ardent support to the editorial, designing and production team. Their endless efforts to recruit the best for this project, has resulted in the accomplishment of this book. They are a veteran in the field of academics and their pool of knowledge is as vast as their experience in printing. Their expertise and guidance has proved useful at every step. Their uncompromising quality standards have made this book an exceptional effort. Their encouragement from time to time has been an inspiration for everyone.

The publisher and the editorial board hope that this book will prove to be a valuable piece of knowledge for researchers, students, practitioners and scholars across the globe.

# List of Contributors

**Scott Murray and Michael N. Ha**
Dalhousie University, Faculty of Medicine, Halifax, Nova Scotia, Canada

**Murali Rajaraman**
Dalhousie University, Faculty of Medicine, Halifax, Nova Scotia, Canada
Department of Radiation Oncology, Capital District Health Authority, Halifax, Nova Scotia, Canada

**Stephanie L. Snow**
Dalhousie University, Faculty of Medicine, Halifax, Nova Scotia, Canada.
Department of Internal Medicine, Division of Medical Oncology, Capital District Health Authority, Halifax, Nova Scotia, Canada

**Kara Thompson**
Dalhousie University, Research Methods Unit, Halifax, Nova Scotia, Canada

**Robert D. Hart**
Dalhousie University, Faculty of Medicine, Halifax, Nova Scotia, Canada.
Department of Surgery, Division of Otolaryngology, Capital District Health Authority, Halifax, Nova Scotia, Canada

**Derrick R. Randall, Phillip S. Park and Justin K. Chau**
Section of Otolaryngology – Head & Neck Surgery, Department of Surgery, University of Calgary, Calgary, Foothills Medical Centre, 1403 - 29 Street NW, Calgary, AB T2N 2T9, Canada

**Brittany Barber, Margaret Nesbitt, Jeffrey Harris, Daniel O'Connell David Côté, Vincent Biron and Hadi Seikaly**
Division of Otolaryngology-Head & Neck Surgery, University of Alberta Hospital, 1E4, Walter Mackenzie Centre, 8440-112 St, Edmonton, AB T6G 2B7, Canada

**Jace Dergousoff2 Nicholas Mitchell**
Department of Psychiatry, University of Alberta Hospital, 1E1, Walter Mackenzie Centre, 8440-112 St, Edmonton, AB T6G 2B7, Canada

**Andrew Foreman, John R. de Almeida, Ralph Gilbert and David P. Goldstein**
Department of Otolaryngology Head and Neck Surgery, University Health Network, Princess Margaret Cancer Centre, University of Toronto, Toronto, ON, Canada

**Michael Roskies1, Michael P. Hier1, Richard J. Payne1, Alex Mlynarek1, Veronique Forest1,Xiaoyang Liu and Mark Levental**
Department of Radiology, Jewish General Hospital & McGill University, Montreal, Quebec, Canada

**Reza Forghani**
Department of Radiology, Jewish General Hospital & McGill University, Montreal, Quebec, Canada
Segal Cancer Centre and Lady Davis Institute for Medical Research, Jewish General Hospital & McGillUniversity, Montreal, Quebec, Canada Full list of author information is available at the end of the article

**Rolina Al-Wassia**
Department of Radiation Oncology, King Abdulaziz University, Abdullah Suleiman Street, P.O Box 80200, 21589 Jeddah, Saudi Arabia

**Siavosh Vakilian and George Shenouda**
Department of Radiation Oncology, McGill University Health Centre, McGill University, Montreal, Québec, Canada

**Crystal Holly**
Department of Clinical Epidemiology, Mc Gill University, Montreal, Québec, Canada

**Khalil Sultanem**
Radiation Oncology, Segal Cancer Centre, Sir Mortimer B. Davis Jewish General Hospital, McGill University, Montreal, Québec, Canada

**Stephanie E. Johnson-Obaseki and Varant Labajian**
Department of Otolaryngology-Head and Neck Surgery, University of Ottawa, S3 – 501 Smyth Road, Ottawa, ON K1H 8L6, Canada

**Martin J. Corsten**
Department of Otolaryngology – Head and Neck Surgery, Aurora Health Care, Aurora St. Luke's Medical Center, 2801 W. Kinnickinnic River Parkway, Suite 630,
Milwaukee, WI 53215, USA

**James T. McDonald**
Department of Economics, University of New Brunswick, PO Box 4400, Fredericton, NB E3B6C4, Canada

**Boban M. Erovic, Manish D. Shah, Guillem Bruch, John R. de Almeida, Patrick J. Gullane, Dale Brown, Ralph W. Gilbert and Jonathan C. Irish**
Department of Otolaryngology-Head and Neck Surgery, Wharton Head and Neck Program, University Health Network, Princess Margaret Cancer Centre, Toronto, ON, Canada

**Meredith Johnston, John Kim and Brian O'Sullivan**
Department of Radiation Oncology, Princess Margaret Cancer Centre, University of Toronto, Toronto, ON, Canada

**David P. Goldstein**
Department of Otolaryngology-Head and Neck Surgery, Wharton Head and Neck Program, University Health Network, Princess Margaret Cancer Centre, Toronto, ON, Canada
Princess Margaret Hospital, Wharton Head and Neck Centre, 610 University Avenue, 3rd Floor, Toronto, ON M5G 2 M9, Canada

**Bayardo Perez-Ordonez and Ilan Weinreb**
Department of Pathology, University Health Network, Princess Margaret Cancer Centre, Toronto, ON, Canada

**Eshetu G. Atenafu**
Department of Biostatistics, University Health Network, Princess Margaret Cancer Centre, Toronto, ON, Canada

**Khalid Hussain AL-Qahtani**
Department of Otolaryngology-Head & Neck Surgery, College of Medicine, King Saud University, Riyadh, Saudi Arabia

**Mushabbab Al Asiri and Mutahir A. Tunio**
Radiation Oncology, Comprehensive Cancer Center, King Fahad Medical City, Riyadh 59046, Saudi Arabia

**Naji J. Aljohani**
Endocrinology and thyroid Oncology, King Fahad Medical City, Riyadh 59046, Saudi Arabia

**Yasser Bayoumi**
Radiation Oncology, NCI, Cairo University, Cairo, Egypt

**Hanadi Fatani**
Histopathology, King Fahad Medical City, Riyadh 59046, Saudi Arabia

**Abdulrehman AlHadab**
Radiation Oncology, King AbdulAziz University, Riyadh 59046, Saudi Arabia

**Jonathan C. Melong, Matthew H. Rigby, Robert D. Hart, Jonathan R.B. Trites and S. Mark Taylor**
Division of Otolaryngology - Head and Neck Surgery, Queen Elizabeth II Health Sciences Centre and Dalhousie University, Halifax, NS, Canada

**Martin Bullock**
Division of Anatomical Pathology, Queen Elizabeth II Health Sciences Centre and Dalhousie University, Halifax, NS, Canada

**M. Elise R. Graham, Robert D. Hart, Fawaz M. Makki, Angela L. Butler, Matthew H. Rigby, Jonathan R. B. Trites and S. Mark Taylor**
Division of Otolaryngology, Queen Elizabeth II Health Sciences Centre and
Dalhousie University, Halifax, NS, Canada

**Susan Douglas, Devanand Pinto and Rama Singh**
NRC Human Health Therapeutics, Oxford Street, Halifax, NS, Canada

**Martin Bullock**
Division of Anatomical Pathology, Queen Elizabeth II Health Sciences Centre and Dalhousie University, Halifax, NS, Canada

**Islam Herzallah**
Department of Otolaryngology, Zagazig University, Zagazig, Egypt

**Bassam Alzuraiqi**
Department of Otolaryngology-Head & Neck Surgery, King Abdullah Medical City, Makkah, Saudi Arabia

**Naif Bawazeer and Osama Marglani**
Department of Otolaryngology-Head & Neck Surgery, Umm Al-Qura University, Makkah, Saudi Arabia

**Ameen Alherabi**
Department of Otolaryngology-Head & Neck Surgery, Umm Al-Qura University, Makkah, Saudi Arabia
P.O.Box 41405, Jeddah 21521, Saudi Arabia

**Sherif K. Mohamed**
Department of Otolaryngology, Ain Shams University, Cairo, Egypt

**Khalid Al-Qahtani**
Department of Otolaryngology-Head and Neck Surgery, King Saud University, Riyadh, Saudi Arabia

**Talal Al-Khatib**
Department of Otolaryngology-Head & Neck Surgery, King Abdulaziz
University, Jeddah, Saudi Arabia

**Abdullah Alghamdi**
Department of Ophthalmology, Umm Al-Qura University, Makkah, Saudi Arabia

**Caiwen Huang**
Department of Electrical and Computer Engineering, Western University,
London, ON, Canada

**Horace Cheng**
Department of Otolaryngology – Head and Neck Surgery, Schulich School of Medicine and Dentistry, Western University, London, ON, Canada

**Yves Bureau**
Lawson Health Research Institute, London, ON, Canada. 5Department of Medical Biophysics, Western University, London, ON, Canada

**Sumit K. Agrawal**
Department of Electrical and Computer Engineering, Western University, London, ON, Canada
Department of Otolaryngology – Head and Neck Surgery, Schulich School of Medicine and Dentistry, Western University, London, ON, Canada
London Health Sciences Centre, Room B1-333, University Hospital, 339 Windermere Rd., London N6A 5A5ON, Canada

**Hanif M. Ladak**
Department of Electrical and Computer Engineering, Western University,London, ON, Canada
Department of Otolaryngology – Head and Neck Surgery, Schulich School of Medicine and Dentistry, Western University, London, ON, Canada
Biomedical Engineering Graduate Program, Western University, London, ON, Canada
Lawson Health Research Institute, London, ON, Canada. 5Department of Medical Biophysics, Western University, London, ON, Canada

**Graeme B. Mulholland, Han Zhang, Hadi Seikaly, Daniel O'Connell, Vincent L. Biron and Jeffrey R. Harris**
Division of Otolaryngology-Head and Neck Surgery, University of Alberta Hospital, 1E4.29 WMC, 8440 – 112 Street, Edmonton, AB T6G 2B7, Canada

**Nhu-Tram A. Nguyen**
Division of Radiation Oncology, McMaster University, Hamilton, Canada

**Nicholas Tkacyzk**
Northern Ontario School of Medicine, Sudbury, Canada

**Khalid Hussain AL-Qahtani**
Department of Otolaryngology-Head & Neck Surgery, College of Medicine, King Saud University, Riyadh, Saudi Arabia

**Mutahir A. Tunio and Khalid Riaz**
Radiation Oncology, King Fahad Medical City, Riyadh, Saudi Arabia

**Mushabbab Al Asiri**
Radiation Oncology, Comprehensive Cancer Center, King Fahad Medical City, Riyadh 59046, Saudi Arabia

**Naji J. Aljohani**
Endocrinology and Thyroid Oncology, King Fahad Medical City, Riyadh 59046, Saudi Arabia

**Yasser Bayoumi**
Radiation Oncology, NCI, Cairo University, Cairo, Egypt

**Wafa AlShakweer**
Histopathology, Comprehensive Cancer Center, King Fahad Medical City, Riyadh 59046, Saudi Arabia

**Russell N. Schwartz**
Faculty of Science, McGill University, 845 Rue Sherbrooke West, Montréal, QC, Canada

**Richard J. Payne**
Department of Otolaryngology-Head and Neck Surgery, Sir Mortimer B. Davis-Jewish General Hospital, McGill University, 3755 Côte Ste-Catherine Road, Montreal, QC, Canada. 3Department of Otorhinolaryngology Adult (Otl) (Ent) (Surgery), Royal Victoria Hospital, McGill University Health Center, 687 Pine Avenue West, Montreal, QC, Canada.

**Véronique-Isabelle Forest and Michael P. Hier**
Department of Otolaryngology-Head and Neck Surgery, Sir Mortimer B. Davis-Jewish General Hospital, McGill University, 3755 Côte Ste-Catherine Road, Montreal, QC, Canada

**Amanda Fanous**
Department of Otolaryngology-Head and Neck Surgery, McGill Executive Institute, McGill University, 1001 Rue Sherbrooke West, Montreal, QC, Canada

**Camille Vallée-Gravel**
Faculty of Medicine, McGill University, 845 Rue Sherbrooke West, Montréal, QC, Canada

**Takafumi Yamano**
Section of Otorhinolaryngology, Department of Medicine, Fukuoka Dental College, 2-15-1 Tamura,Sawara-ku, Fukuoka 814-0193, Japan Department of Otorhinolaryngology, Fukuoka University School of Medicine, Jounan-ku Nanakuma 7-45-1, Fukuoka 814-0180, Japan

**Hitomi Higuchi and Takashi Nakagawa**
Department of Otorhinolaryngology, Fukuoka University School of Medicine, Jounan-ku Nanakuma 7-45-1, Fukuoka 814-0180, Japan

**Tetsuo Morizono**
Nishi Fukuoka Hospital, Nishi-ku Ikino-matsubara 3-18-8, Fukuoka 819-8555, Japan

**Khalid Hussain AL-Qahtani**
Department of Otolaryngology-Head & Neck Surgery, College of Medicine, King Saud University, Riyadh, Saudi Arabia

**Yasser Bayoumi**
Radiation Oncology, NCI, Cairo University, Cairo, Egypt

**Mutahir A. Tunio and Venkada Manickam Gurusamy**
Radiation Oncology, King Fahad Medical City, Riyadh 59046, Saudi Arabia

**Fahad Ahmed A. Bahamdain**
Faculty of Medicine, King AbdulAziz University, Riyadh 59046, Saudi Arabia

**Hanadi Fatani**
Histopathology, Comprehensive Cancer Center, King Fahad Medical City, Riyadh 59046, Saudi Arabia

**Brian W. Rotenberg**
Department of Otolaryngology–Head and Neck Surgery, Western University, London, Ontario, Canada
St. Joseph's Hospital, Room B2-501, 268 Grosvenor Street, London, ON N6A 4V2, Canada

**Claudio Vicini**
Head & Neck Department, ASL of Romagna, ENT and Oral Surgery Unit, Morgagni-Pierantoni Hospital (Forlì), Ospedale degli Infermi (Faenza), Forlì, Italy

**Edward B. Pang and Kenny P. Pang**
Asia Sleep Centre, Paragon, Singapore

**John Henry Owen, Christine M. Komarck and Martin P. Graha**
Department of Otolaryngology/Head Neck Surgery, University of Michigan School of Medicine, Ann Arbor, MI 48109-5616, USA

**Shannon F. Rudy**
Department of Otolaryngology/Head Neck Surgery, University of MichiganSchool of Medicine, Ann Arbor, MI 48109-5616, USA.
Department of Otolaryngology/Head Neck Surgery, Stanford University, Stanford, CA 94305, USA

**J. Chad Brenner, Carol R. Bradford, Mark EP Prince and Thomas E. Carey**
Department of Otolaryngology/Head Neck Surgery, University of Michigan School of Medicine, Ann Arbor, MI 48109-5616, USA
Comprehensive Cancer Center, University of Michigan School of Medicine, Ann Arbor, MI 48109-5616, USA

**Emily L. Bellile**
Cancer Center Biostatistics Core, University of Michigan School of Medicine, Ann Arbor, MI 48109-5616, USA

**Jennifer L. Harris, Jun Liu and Jianwei Che**
Genomics Institute of the Novartis Research Foundation, 10675 John Jay Hopkins Drive, San Diego, CA 92121, USA

**Megan V. Scott**
Wayne State University School of Medicine, Detroit, MI 48201, USA

**S. Hosseini**
Faculty of Medicine, McGill University, Montreal, QC, Canada

**R. J. Payne, A. Mlynarek, M. P. Hier and V. I. Forest**
Department of Otolaryngology – Head and Neck Surgery, McGill University, Montreal, QC, Canada
Department Otolaryngology - Head and Neck Surgery, King Abdulaziz University, Jeddah, Saudi Arabia

**F. Zawawi**
Department of Otolaryngology – Head and Neck Surgery, McGill University, Montreal, QC, Canada
Department Otolaryngology - Head and Neck Surgery, King Abdulaziz University, Jeddah, Saudi Arabia

**M. Tamilia**
Division of Endocrinology, Jewish General Hospital, McGill University, Montreal, QC, Canada

**Lisa Singer**
Department of Radiation Oncology, University of California, San Francisco, 1600 Divisadero St, Suite H-1031, San Francisco, CA 94143 - 1708, USA

**Sarah M. Calkins2, Andrew E. Horvai**
Department of Pathology, University of California, San Francisco, San Francisco, CA, USA

**William R. Ryan**
Department of Otolaryngology, University of California, San Francisco, 1600 Divisadero St, Suite H-1031, San Francisco, CA 94143 - 1708, USA

**Sue S. Yom**
Department of Radiation Oncology, University of California, San Francisco, 1600 Divisadero St, Suite H-1031, San Francisco, CA 94143 - 1708, USA
Department of Otolaryngology, University of California, San Francisco, 1600 Divisadero St, Suite H-1031, San Francisco, CA 94143 - 1708, USA

**A. Butler, M. H. Rigby, J. Scott, J. Trites, R. Hart and S. M. Taylor**
Dalhousie University, Halifax, Canada

**Sarah Khalife and Sarah Bouhabel**
Department of Otolaryngology-Head and Neck Surgery, McGill University Health Centre, 1001 Boulevard Decarie, Montreal, QC, Canada

**Richard J. Payne**
Department of Otolaryngology-Head and Neck Surgery, McGill University Health Centre, 1001 Boulevard Decarie, Montreal, QC, Canada
Department of Otolaryngology-Head and Neck Surgery, Sir Mortimer B. Davis Jewish General Hospital, McGill University, 3755 Côte Ste-Catherine Road, Montreal, QC, Canada

**Veronique-Isabelle Forest and Michael P. Hier**
Department of Otolaryngology-Head and Neck Surgery, Sir Mortimer B. Davis-Jewish General Hospital, McGill University, 3755 Côte Ste-Catherine Road, Montreal, QC, Canada

**Louise Rochon**
Department of Pathology, Sir Mortimer B. Davis-Jewish General Hospital, McGill University, 3755 Côte Ste-Catherine Road, Montreal, QC, Canada

**Michael Tamilia**
Department of Endocrinology and Metabolism, Sir Mortimer B. Davis-Jewish General Hospital, McGill University, 3755 Côte Ste-Catherine Road, Montreal, QC, Canada

**Gordon Fung-Zak Tsang**
Department of Otolaryngology-Head & Neck Surgery, University of Toronto,Toronto, ON, Canada.

**John M. Lee**
Department of Otolaryngology-Head & Neck Surgery, University of Toronto,Toronto, ON, Canada
Department of Otolaryngology-Head & Neck Surgery, St. Michael's Hospital, Toronto, ON, Canada

**Carmen L. McKnight**
Department of Otolaryngology-Head & Neck Surgery, St. Michael's Hospital, Toronto, ON, Canada

**Laura Minhui Kim**
Faculty of Medicine, University of Toronto, Toronto, ON, Canada

**Eugene L. Son, Michael P. Underbrink and Vicente A. Resto**
Department of Otolaryngology - Head and Neck Surgery, University of Texas
Medical Branch, 301 University Boulevard, Galveston, TX 77555, USA

**Suimin Qiu**
Department of Pathology, University of Texas Medical Branch, 301 University Boulevard, Galveston, TX 77555, USA

**Woo Jin Kim, Byung-Guk Kim and Ki-Hong Chang**
Department of Otorhinolaryngology-Head and Neck Surgery, College of Medicine, The Catholic University of Korea, Seoul, Korea

**Jeong-Hoon Oh**
Department of Otorhinolaryngology-Head and Neck Surgery, College of
Medicine, The Catholic University of Korea, Seoul, Korea
Department of Otorhinolaryngology-Head and Neck Surgery, The Catholic
University of Korea, 180 Wangsan-Ro, Dongdaemun-Gu, Seoul 130-709, South Korea

**Vinay T. Fernandes**
Department of Otolaryngology-Head & Neck Surgery, University of Toronto,Toronto, Canada

**Robert J. De Santis**
Sunnybrook Health Sciences Centre, 2075 Bayview Avenue, Suite M1 102, Toronto, ON M4N 3 M5, Canada

**Danny J. Enepekides and Kevin M. Higgins**
Department of Otolaryngology–Head & Neck Surgery, University of Toronto, Sunnybrook Health Sciences Centre, 2075 Bayview Avenue, Suite M1 102, Toronto, ON M4N 3 M5, Canada

**E. Newton**
1University of Ottawa, Ottawa, ON, Canada

**A. Lasso, W. Petrcich**
Department of Otolaryngology - Head and Neck Surgery, University of Ottawa, Ontario, Canada

**S. J. Kilty**
Ottawa Hospital Research Institute (OHRI), Ottawa, ON, Canada

**Hisham Wasl, Jessica McGuire and Darlene Lubbe**
Division of Otolaryngology, University of Cape Town, Cape Town, South Africa

**Rodrigo Salazar-Gamarra**
UNIP Postgraduate Dental School, Universidade Paulista, Rua Afonso Braz, 525 - Cj. 81 Vila Nova Conceição, São Paulo CEP 04511-011, SP, Brazil

**Rosemary Seelaus**
The Craniofacial Center, University of Illinois at Chicago, 811 S Paulina St, Chicago, IL 60612, USA

**Jorge Vicente Lopes da Silva**
Division of the Centro Tecnológico da Informação Renato Archer, Rodovia Dom Pedro I, Km 143, 6 - Amarais, Campinas, SP 13069-901, Brazil

**Airton Moreira da Silva**
Centro Tecnológico da Informação Renato Archer Campinas, Rodovia Dom Pedro I, Km 143, 6 - Amarais, Campinas, SP 13069-901, Brazil

**Luciano Lauria Dib**
UNIP Postgraduate Dental School, Universidade Paulista, Rua Afonso Braz, 525 - Cj. 81 Vila Nova Conceição, São Paulo CEP 04511-011, SP, Brazil
Oncology Center, Hospital Alemão Oswaldo Cruz, Rua Afonso Braz, 525 - Cj. 81 Vila Nova Conceição, São Paulo CEP 04511-011, SP, Brazil

# Index